OB/GYN

SECRETS

D1336304

OB/GYN

SECRETS

FOURTH EDITION

AMANDA MULARZ, MD
Clinical Instructor
David Geffen School of Medicine at UCLA
Los Angeles, California;
Maternal-Fetal Medicine Fellow
Department of Obstetrics and Gynecology
Ronald Reagan-UCLA Medical Center
Los Angeles, California

STEVEN DALATI, MD
Assistant Clinical Professor of Obstetrics and Gynecology
David Geffen School of Medicine at UCLA
Los Angeles, California;
Department of Obstetrics and Gynecology
Olive View-UCLA Medical Center
Sylmar, California

RYAN PEDIGO, MD
Assistant Professor
David Geffen School of Medicine at UCLA
Los Angeles, California;
Attending Physician and Clerkship Director
Department of Emergency Medicine
Harbor-UCLA Medical Center
Torrance, California

ELSEVIER

ELSEVIER

1600 John F. Kennedy Blvd.
Ste 1800
Philadelphia, PA 19103-2899

OB/GYN SECRETS   ISBN: 978-0-323-39922-7

Notices

Knowledge and best practice in this field are constantly changing. As new research and experience broaden our understanding, changes in research methods, professional practices, or medical treatment may become necessary.

Practitioners and researchers must always rely on their own experience and knowledge in evaluating and using any information, methods, compounds, or experiments described herein. In using such information or methods they should be mindful of their own safety and the safety of others, including parties for whom they have a professional responsibility.

With respect to any drug or pharmaceutical products identified, readers are advised to check the most current information provided (i) on procedures featured or (ii) by the manufacturer of each product to be administered, to verify the recommended dose or formula, the method and duration of administration, and contraindications. It is the responsibility of practitioners, relying on their own experience and knowledge of their patients, to make diagnoses, to determine dosages and the best treatment for each individual patient, and to take all appropriate safety precautions.

To the fullest extent of the law, neither the Publisher nor the authors, contributors, or editors, assume any liability for any injury and/or damage to persons or property as a matter of products liability, negligence or otherwise, or from any use or operation of any methods, products, instructions, or ideas contained in the material herein.

Library of Congress Cataloging-in-Publication Data

Ob/gyn secrets (Frederickson)
Ob/gyn secrets / [edited by] Amanda Mularz, Steven Dalati, Ryan Pedigo.-- Fourth edition.
    p. ; cm. -- (Secrets series)
Includes bibliographical references and index.
ISBN 978-0-323-39922-7 (pbk. : alk. paper)
    I. Mularz, Amanda, editor. II. Dalati, Steven, editor. III. Pedigo, Ryan, editor. IV. Title. V. Series:
Secrets series.
    [DNLM: 1. Genital Diseases, Female--Examination Questions. 2. Pregnancy Complications--Examination
Questions. 3. Pregnancy. WP 18.2]
RG111
618.076--dc23
                2015036610

Executive Content Strategist: James Merritt
Content Development Specialist: Margaret Nelson
Publishing Services Manager: Patricia Tannian
Project Manager: Stephanie Turza
Book Designer: Ryan Cook

Printed in United States of America

Last digit is the print number: 9   8   7   6   5   4   3   2   1

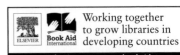

Working together
to grow libraries in
developing countries

www.elsevier.com • www.bookaid.org

*To my husband, and all who contributed their time and effort
to make this possible; many thanks.*

A.M.

*To my colleagues, friends, and amazing wife, whose effort
and energy made this publication possible.*

S.D.

*To all of my mentors and teachers throughout my journey
who have always been there to support me, guide me,
and drive me to be better.*

R.P.

CONTENTS

VI   LABOR, DELIVERY, AND POSTPARTUM

CONTRIBUTORS

Alin Lina Akopians, MD, PhD
Reproductive Endocrinology and Infertility Fellow
Department of Obstetrics and Gynecology
Ronald Reagan-UCLA Medical Center
Los Angeles, California

Shant Ashdjian, MD
Attending Physician
Department of Obstetrics and Gynecology
Kaiser Permanente Downey Medical Center
Downey, California

Mary Anne M. Baquing, MD
Resident Physician
Department of Obstetrics and Gynecology
Harbor-UCLA Medical Center
Torrance, California

Kelly A. Best, MD
Program Director and Attending Physician
Department of Obstetrics and Gynecology
University of Florida College of Medicine
Jacksonville, Florida

Antonio Bonet, MD
Assistant Professor
Division of Pulmonary and Critical Care
Department of Medicine
Olive View-UCLA Medical Center
Sylmar, California;
Fellowship in Pulmonary and Critical Care Medicine
Department of Medicine
Cedars-Sinai Medical Center
Los Angeles, California

Erin Burnett, MD
Assistant Professor
Program Director, Ultrasound and Prenatal Diagnosis
Department of Obstetrics and Gynecology
University of Florida Medical Center
Jacksonville, Florida;
Fellowship in Maternal and Fetal Medicine
Emory University School of Medicine
Atlanta, Georgia

Paul Buzad, MD
Associate Professor
David Geffen School of Medicine at UCLA
Los Angeles, California;
Attending Physician
Department of Obstetrics and Gynecology
Olive View-UCLA Medical Center
Sylmar, California

Jacob Casey, MD
Resident Physician
Department of Obstetrics and Gynecology
Los Angeles County/University of Southern
California Medical Center
University of Southern California
Los Angeles, California

Anna Karina Celaya, MD
Assistant Professor
David Geffen School of Medicine at UCLA
Los Angeles, California;
Attending Physician
Department of Obstetrics and Gynecology
Harbor-UCLA Medical Center
Torrance, California

Zaid Q. Chaudhry, MD
David Geffen School of Medicine at UCLA
Department of Obstetrics and Gynecology
Division of Female Pelvic Medicine and
Reconstructive Surgery
Los Angeles, California

Judy H. Chen, MD
Assistant Clinical Professor
Department of Obstetrics and Gynecology
Los Angeles County/University of Southern
California Medical Center
Los Angeles, California

Erin C. Chong, MD
Resident Physician
Department of Obstetrics and Gynecology
Harbor-UCLA Medical Center
Torrance, California

Lee Coleman, MD
Assistant Professor
Assistant Program Director for Obstetric
Anesthesiology
Department of Anesthesiology
Cedars Sinai Medical Center
Los Angeles, California

Laurin Cristiano, MD
Resident Physician
Department of Obstetrics and Gynecology
Ronald Reagan-UCLA Medical Center
Los Angeles, California

Christine Djapri, MD
Resident Physician
Department of Obstetrics and Gynecology
University of Florida Medical Center
Jacksonville, Florida

Hai-Lang Duong, MD
Visiting Assistant Professor of Obstetrics and
  Gynecology
David Geffen School of Medicine at UCLA
Los Angeles, California;
Chief, Section of Maternal-Fetal Medicine
Department of Obstetrics and Gynecology
Olive View-UCLA Medical Center
Sylmar, California

Ramy Eskander, MD
Assistant Professor
David Geffen School of Medicine at UCLA
Los Angeles, California;
Attending Physician
Department of Obstetrics and Gynecology
Harbor-UCLA Medical Center
Torrance, California

Kristina Galyon, DO
Maternal Fetal Medicine Fellow
Department of Obstetrics and Gynecology
Harbor-UCLA Medical Center
Torrance, California

Lisa Garcia, MD
Assistant Professor of Clinical Obstetrics and
  Gynecology
David Geffen School of Medicine at UCLA
Los Angeles, California;
Department of Obstetrics and Gynecology
Olive View-UCLA Medical Center
Sylmar, California

Rebecca M. Geer, MD
Resident Physician
Department of Obstetrics and Gynecology
Harbor-UCLA Medical Center
Torrance, California

Carrie E. Jung, MD
Resident Physician
Department of Obstetrics and Gynecology
Los Angeles County/University of Southern
  California Medical Center
Los Angeles, California

Daniela Karagyozyan, MD
Fellow
Obstetric Anesthesiology
Cedars-Sinai Medical Center
Los Angeles, California

Lirona Katzir, MD
Visiting Assistant Professor
Department of Obstetrics and Gynecology
Olive View-UCLA Medical Center
Sylmar, California

Enid T. Kuo, MD
Associate Residency Program Director
Kaiser Permanente Los Angeles Medical Center
Los Angeles, California

Debra Linker, MD
Physician
Department of Obstetrics and Gynecology
Palo Alto Foundation Medical Group
Palo Alto Foundation Medical Clinics and the Sutter
  Health System
Mountain View, California

Elena Martinez, MD
Program Director and Attending Physician
Kaiser Permanente Los Angeles Medical Center
Los Angeles, California

Travis W. McCoy, MD
Piedmont Reproductive Endocrinology Group
Asheville, North Carolina;
Fellowship in Reproductive Endocrinology and
  Infertility
University of Louisville
Louisville, Kentucky

Kristen M. McMaster, MD
Maternal-Fetal Medicine Fellow
University of Mississippi Medical Center
Jackson, Mississippi

Erin Mellano, MD
Department of Obstetrics and Gynecology
Division of Female Pelvic Medicine and
  Reconstructive Surgery
David Geffen School of Medicine at UCLA
Los Angeles, California

Hannah Newmark, MD
Resident Physician
Department of Obstetrics and Gynecology
Harbor-UCLA Medical Center
Torrance, California

Maiuyen Nguyen, MD
Attending Physician
Department of Obstetrics and Gynecology
Kaiser Permanente Downey Medical Center
Downey, California

Tina A. Nguyen, MD
Assistant Professor
Maternal-Fetal Medicine
Department of Obstetrics and Gynecology
David Geffen School of Medicine at UCLA
Los Angeles, California

Michelle S. Özcan, MD
Assistant Professor
Associate Residency Program Director
Department of Obstetrics and Gynecology
University of Florida College of Medicine
Jacksonville, Florida

Susan Park, MD
Assistant Clinical Professor
Division of Gynecology Oncology
Department of Obstetrics and Gynecology
University of California–Riverside
Riverside, California

Ryan Pedigo, MD
Assistant Professor
David Geffen School of Medicine at UCLA
Los Angeles, California;
Attending Physician and Clerkship Director
Department of Emergency Medicine
Harbor-UCLA Medical Center
Torrance, California

Tiffany Pedigo, MD
Chief Resident Physician
Department of Pediatrics
Ronald Reagan-UCLA Medical Center
Los Angeles, California

Carlos Rangel, MD
Physician
Adventist Health Central Valley
Hanford, California

Maricela Rodriguez-Gutierrez, MD
Physician
Department of Obstetrics and Gynecology
Kaiser Permanente;
Adjunct Clinical Assistant Professor
Department of Obstetrics and Gynecology
Keck School of Medicine of University of Southern
    California
Los Angeles, California

Jared Roeckner, MD
Resident Physician
Department of Obstetrics and Gynecology
University of Florida Medical Center
Jacksonville, Florida

Rachel Rosenheck, MD
Physician
Los Angeles County/University of Southern
    California Medical Center
Los Angeles, California

Alyssa Scott, MD
Attending Physician
Department of Emergency Medicine
St. Francis Medical Center
Lynwood, California

Whitney Sigala, MD
Resident Physician
Department of Obstetrics and Gynecology
Harbor-UCLA Medical Center
Torrance, California

Manpreet Singh, MD
Ultrasound Fellow
Department of Emergency Medicine
Harbor-UCLA Medical Center
Torrance, California

Ella Speichinger, MD
Assistant Professor
David Geffen School of Medicine at UCLA
Los Angeles, California;
Attending Physician
Department of Obstetrics and Gynecology
Olive View-UCLA Medical Center
Sylmar, California

Lauren W. Sundheimer, MD
Fellow, Reproductive Endocrinology and Infertility
Department of Obstetrics and Gynecology
David Geffen School of Medicine at UCLA
Cedars-Sinai Medical Center
Los Angeles, California

Julia Switzer, MD
Clinical Instructor
University of Illinois at Chicago School of
    Medicine
Chicago, Illinois

Bao Tran, MD
Chief Cardiology Fellow
Department of Medicine
Division of Cardiology
Ronald Reagan-UCLA Medical Center
Los Angeles, California

Stephanie G. Valderramos, MD, PhD
Fellow and Clinical Instructor
Division of Maternal-Fetal Medicine
Department of Obstetrics and Gynecology
University of California–Los Angeles School of
    Medicine
Los Angeles, California

Isha Wadhawan, MD
Resident Physician
Department of Obstetrics and Gynecology
Ronald Reagan-UCLA Medical Center
Los Angeles, California

Alexandra Walker, DO
Resident Physician
Department of Obstetrics and Gynecology
University of Florida Medical Center
Jacksonville, Florida

Cecilia K. Wieslander, MD
Associate Professor
David Geffen School of Medicine at UCLA
Los Angeles, California;
Attending Physician
Department of Obstetrics and Gynecology
Olive View-UCLA Medical Center
Sylmar, California

Stacy M. Yadava, MD
Resident Physician
Department of Obstetrics and Gynecology
Santa Clara Valley Medical Center
San Jose, California

Danny Younes, MD
Resident Physician
Department of Obstetrics and Gynecology
Harbor-UCLA Medical Center
Torrance, California

Mae Zakhour, MD
Fellow and Clinical Instructor
Division of Gynecologic Oncology
Department of Obstetrics and Gynecology
University of California-Los Angeles/Cedars-Sinai
    Medical Center
Los Angeles, California

Mark Zakowski, MD
Chief of Obstetric Anesthesiology
Cedars-Sinai Medical Center;
Adjunct Associate Professor
Charles R. Drew University of Medicine and Science
Los Angeles, California

PREFACE

We are pleased to have the opportunity to provide you with the fourth edition of *OB/GYN Secrets*, which has been completely revamped. The field of obstetrics and gynecology has rapidly evolved in the past 11 years since the last edition; cervical cancer screening alone has been revised multiple times! Our goal in this edition is to provide the most up-to-date, evidence-based medicine available in an easy-to-read format designed for students on their OB/GYN rotation, OB/GYN residents, and allied health professionals interested in learning more about the specialty.

We hope this book will assist learners in preparing for their examinations as well as their care of patients. We would like to acknowledge all of the contributors to the prior three editions of this text and thank them for setting the groundwork for this important subject. In addition, we are indebted to the many authors who lent their time and expertise to making this edition possible. A special thanks to our section editors, Dr. Travis McCoy and Dr. Lejla Delic, for their efforts and time spent making this publication exceptional.

We hope you enjoy the newest *OB/GYN Secrets!*

Sincerely,

Amanda Mularz, MD

Steven Dalati, MD

Ryan Pedigo, MD

TOP 100 SECRETS

These secrets summarize the concepts, principles, and most salient details of obstetrics and gynecology.

1. Combination oral contraceptives (OCPs) work primarily by inhibiting ovulation through suppression of LH and FSH.

2. OCPs decrease the risk of ovarian and endometrial cancers.

3. Symptoms of menopause include irregular then absent menses, hot flashes, and vaginal atrophy or dryness.

4. Midcycle surge of luteinizing hormone (LH) predicts impending ovulation.

5. The order of puberty is: growth spurt, thelarche, adrenarche, peak growth, then menarche.

6. The three most common causes of primary amenorrhea are gonadal dysgenesis, müllerian agenesis, and androgen insensitivity.

7. The most common cause of secondary amenorrhea is pregnancy.

8. Androgen insensitivity and müllerian agenesis are two syndromes characterized by breast development and the absence of a uterus; they can be differentiated by obtaining a karyotype.

9. Premenstrual syndrome (PMS) is defined as emotional and physical symptoms that occur at the same time each month prior to the menstrual cycle.

10. Fibroids are estrogen-sensitive, fibromuscular, benign tumors that are thought to originate from a monoclonal cell line. They can cause abnormal uterine bleeding, dysmenorrhea, pelvic pressure, and even bladder and bowel symptoms.

11. Fibroids can be treated medically, surgically, or with uterine artery embolization.

12. The phases of the sexual response cycle are excitement, plateau, orgasm, and resolution.

13. Genito-pelvic pain/penetration disorder is often associated with a history of sexual abuse or trauma.

14. Polycystic ovarian syndrome (PCOS) is a diagnosis of exclusion and requires two or more of the following: anovulation or oligo-ovulation, clinical or biochemical evidence of hyperandrogenism, and polycystic ovaries on ultrasound.

15. Endometriosis is endometrial tissue outside the uterus; it can cause pelvic pain, dyspareunia, and infertility.

16. Adenomyosis is endometrial tissue in the myometrium; it can cause heavy menstrual bleeding and dysmenorrhea.

17. Not all pelvic pain is gynecologic in origin.

18. The ulcer of primary syphilis is usually single and painless, while the ulcer of herpes is usually multiple and painful.

19. Trichomoniasis and candidiasis are diagnosed with microscopy by visualizing the organisms in vaginal discharge; bacterial vaginosis is diagnosed by the "whiff test" and the presence of "clue cells."

20. Although PID is usually a polymicrobial infection, it generally begins with infection with either *N. gonorrhoeae* or *C. trachomatis*.

21. Approximately 8-20% of clinically recognized pregnancies and 13-26% of unrecognized pregnancies end in miscarriage.

22. Autosomal trisomies are the most common chromosomal abnormality in miscarriages, but the most common *single* karyotype is monosomy X.

23. Legalization of abortion has significantly reduced the number of women hospitalized with abortion-related complications.

24. An initial infertility evaluation should include a menstrual calendar, ultrasound to evaluate uterine anatomy, luteal phase progesterone level to assess for ovulation, and semen analysis.

25. Risks of ovulation induction include multiple gestation and ovarian hyperstimulation.

26. In vitro fertilization (IVF), can be used to overcome tubal disease or male factor infertility; it involves ovarian stimulation with injectable gonadotropins, egg retrieval, fertilization, and subsequent embryo transfer.

27. Stress incontinence is loss of urine due to increased intra-abdominal pressure, urethral hypermobility, or intrinsic sphincter deficiency.

28. Urge incontinence is loss of urine due to detrusor instability.

29. Women are almost nine times more likely to be killed by a current or former intimate partners than by a stranger.

30. The incidence of intimate partner violence is variable during pregnancy and postpartum.

31. High-risk strains of human papillomavirus (HPV) cause genital dysplasia and may lead to invasive cancer.

32. Regular screening with Pap smears has led to a significant decrease in the incidence of cervical cancer.

33. Cervical cancer is clinically staged (i.e., it does not involve surgical exploration).

34. Treatment of cervical cancer depends on stage; surgery is usually appropriate up to Stage IIA.

35. Vulvar cancer is predominantly squamous; spread to superficial inguinal nodes occurs via lymphatic channels.

36. Paget's disease of the vulva may be associated with underlying adenocarcinoma, and excision is recommended.

37. Important risk factors for endometrial cancer include obesity, anovulation, and use of tamoxifen.

38. Endometrial cancer most commonly presents with abnormal uterine bleeding, especially postmenopausal bleeding.

39. Sex cord and germ cell tumors are usually diagnosed at early stages and are highly curable; epithelial ovarian cancer usually presents at late stages.

40. Epithelial ovarian cancer is surgically staged and treated with a combination of cytoreductive surgery and chemotherapy.

41. In a normal pregnancy, beta-hCG levels increase by approximately 50-100% every 48 hours.

42. The discriminatory zone is the beta hCG level at which an intrauterine pregnancy should be seen on ultrasound; it is generally considered to be between 1,500 and 2,500 mIU/mL.

43. Ectopic pregnancies usually present with abdominal pain and abnormal vaginal bleeding.

44. A woman with a history of a child with a neural tube defect should take 4 mg of folic acid on a daily basis, but only 400 mcg daily is recommended for those without such a history.

45. Advanced maternal age is associated with increased risks of chromosomal abnormalities, first-trimester losses, and obstetric complications.

46. Pregnancy is a state of compensated respiratory alkalosis.

47. Plasma volume increases by as much as 45%, but red blood cell mass increases by only 20-30%; this results in dilutional anemia.

48. During pregnancy, increased renal plasma flow and increased glomerular filtration rate lead to decreased serum BUN and creatinine.

49. Pregnancy increases the risk of pyelonephritis due to anatomic changes and decreased ureteral motility.

50. Cardiac output increases by 30-50% in pregnancy due to increases in heart rate and stroke volume.

51. Labor and delivery can be a critical time for women with cardiac disease due to dramatic fluctuations in hemodynamic and volume status.

52. Pregnancy is a hypercoagulable state due to increased clotting factors and venous stasis.

53. Pulmonary embolism is the leading cause of maternal mortality in developed countries.

54. Group B streptococcal (GBS) infection is a cause of neonatal sepsis and carries a high neonatal mortality and morbidity, especially in premature neonates. The CDC recommends maternal screening via vaginal and rectal cultures in the late third trimester and prophylaxis with antibiotics during labor for those who test positive.

55. All pregnant women should be screened for HIV.

56. Maternal parvovirus infection can cause fetal anemia, hydrops, and even intrauterine demise.

57. Maternal systemic lupus erythematosus can cause congenital heart block, which is nonreversible.

58. The risk of major and minor congenital anomalies in women on anticonvulsants is 4-6%, compared to the baseline population risk of 2-3%.

59. Although lithium has been associated with cardiac malformations—especially Ebstein's anomaly—the extent of the risk is unclear.

60. There is no safe level of alcohol consumption in pregnancy; the best advice is not to drink alcohol at all.

61. The recommended weight gain in pregnancy for women of normal weight is 25-35 pounds.

62. Nausea and vomiting of pregnancy (NVP) usually resolves prior to 20 weeks gestation.

63. The only cure for preeclampsia is delivery.

64. Magnesium sulfate should be given to women with severe preeclampsia during labor and for 24 hours after delivery to reduce the risk of seizures.

65. A nonfasting, 1-hour, 50-gm glucose challenge test is used to screen for gestational diabetes; a fasting, 3-hour, 100-gm glucose tolerance test is then used to confirm the diagnosis.

66. Gestational diabetes increases a woman's risk of developing type 2 diabetes later in life.

67. in patients with insulin-dependent diabetes mellitus (IDDM), good glycemic control should be achieved prior to conception in order to decrease the risk of congenital malformations.

68. Although an increase in thyroid-binding globulin during pregnancy causes total circulating T4 and T3 to increase, free levels are not changed.

69. The treatment of asthma in pregnancy is essentially the same as that for nonpregnant women.

70. Women with genital herpes lesions or prodromal symptoms at the onset of labor should deliver by cesarean delivery to prevent vertical transmission.

71. Placental abruption and stillbirth occur in 8% of pregnant cocaine users.

72. Postpartum blues occur in 50-80% of women, depression in 8-15%, and psychosis in 1-2/1000.

73. Special considerations for general anesthesia in the pregnant woman include aspiration risk, physiologic respiratory changes, hypercoagulability, and compression of the inferior vena cava by the gravid uterus.

74. The initial evaluation of a pregnant trauma patient is the same for nonpregnant woman; stabilize the mother before evaluating the fetus.

75. After 4 minutes of CPR in a pregnant woman, a perimortem cesarean should be performed if there is no return of spontaneous circulation.

76. Preterm labor and delivery are common in multiple gestations; mean gestational lengths are 35 weeks for twins, 33 weeks for triplets, and 31 weeks for quadruplets.

77. Twin-to-twin transfusion syndrome can occur in monozygotic pregnancies; it is caused by an irregular distribution of placental vascular anastomosis between the fetuses.

78. Fetal hemolytic disease can occur when a pregnant woman produces antibodies against fetal red blood cell antigens.

79. Rhogam is anti-D immunoglobulin; it is given to Rh-negative women at 28 weeks, at any other time when there is risk for fetomaternal hemorrhage, and postpartum.

80. In the first trimester, gestational dating is determined by measuring the crown-rump length. In the second and third trimesters, it is determined by measuring the biparietal diameter, head circumference, femur length, and abdominal circumference.

81. Intrauterine growth restriction (IUGR) is generally defined as an estimated fetal weight less than the tenth percentile; however, most adverse perinatal outcomes occur at estimated weights less than the fifth percentile.

82. Fetal urine is the major source of amniotic fluid production after the first trimester, and fetal swallowing is the major mode of resorption.

83. Although many cases of polyhydramnios are associated with maternal diabetes, the majority of cases are idiopathic.

84. Human chorionic gonadotropin (HCG) is produced by the syncytiotrophoblast; it maintains the production of progesterone by the corpus luteum in early pregnancy.

85. Abnormal placentation may occur over the internal cervical os (previa), be adherent to the myometrium (accreta), invade into the myometrium (increta), or invade through the myometrium (percreta).

86. Placenta previa classically presents as *painless* third-trimester vaginal bleeding; placental abruption presents as painful vaginal bleeding.

87. Bed rest, pelvic rest, and/or restricted activity have not been proven to be effective in reducing preterm delivery.

88. Cervical cerclage is indicated for the treatment of cervical insufficiency in singleton pregnancies.

89. At the time of an exam, premature rupture of membranes (PROM) is confirmed by pooling of fluid in the vaginal vault, a positive nitrazine test, and ferning of vaginal fluid on a microscope slide.

90. External cephalic version is a technique where one or two people attempt to maneuver a fetus from breech to cephalic presentation using directed pressure on the maternal abdomen.

91. A non-stress test assesses fetal heart rate baseline, variability, and accelerations. It is used to test for fetal well-being, and has a high negative predictive value.

92. Intrapartum fetal heart rate monitoring has been shown to decrease the number of neonatal seizures, but it increases the number of cesarean deliveries without changing the rate of long-term neurologic sequelae or cerebral palsy.

93. Fetal heart rate decelerations are defined by their relationship in time to contractions — variable (caused by cord compression), early (head compression), and late (uteroplacental insufficiency)

94. There are three stages of labor: onset of contractions to complete dilation, complete dilation to delivery of fetus, and delivery of fetus to delivery of placenta.

95. There are seven cardinal movements of labor: engagement, descent, flexion, internal rotation, extension, external rotation, and expulsion.

96. The most concerning complication of trial of labor after cesarean (TOLAC) is uterine rupture; the type and number of previous uterine incision determines the degree of risk.

97. Unlike adults, neonatal resuscitation utilizes the "ABCs" (airway, breathing, and circulation).

98. Postpartum hemorrhage is defined as blood loss > 500 mL for a vaginal delivery and > 1000 mL for a cesarean; the most common cause is uterine atony.

99. The most common complication of cesarean delivery is infection.

100. The most common cause of postpartum fever is endometritis, and the greatest risk factor for this infection is cesarean delivery.

THE MENSTRUAL CYCLE

Jacob Casey, MD, and Judy H. Chen, MD

1. **At what ages do women begin and stop menstruating?**
   In the United States, menarche (the first menstruation) begins between the ages of 10 and 12 years old; menopause (the last menstruation) can vary widely for each woman but generally occurs between 45 and 55 years of age.

2. **What are the phases of the menstrual cycle, and which portions of the reproductive system do they affect?**
   The menstrual cycle affects both the ovary and the endometrium, with two phases in each. Within the ovary, the phases are follicular and luteal. Within the endometrium are proliferative and secretory phases.
   In the ovary, the follicular phase matures the ovum in preparation for ovulation. The luteal phase occurs after ovulation and is maintained by the corpus luteum; it is when the ovum moves through the oviducts and prepares for fertilization and implantation.
   In concert with the changes in the ovary, the endometrium matches the follicular phase of the ovary with its own proliferative phase. During this time, the rising estrogen stimulates the endometrium to increase the number of glands, amount of stromal cells, and vasculature. The secretory phase mirrors the luteal phase of the ovary and is mediated by the presence of progesterone; its purpose is to prepare for implantation (Fig. 1-1).

3. **What is the role of the hypothalamic-pituitary-ovarian (HPO) axis?**
   The HPO axis must be intact for the menstrual cycle to function properly; any disruption has an impact. For example, improper maturation of gonadotropin-releasing hormone (GnRH) neurons at the level of the hypothalamus can cause amenorrhea, as seen in **Kallmann syndrome.**

4. **What are the two main hormones released by the pituitary gland during the menstrual cycle?**
   Follicle-stimulating hormone (FSH) and luteinizing hormone (LH), which are two glycoproteins that have identical alpha-subunits. (This alpha-subunit is also shared by thyroid-stimulating hormone [TSH] and human chorionic gonadotropin [hCG].)

5. **When is the number of germ cells in the ovaries highest?**
   Primordial germ cells begin to form at 5 to 6 weeks of gestation, and they multiply to reach the maximum amount of cells by 20 weeks (approximately 6 to 7 million per ovary). At birth, only approximately 2 million germ cells remain, as a result of atresia and apoptosis.
   Women have approximately 300,000 germ cells per ovary at the time of puberty; by menopause, fewer than 100,000 remain.

6. **What are the two main layers of the endometrium?**
   The basal layer and the functional layer.
   The basal layer overlies the myometrium and consists of glands and stroma that are not hormonally sensitive (i.e., they are not shed during menstruation).
   The functional layer overlies the basal layer and is exposed to the uterine cavity. It is the site of blastocyst implantation, it is sensitive to hormones, and it is shed during menstruation. During the secretory phase, vacuoles within its glandular cells move from an intracellular to an intraluminal location and are the reason for this phase's name.

7. **What is the mean duration of a menstrual cycle?**
   The **mean** duration is 28 ± 2 days. However, the **normal range** is between 21 and 35 days (28 ± 7 days). A cycle shorter than 21 days is called polymenorrhea, and a cycle longer than days 35 is called oligomenorrhea.

8. **When are the two most common times in a woman's life for irregular menstrual cycles to occur?**
   Two years after puberty and 3 years before menopause.

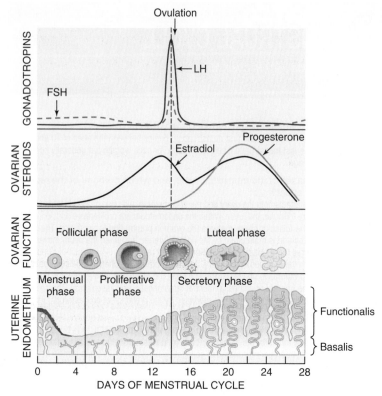

Figure 1-1. Hormone levels during a normal menstrual cycle. *(Modified from Gambone JC: Female reproductive physiology. In Hacker NF, Gambone JC, Hobel CJ, eds. Hacker and Moore's Essentials of Obstetrics and Gynecology. 5th ed. Philadelphia: Saunders, 2010.)*

9. **What is a primordial follicle?**
   An oocyte arrested in the diplotene phase of meiosis I.
   Primordial follicles are encompassed by a layer of granulosa cells that aid in the growth of the follicle to become a primary (preantral) follicle and then a secondary (antral) follicle.

10. **What are the three stages of the follicular phase?**
    1. Recruitment of antral follicles
    2. Selection of a dominant follicle
    3. Growth of the dominant follicle

11. **What is the primary hormone responsible for follicular growth during the follicular phase?**
    FSH, which provides the signal for further cell growth and rescues the follicle from atresia. An increase in the FSH/LH ratio can be seen at the start of each follicular phase.

12. **What two cell layers in the ovary are hormonally sensitive and important for the maturation of a dominant follicle?**
    The granulosa cell layer and the theca cell layer.
    The granulosa cell layer contains FSH receptors and is responsible for estrogen synthesis by increasing the production of the enzyme **aromatase.**
    The theca cell layer, which forms during follicular maturation, contains LH receptors and is responsible for the production of androgens. Androgens from the theca cell layer diffuse back into the granulosa cells and are converted into estrogen by aromatization.

13. How is a dominant follicle selected from a group of antral follicles, and at what point in the cycle does this occur?
Although the exact mechanism is not known, dominant follicles have a greater sensitivity to FSH compared with other follicles.
Dominant follicles are generally selected by day 6 to 9 of the menstrual cycle.

14. Approximately how many dominant follicles are formed in a woman's lifetime?
Approximately 400.

15. What happens to the follicles not selected to become dominant?
They undergo apoptosis.

16. What is the LH surge, and what causes it?
The LH surge is an acute rise in LH that triggers ovulation. It is primarily driven by rising estrogen production from the dominant follicle, which peaks approximately 24 to 36 hours before ovulation (see Fig. 1-1).

17. When is ovulation most likely to occur?
Approximately 32 hours after luteinizing hormone (LH) starts to rise or approximately 16 hours after it peaks (see Fig. 1-1).

18. How is the oocyte released from the ovary?
The LH surge induces an inflammatory-like response in which prostaglandins and proteases work to break down the cell layers of the dominant follicle and allow for the oocyte to be released. Blood flow to the follicle also increases during this time.

19. What happens to the oocyte on being released from the ovary?
The oocyte is now signaled to continue meiosis, in which it progresses from the diplotene stage of meiosis I to arrest at the metaphase stage of meiosis II. At this point, the first polar body can be seen. Meiosis II is completed only if fertilization occurs.

20. What does the remainder of the dominant follicle become after ovulation?
The remaining cell layers form a new structure called the corpus luteum and produce progesterone, a key component of the luteal phase.

21. What are three major effects of progesterone during the luteal phase?
1. Negative feedback at the level of the hypothalamus decreases GnRH, which reduces secretion of FSH and LH secretion.
2. Progesterone causes the hypothalamus to increase basal body temperature.
3. Progesterone increases the number of subnuclear vacuoles in the endometrium to prepare for implantation.

22. When does the level of progesterone peak?
Approximately 8 days after the LH surge.
At this time the corpus luteum is still producing aromatase, which converts progesterone to estrogen and causes a synchronous rise in both hormones (see Fig. 1-1).

23. How long does the luteal phase last?
The corpus luteum has a limited lifespan of 14 days; the start of the next menses therefore provides information when ovulation occurred by counting backwards. However, there is increasing evidence that there may be greater variability during this phase than previously believed.

24. What happens to the corpus luteum if fertilization occurs?
hCG produced by the blastocyst prevents degradation and allows for the continued production of progesterone. Eventually, the placenta begins to synthesize enough progesterone to maintain the pregnancy.

25. When should intercourse occur for the greatest chance of fertilization?
One to 2 days before ovulation.
Sperm can survive up to 5 days in the female genital tract, and the oocyte can survive up to 24 hours after ovulation.

26. When does implantation occur?
Implantation occurs 6 to 9 days after ovulation.

27. What triggers menstruation at the end of the cycle?

In the absence of implantation and subsequent hCG production, the functional layer of the endometrium is shed; endometrial glands and stroma are broken down by matrix metalloproteinases and proteolytic enzymes.

28. How does cervical mucus change during the menstrual cycle?

During the follicular phase, estrogen causes thin, watery, or stringy mucus to facilitate sperm transport. After ovulation, progesterone causes the mucus to thicken and act as a barrier to ascending infection.

KEY POINTS: MENSTRUAL CYCLE

1. FSH signals follicular recruitment and increases LH receptor expression.
2. LH midcycle surge predicts impending ovulation.
3. The lifespan of the corpus luteum requires tonic LH secretion or stimulation by hCG.
4. The phases of the menstrual cycle are as follows:
   Ovary: follicular, ovulation, luteal
   Endometrium: proliferative, secretory, menstrual

BIBLIOGRAPHY

1. Hacker NF, Gambone JC, Hobel CJ. *Hacker & Moore's Essentials of Obstetrics and Gynecology.* 5th ed. Philadelphia: Saunders; 2009.
2. Lentz GM, Lobo RA, Gershenson DM, Katz VL. *Comprehensive Gynecology.* 6th ed. Philadelphia: Mosby; 2013.
3. Speroff L, Fritz MA. *Clinical Gynecologic Endocrinology and Infertility.* 7th ed. Philadelphia: Lippincott Williams & Wilkins; 2005.

PREMENSTRUAL SYNDROME AND DYSMENORRHEA

Alin Lina Akopians, MD, PhD

CHAPTER 2

1. **What is premenstrual syndrome (PMS)?**
   Cyclic physical and behavioral symptoms that appear in the days preceding menses and interfere with work or lifestyle, followed by a symptom-free interval. Symptoms typically occur during the luteal phase of the menstrual cycle and abate by day 4 of menstruation.

2. **What symptoms are associated with PMS?**
   Symptoms may be psychological, somatic, and/or behavioral. The most common symptoms are irritability, anxiety, depression, mood swings, bloating, abdominal discomfort, weight gain, acne, breast pain, headache, fatigue, and increased appetite with food cravings (particularly for sweets).

3. **Do we know what causes PMS?**
   No. Numerous theories have been postulated, all of which have to do with various hormonal alterations: ovarian hormones (estrogen and progesterone), fluids and electrolytes (aldosterone, renin and angiotensin, and vasopressin), neurotransmitters (γ-aminobutyric acid [GABA] and serotonin), and other hormones (endorphins, androgens, and glucocorticoids). The pathogenesis is likely related to changes in gonadal steroid production during the luteal phase and their subsequent effect on neurotransmitters such as GABA and serotonin in the central nervous system (CNS).

4. **What is the incidence of PMS?**
   PMS affects 20% to 40% of women, with up to 20% experiencing moderate symptoms and up to 40% having mild symptoms. From 2% to 10% of women are severely affected, thus making the incidence of severe PMS approximately 6 in 1000 to 40 in 1000 women.

5. **How is PMS diagnosed?**
   No specific tests or published diagnostic guidelines are available. However, the following criteria are widely accepted among physicians:
   1. Cyclic symptoms documented for at least two cycles, as a prospective diary of severity of symptoms.
   2. Symptoms occurring only during the luteal phase, approximately 2 weeks before menstruation.
   3. Symptoms relieved by day 4 of menses.

6. **What is premenstrual dysphoric disorder (PMDD)?**
   A severe form of premenstrual disorder affecting approximately 5% to 8% of women. Recognized by the American Psychiatric Association and described in the *Diagnostic and Statistical Manual of Mental Disorders,* fifth edition (DSM-5), the diagnosis requires five premenstrual symptoms with at least one being a moderately to severely disabling affective symptom.

7. **How is PMS treated?**
   Treatment is mainly directed toward the predominant bothersome symptoms. Education and understanding alone may be sufficient for many patients. Stress management and lifestyle changes (e.g., weight loss, exercise, smoking cessation, and restriction of caffeine and alcohol consumption) may improve symptoms, as well as calcium supplementation. Various medications have also been shown to be effective and include selective serotonin reuptake inhibitors (SSRIs), alprazolam, gonadotropin-releasing hormone (GnRH) agonists, oral contraceptive pills (OCPs), and spironolactone.

8. **How is severe PMS or PMDD treated?**
   The American Congress of Obstetricians and Gynecologists (ACOG) currently recommends SSRIs (fluoxetine and sertraline) as the drugs of choice for treatment of severe PMS or PMDD. Treatment can be either continuous or confined to the luteal phase. The exact mechanism of symptom improvement is unknown.

11

9. **Do GnRH agonists have a role in treatment?**
   Treatment with a GnRH agonist causes "medical menopause" and has been shown to improve PMS symptoms. However, the resulting hypoestrogenic state has many unfavorable side effects, such as depression, anxiety, irritability, vasomotor symptoms, vaginal dryness, and muscle aches. A long-term risk of osteoporosis also exists.

10. **Do OCPs have a role in treatment?**
    OCPs eliminate the hormonal fluctuations observed during normal menstrual cycles and have been proven to be effective in treating PMDD. OCPs containing the progestogen drospirenone may help ameliorate symptoms of water retention, bloating, weight gain, and breast tenderness because drospirenone is derived from an analogue of spironolactone and has both antiandrogenic and antimineralocorticoid properties.

11. **Does spironolactone have a role in treatment?**
    The physical symptoms of fluid retention (e.g., weight gain and breast tenderness), as well as some emotional symptoms, may be related to elevations in renin and angiotensin and in aldosterone and are alleviated by spironolactone.

12. **Can sterilization be used to treat PMS?**
    Sterilization by tubal ligation has not been shown to reduce PMS symptoms. In extraordinary circumstances, women with severe, debilitating disease can be treated with a total hysterectomy and bilateral oophorectomy.

KEY POINTS: PREMENSTRUAL SYNDROME

1. PMS describes emotional and physical symptoms that occur at the same time in the menstrual cycle each month.
2. Although no one cause of PMS has been established, treatments correlate with possible causes, such as progesterone supplementation, SSRIs, and nonsteroidal antiinflammatory drugs (NSAIDs).

---

13. **What is dysmenorrhea?**
    Pelvic pain associated with menstrual periods. It is classified as either primary or secondary, and the pain is usually described as cramping. The pain can also be felt outside the pelvis and may manifest as backaches, headaches, and extremity pain. Dysmenorrhea can be accompanied by a variety of systemic symptoms such as lightheadedness, insomnia, nausea, vomiting, and diarrhea.

14. **What is the difference between primary and secondary dysmenorrhea?**
    Primary dysmenorrhea is pain resulting from myometrial contraction during ovulatory cycles with no associated identifiable pathologic process. Secondary dysmenorrhea is pain caused by other gynecologic conditions. The most common conditions associated with secondary dysmenorrhea are uterine leiomyomas, adenomyosis, and endometriosis.

15. **What is the incidence of dysmenorrhea?**
    As many as 72% of women experience some discomfort associated with their menses. In a small but significant percentage, symptoms are severe enough to interfere with daily activities or cause absence from work or school. In adolescent girls, the prevalence of primary dysmenorrhea is thought to be as high as 60% to 90%. Dysmenorrhea is less common and less severe in women who have previously given birth.

16. **Is dysmenorrhea considered to be a form of chronic pelvic pain?**
    No. Even though women with dysmenorrhea (particularly secondary dysmenorrhea) can have pelvic symptoms between menstrual periods, dysmenorrhea is characterized by the onset or exacerbation of symptoms in association with menses.

17. **How is dysmenorrhea evaluated?**
    Primary dysmenorrhea is a clinical diagnosis. A thorough patient history is essential to rule out other gynecologic or nongynecologic (e.g., urologic or gastrointestinal) causes of pelvic pain and connect the timing or exacerbation of the symptoms to menstruation.

18. **What causes the pain of primary dysmenorrhea?**
    Primary dysmenorrhea is likely associated with myometrial ischemia secondary to frequent and prolonged uterine contraction. The principal cause seems to be increased production of prostaglandin $F_{2\alpha}$ that stimulates uterine contraction. Prostaglandin $F_{2\alpha}$ can also contribute to systemic symptoms (e.g., nausea, diarrhea, and headaches).

19. **How is dysmenorrhea treated?**
    Both primary and secondary dysmenorrhea can be treated with NSAIDs or OCPs, or both. NSAIDs decrease prostaglandin production and can provide symptom relief in 70% to 90% of patients. In primary amenorrhea, OCPs are considered a first-line agent in sexually active female patients. These drugs cause atrophy of the endometrium, which is the principal site of prostaglandin production. They can also reduce the amount and duration of bleeding.

    In secondary dysmenorrhea, treatment may be directed at the underlying pathologic process, once it has been identified. In the case of uterine myomas or endometriosis, surgical management may be considered. However, medical therapy is usually attempted before resorting to surgical intervention.

20. **What nonmedical options exist for treatment of dysmenorrhea?**
    A vegetarian diet, vitamin E, exercise, and the direct application of a heating pad to the lower abdomen may be helpful for some women. Evidence is insufficient to recommend dietary changes for all women with dysmenorrhea, but two clinical trials have shown improvement of symptoms with use of a heated abdominal patch or wrap for 8 to 12 hours compared with placebo.

21. **What should be done when the response to medical therapy is inadequate?**
    Women with secondary dysmenorrhea should be offered treatment of the underlying pathologic process; this often involves surgical intervention. Women with primary dysmenorrhea should be offered a more extensive workup to see whether their symptoms have a previously unrecognized cause. This investigation can involve pelvic ultrasound examination, hysteroscopy, or laparoscopy.

BIBLIOGRAPHY

1. Andersch B, Milsom I. An epidemiologic study of young women with dysmenorrhea. *Am J Obstet Gynecol.* 1982;144:655–660.
2. Brandenburg S, Tuynman-Qua H, Verheij R, Pepplinkhuizen L. Treatment of premenstrual syndrome with fluoxetine: an open study. *Int Clin Psychopharmacol.* 1993;8:315–317.
3. Casper RF, Hearn MT. The effect of hysterectomy and bilateral oophorectomy in women with severe premenstrual syndrome. *Am J Obstet Gynecol.* 1990;162:105–109.
4. Chan AF, Mortola JF, Wood SH, et al. Persistence of premenstrual syndrome during low-dose administration of the progesterone antagonist RU 486. *Obstet Gynecol.* 1994;84:1001–1005.
5. Ford O, Lethaby A, Roberts H, et al. Progesterone for pre-menstrual syndrome. *Cochrane Database Syst Rev.* 2009;2:CD003415.
6. Frank RT. The hormonal causes of premenstrual tension. *Arch Neurol Psychiatry.* 1931;26:1052.
7. Freeman E, Rickels K, Sondheimer S, Polanski M. Ineffectiveness of progesterone suppository treatment for premenstrual syndrome. *JAMA.* 1990;264:349–353.
8. Freeman E, Rickels K, Sondheimer S, Polansky M. A double-blind trial of oral progesterone, alprazolam, and placebo in treatment of severe PMS. *JAMA.* 1995;274:51–57.
9. Fritz MA, Speroff L. Menstrual disorders. In: *Clinical Gynecologic Endocrinology and Infertility.* 8th ed. Philadelphia: Lippincott Williams & Wilkins; 2011:567–589.
10. Ginsburg KA. Some practical approaches to treating PMS. *Contemp Obstet Gynecol.* 1995;40:24.
11. Green R, Dalton K. The premenstrual syndrome. *Br Med J.* 1953;1:1007.
12. Mark AS, Hricak H, Heinrichs LW, et al. Adenomyosis and leiomyoma: differential diagnosis with MR imaging. *Radiology.* 1987;163:527–529.
13. Morrison BW, Daniels SE, Kotey P, et al. Rofecoxib, a specific cyclooxygenase-2 inhibitor, in primary dysmenorrhea: a randomized controlled trial. *Obstet Gynecol.* 1999;94:504–508.
14. Pearlstein TB, Bachmann GA, Zacur HA, et al. Treatment of premenstrual dysphoric disorder with a new drospirenone-containing oral contraceptive formulation. *Contraception.* 2005;72:414–421.
15. Rapkin AJ, Akopians AL. Pathophysiology of premenstrual syndrome and premenstrual dysphoric disorder. *Menopause Int.* 2012;18:52–59.
16. Rapkin AJ, Winer SA. The pharmacologic management of pre-menstrual dysphoric disorder. *Expert Opin Pharmacother.* 2008;9:429–445.
17. Smith S, Rinehart JS, Ruddock VE, Schiff I. Treatment of premenstrual syndrome with alprazolam: results of a double-blind, placebo-controlled, randomized crossover clinical trial. *Obstet Gynecol.* 1987;70:37–42.

18. Sundell G, Milsom I, Andersch B. Factors influencing the prevalence and severity of dysmenorrhea in young women. *Br J Obstet Gynecol.* 1990;97:588–594.
19. Thys-Jacobs S, Starkey P, Bernstein D, et al. Calcium carbonate and the premenstrual syndrome: effects on premenstrual and menstrual symptoms. Premenstrual Syndrome Study Group. *Am J Obstet Gynecol.* 1998;179:444–452.
20. Yonkers KA, Brown C, Pearlstein TB, et al. Efficacy of a new low-dose oral contraceptive with drospirenone in premenstrual dysphoric disorder. *Obstet Gynecol.* 2005;106:492–501.

ABNORMAL UTERINE BLEEDING

Hannah Newmark, MD

1. **What is a normal menstrual cycle and a normal amount of uterine bleeding?**
   A normal menstrual cycle averages 28 days but can range from 21 to 35 days, and menses last for an average of 4 days. Normal blood loss is approximately 35 mL.

2. **What is abnormal uterine bleeding (AUB)?**
   AUB is bleeding from the uterine corpus that is abnormal in regularity, volume, frequency, or duration in the absence of pregnancy. It is usually subjective (i.e., a patient's bleeding pattern or amount changes from what she considers normal).

3. **Is AUB common?**
   Yes. Thirty-three percent of gynecologist office visits and up to 70% of gynecology consultations for perimenopausal and postmenopausal women are for AUB.

4. **How is AUB categorized?**
   Categorization is necessary to define the underlying cause and help direct treatment. Historically, terms such as menorrhagia (>80 mL of blood loss per menses) and metrorrhagia (bleeding between periods) were used. However, these terms have been replaced by heavy menstrual bleeding (HMB) and intermenstrual bleeding (IMB), which can be further classified using the PALM-COIEN mnemonic system (Table 3-1). Oligomenorrhea and polymenorrhea have also been discarded in favor of more descriptive terms (e.g., AUB-HMB/IMB with bleeding every 2 weeks, AUB with no bleeding for 6 months followed by 29 days of bleeding).

Table 3-1. Categorization of Abnormal Uterine Bleeding and the PALM-COIEN Mnemonic System

TYPE OF BLEEDING	STRUCTURAL CAUSES (PALM)	NONSTRUCTURAL CAUSES (COEIN)
Abnormal uterine bleeding (AUB)	Polyp	Coagulopathy
Heavy menstrual bleeding (HMB)	Adenomyosis	Ovulatory dysfunction
Intermenstrual bleeding (IMB)	Leiomyoma	Endometrial
Postmenopausal bleeding (PMB)	Malignancy/hyperplasia	Iatrogenic
		Not yet classified

Structural causes (mnemonic PALM):

Polyp: Overgrowth of endometrium into the uterine cavity. Usually benign, but up to 5% of polyps in postmenopausal women can contain malignant cells. Can be seen and potentially removed using hysteroscopy.

Adenomyosis: Growth of endometrial glands into the muscular layer of the uterus (myometrium). Can cause painful periods and make the uterus globular and enlarged.

Leiomyoma: Benign smooth muscle tumors, present in up to 70% of women. Also referred to as fibroids. Mainly seen in reproductive years and thought to be hormonally driven, although their exact cause is unknown. Range in size from 0.5 cm to massive (filling entire abdomen); symptoms generally depend on location.
  - Submucosal: Partially inside endometrial cavity, can cause heavy bleeding. Can be seen and potentially removed using hysteroscopy.
  - Other: Subserosal, intramural or pedunculated; less likely to cause bleeding but can cause pain and pressure symptoms.

15

For more information on leiomyoma classification, see Chapter 5, Figure 5-1.

Malignancy and hyperplasia: Usually manifest in perimenopausal or postmenopausal women, most often as painless postmenopausal bleeding. Can manifest as AUB in premenopausal women.

Nonstructural causes (mnemonic COEIN):

Coagulopathy: Most commonly resulting from von Willebrand disease (note: although up to 1% of women have von Willebrand disease, only 1 in 10,000 women has symptoms)

Ovulatory dysfunction: Many causes (e.g., perimenopause, polycystic ovarian syndrome, pregnancy, lactation, anorexia, pituitary dysfunction, and premature ovarian failure)

Endometrial: Primary endometrial dysfunction; a diagnosis of exclusion

Iatrogenic: Many causes (e.g., instrumentation, anticoagulation, other therapies)

Not yet classified: Used to indicate that a workup has not been completed or the cause is uncertain

5. **What elements of a history and physical examination can help elucidate the cause of AUB?**

History:
- What is a normal bleeding pattern for the patient, and when did it change?
- Age of menarche? Menopause?
- Associated symptoms? (Pain can indicate infection; bruising or bleeding can indicate coagulopathy; lightheadedness can be a symptom of anemia or thyroid disease; hot flashes can indicate perimenopause or menopause.)
- Medical conditions or medications (e.g., anticoagulation, high-dose nonsteroidal anti-inflammatory drugs [NSAIDs], oral contraceptives).
- Medical and surgical history.
- Family history or symptoms concerning for bleeding disorder.

Physical examination:
- Look for signs of anemia or a bleeding disorder (bleeding or bruising, pallor), hypothyroidism or hyperthyroidism (fine tremor, goiter, delayed deep tendon reflexes), and hyperandrogenism (acanthosis nigricans, hirsutism, central obesity).
- Speculum examination: Assess for a cervical mass or polyps or a prolapsing leiomyoma.
- Bimanual examination: Assess the size of the uterus and the presence or absence of pain.

6. **Do the common causes of AUB vary with age?**

Yes. The differential diagnosis is affected by the patient's stage of her reproductive lifespan.
- Ages 13 to 18 years: Many adolescents do not have a fully mature hypothalamic pituitary axis and can experience anovulatory cycles for up to 2 years after menarche. Have a strong suspicion of an underlying bleeding disorder if hospitalization or transfusion is required. Other common causes are imperfect hormonal contraceptive use, pregnancy, or infection.
- Ages 19 to 39 years: Common causes include pregnancy, structural lesions such as polyps or fibroids, anovulatory cycles (most commonly from polycystic ovarian syndrome), or endometrial hyperplasia or malignant disease.
- Age 40 years to menopause: Anovulatory cycles can occur during perimenopause. Other common causes are structural lesions, endometrial hyperplasia, and malignant disease.

7. **What laboratory tests should be ordered in a patient with AUB?**
- All women with abnormal bleeding should be tested for pregnancy.
- A complete blood count (CBC) can rule out anemia and thrombocytopenia.
- A thyroid-stimulating hormone (TSH) level can assess thyroid function.
- If a bleeding disorder is suspected, prothrombin time (PT), partial thromboplastin time (PTT), von Willebrand factor, ristocetin cofactor activity, and factor VIII levels should be ordered. Bleeding time is neither sensitive nor specific and should not be obtained.
- Other laboratory tests to consider are prolactin (if concern exists for a prolactinoma), hemoglobin A1c (if signs of insulin resistance or polycystic ovarian syndrome are present), and follicle-stimulating hormone (FSH) (if patient is perimenopausal or concern for primary ovarian insufficiency exists).

8. **What types of imaging can be used to evaluate AUB?**

Transvaginal ultrasound is the most commonly used technique and can detect larger structural abnormalities. An intracavitary lesion (endometrial polyp or submucosal leiomyoma) can be identified with a **saline-infused sonogram**, in which saline is injected into the uterus at the time of an ultrasound examination. Hysteroscopy can also be performed. Magnetic resonance imaging (MRI) is not considered a first-line study but can be used when knowledge of the precise location and size of fibroids is important.

9. **When and how can AUB be treated empirically?**

If a patient is not at risk for hyperplasia or malignant disease, a trial of medical management may be appropriate. If it is not successful, further evaluation is required. Treatment options include NSAIDs, progestin analogues, oral contraceptives, the levonorgestrel intrauterine device, and depot medroxyprogesterone acetate.

10. **How can AUB caused by structural lesions be treated?**

If a structural abnormality is found, surgical treatment may be required. For intramural, subserosal, and pedunculated leiomyomas, surgical options include myomectomy (laparoscopic or abdominal) and hysterectomy. Another option is treatment with a gonadotropin-releasing hormone agonist, which induces a menopause-like state. Amenorrhea results, and the leiomyomas decrease in size. Because of side effects, this treatment is best used as a temporary bridge to surgical management.

For intracavitary lesions, operative hysteroscopy can be performed. This minimally invasive option can allow many patients to avoid hysterectomy, and small lesions can even be removed in a clinic without general anesthesia. Larger lesions (up to 5 cm) are generally removed in the operating room.

11. **What is endometrial ablation, and when it performed?**

Endometrial ablation is a procedure designed to destroy the outer layer of the endometrium. It can be done in either the clinic or the operating room, and it is an option for women who have completed childbearing and are not at risk for hyperplasia. Many different techniques are available: freezing, instillation of hot water, thermal balloon use, electrocautery, microwaves, or radio waves. Success rates are similar, and up to 85% of patients will achieve long-term resolution of their AUB.

12. **Which patients with AUB should be screened for endometrial cancer?**

Endometrial biopsy to rule out hyperplasia and malignant disease should be performed in women who are more than 45 years old, or at any age if risk factors (obesity, chronic anovulation, or poor response to medical management) are present.

KEY POINTS: ABNORMAL UTERINE BLEEDING

1. A normal menstrual cycle averages 28 days; normal menses last 4 days, and blood loss is approximately 35 mL.
2. AUB is categorized by cause.
3. For women with AUB, endometrial biopsy should be performed to rule out hyperplasia and malignant disease in those who are more than 45 years old or who have risk factors.
4. If a patient is not at risk for hyperplasia or malignant disease, a trial of medical management may be appropriate.
5. Surgical treatments for abnormal uterine bleeding include endometrial ablation, operative hysteroscopy, myomectomy, and hysterectomy.

BIBLIOGRAPHY

1. American College of Obstetricians and Gynecologists. Diagnosis of abnormal uterine bleeding in reproductive-aged women. ACOG practice bulletin no. 128. *Obstet Gynecol.* 2012;120:197–206.
2. American College of Obstetricians and Gynecologists. Management of abnormal uterine bleeding associated with ovulatory dysfunction. ACOG practice bulletin no. 136. *Obstet Gynecol.* 2013;122:176–185.

CHAPTER 4

ENDOMETRIOSIS AND ADENOMYOSIS

Julia Switzer, MD

1. **What is endometriosis?**
   Endometriosis is a chronic, inflammatory condition in which hormonally responsive endometrial glands and stroma are present outside the uterine cavity.

2. **How common is endometriosis?**
   The true prevalence is unknown. It is thought to occur in 6% to 10% of women of reproductive age. It is more frequent among women with chronic pelvic pain (50% to 87%) and infertility (20% to 50%). Having a first-degree relative with endometriosis is considered a risk factor.

3. **How does endometriosis develop?**
   Several theories have been proposed, although the true pathogenesis is uncertain and is likely multifactorial.
   1. Retrograde menstruation (Sampson's theory): Endometriosis is the result of retrograde menstruation; endometrial tissue is carried through the fallopian tubes into the peritoneal cavity, where it implants and proliferates. Support for this theory includes the common finding of endometrial lesions in dependent areas of the peritoneal cavity, direct visualization of menstrual fluid extravasating from the fallopian tubes at time of laparoscopy, and increased incidence of endometriosis in women with uterine outlet obstruction.
   2. Coelomic metaplasia (Meyer's theory): Endometriosis is caused by transformation of pluripotent peritoneal cells into endometrial cells.
   3. Lymphatic or hematologic spread (Halban's theory): Endometrial tissue metastasizes to extrauterine sites through the lymphatic or vascular system. Support for this theory includes the presence of endometriosis outside the peritoneal cavity, including lymph nodes.
   4. Induction theory: Certain hormonal, immunologic, or inflammatory factors stimulate differentiation into endometrial tissue and/or allow ectopic endometrial cells to implant and proliferate. Support for this theory includes the finding of increased numbers of activated macrophages and proinflammatory cytokines (interleukin-6 [IL-6], IL-8, and tumor necrosis factor-α [TNF-α]) in the peritoneum, local production of prostaglandins in endometrial lesions, and local production of estrogen in endometrial lesions stimulated by increased aromatase activity.

4. **What are the symptoms of endometriosis?**
   The classic symptoms are cyclic pelvic pain beginning just before the menses, infertility, and dyspareunia. Patients may also present with noncyclic chronic pelvic pain, dysuria, pain with defecation (dyschezia), or an endometrioma (a type of adnexal mass in patients with endometriosis).

5. **What are the physical examination findings associated with endometriosis?**
   Patients may have diffuse pelvic pain, uterosacral nodularity or tenderness, an adnexal mass, or a fixed, retroverted uterus. Other patients may have no distinct examination findings.

6. **How is endometriosis diagnosed?**
   In symptomatic patients, the diagnosis can be made clinically based on history and physical exam and empiric medical therapy can be initiated. Endometriomas can be identified on transvaginal pelvic ultrasound by their classic "ground glass" appearance. Visual recognition of characteristic lesions (black, blue, red, white, or clear vesicular lesions and associated findings of scarring or fibrosis) at the time of laparoscopy is possible. Definitive diagnosis is made by laparoscopy with peritoneal biopsy and histopathologic confirmation of endometrial glands and stroma or hemosiderin-laden macrophages. Endometriomas can also be identified at the time of surgical intervention by visualization of their hallmark brown cyst fluid ("chocolate cysts").

7. **What are the most common anatomic sites of endometriosis?**
   Endometrial lesions are commonly found on the ovary, uterosacral ligaments, fallopian tubes, rectosigmoid colon, pelvic peritoneum, and posterior cul-de-sac. Endometriosis has also been reported at distant anatomic sites including the lung and incisional sites.

8. **How is endometriosis staged?**
   Although no clear correlation exists between the extent of disease and symptoms, the American Society of Reproductive Medicine staging system describes the location and type of disease and ranges from 1 to 4 (minimal to severe). This system is used to record operative findings and compare results of different therapies.

9. **What medical treatments are available?**
   Treatment of pain associated with endometriosis is aimed at downregulating estradiol production by inhibiting ovulation, which induces endometrial atrophy and counteracts the chronic inflammatory state.

   - Combined oral contraceptive pills (OCPs) induce decidualization and atrophy of endometrial tissue by suppressing ovarian estradiol production. They are effective for many (60% to 85%) patients; continuous use (skipping placebo pills) can be helpful if women experience symptoms during menses.
   - Gonadotropin-releasing hormone (GnRH) agonists suppress pituitary function by downregulating pituitary (GnRH) receptors, thus leading to anovulation and endometrial atrophy. Treatment is generally limited to 6-month intervals to avoid long-term consequences of hypoestrogenism on bone metabolism and cardiovascular health. Side effects (hot flashes, vaginal dryness, headache, insomnia, libido changes, fatigue, bone loss) can be ameliorated with "add-back therapy" using a progestogen or combined OCP.
   - Progestins induce decidualization and atrophy of endometrial tissue by suppressing luteinizing hormone (LH), which inhibits ovulation. More than 80% of women will have some pain relief. The levonorgestrel-releasing intrauterine device (IUD) has been shown to improve pelvic pain and dyspareunia in patients with endometriosis.
   - Aromatase inhibitors decrease circulating estrogen levels by 50% and appear to regulate local estrogen production within endometriotic lesions.
   - Danazol, a derivative of 17α-ethinyltestosterone, suppresses LH and follicle-stimulating hormone (FSH), thereby causing anovulation and hyperandrogenism. Although it has been shown to be effective in relieving pain, it is rarely used because of its androgenic side effects (acne, deepening of voice, weight gain, hair growth, decreased breast size).
   - Nonsteroidal antiinflammatory drugs (NSAIDs) may inhibit prostaglandin production in ectopic endometrial tissue and effectively treat dysmenorrhea.

10. **What surgical treatments are available?**
    - Conservative: laparoscopic excision or ablation of endometrial implants or laparoscopic removal of an endometrioma. This is the treatment of choice for women in whom medical therapy has failed but who desire future fertility. Although pain relief after 1 year ranges between 50% and 95%, many patients eventually develop recurrent symptoms. Ablation is performed with unipolar cautery, bipolar cautery, laser, or ultrasonic coagulation. Excision requires removal of tissue. No evidence indicates that one surgical technique is superior to another. Laparoscopic uterosacral nerve ablation and presacral neurectomy may decrease midline dysmenorrhea, but these procedures are less commonly performed.
    - Definitive: hysterectomy with or without bilateral salpingo-oophorectomy. If the ovaries are removed, surgical menopause occurs and leads to atrophy of ectopic endometrial tissue.

11. **How does endometriosis lead to infertility?**
    The inflammatory nature of endometriosis is thought to contribute to infertility by altering folliculogenesis leading to poor quality oocytes, decreasing endometrial receptivity, damaging tubal motility or patency, and impairing sperm function.

12. **What is the relationship between endometriosis and malignant disease?**
    The rate of clear cell and endometrioid-type epithelial ovarian carcinoma is higher in women with endometriosis compared with the general population. However, ovarian carcinoma associated with endometriosis is usually diagnosed at an earlier stage and lower grade, and it is associated with a better overall survival rate.

KEY POINTS: ENDOMETRIOSIS

1. Endometriosis, endometrial tissue outside the uterus, causes pelvic pain, dyspareunia, and infertility.
2. Theories about the etiology of endometriosis include metastasis and metaplasia.
3. Endometriosis is typically diagnosed by laparoscopy, but the visible extent may not correlate with the degree of symptoms.
4. Common therapies are NSAIDs and OCPs for milder disease and GnRH agonists or surgical intervention for more severe disease.

13. **What is adenomyosis?**
    Adenomyosis is a chronic condition characterized by invasion of endometrial glands and stroma into the myometrium which induces hypertrophy and hyperplasia.

14. **What are the symptoms of adenomyosis?**
    Classic symptoms of adenomyosis are dysmenorrhea and heavy, prolonged menstrual bleeding.

15. **What physical findings are associated with adenomyosis?**
    Patients with adenomyosis often have an enlarged, globular uterus.

16. **How is adenomyosis diagnosed?**
    Definitive diagnosis is made on histologic examination of a hysterectomy specimen. On magnetic resonance imaging (MRI), a thickened junctional zone is suggestive of adenomyosis.

17. **What treatments are available for adenomyosis?**
    Definitive therapy is total hysterectomy. The levonorgestrel-releasing IUD, GnRH agonists, NSAIDs, and OCPs are options for medical management.

KEY POINTS: ADENOMYOSIS

1. Adenomyosis, endometrial tissue in the myometrium, causes abnormal uterine bleeding and dysmenorrhea.
2. It is often suggested by MRI (thickened junctional zone), but definitive diagnosis is made only by microscopic uterine inspection after hysterectomy.
3. Adenomyosis can be treated initially with NSAIDs and OCPs or cyclic progesterone, but it may require hysterectomy for persistent symptoms.

BIBLIOGRAPHY

1. American College of Obstetricians and Gynecologists. Management of Endometriosis. ACOG practice bulletin no. 114. Washington, DC: American College of Obstetricians and Gynecologists; 2010.
2. American Society for Reproductive Medicine. Revised American Society for Reproductive Medicine classification of endometriosis. 1996. *Fertil Steril.* 1997;67:817–821.
3. Benagiano G, Habiba M. Brosens, I. The pathophysiology of adenomyosis: an update. *Fertil Steril.* 2012;98:572–579.
4. Fritz M, Speroff L. *Clinical Gynecologic Endocrinology and Infertility.* 8th ed. Philadelphia: Lippincott Williams & Wilkins; 2011.
5. Hoffman B, Schorge J, Schaffer J, et al., eds. *Williams Gynecology.* 2nd ed. New York: McGraw-Hill; 2012.
6. Levgur M. Diagnosis of adenomyosis: a review. *J Reprod Med.* 2007;52:177–193.
7. Practice Committee of the American Society for Reproductive Medicine. Treatment of pelvic pain associated with endometriosis. *Fertil Steril.* 2008;90:S260–S269.
8. Practice Committee of the American Society for Reproductive Medicine. Endometriosis and infertility: a committee opinion. *Fertil Steril.* 2012;98:591–598.
9. Vlahos NF, Kalampokas T, Fotiou S. Endometriosis and ovarian cancer: a review. *Gynecol Endocrinol.* 2010;26:213–219.
10. Wong AY, Tang LC, Chin RK. Levonorgestrel-releasing intrauterine system (Mirena) and depot medroxyprogesterone acetate (Depo-Provera) as long-term maintenance therapy for patients with moderate to severe endometriosis: a randomized controlled trial. *Aust N Z J Obstet Gynaecol.* 2010;50:273–279.

CHAPTER 5

LEIOMYOMATOUS UTERUS

Elena Martinez, MD

1. **What is a leiomyoma?**

   Leiomyomas are benign, monoclonal tumors of the smooth muscle cells of the myometrium. They are composed of large amounts of extracellular matrix containing collagen, fibronectin, and proteoglycan. Collagen type I and type III are abundant, but the fibrils are formed abnormally and in disarray. Leiomyomas are also called fibroids, fibromyomas, or myomas.

2. **How common are leiomyomas?**

   Leiomyomas are the most common tumors in women of reproductive age. Rarely observed before puberty, these tumors are most prevalent during the reproductive years and regress after menopause. In white women, the incidence of leiomyomas is thought to be as high as 43% by age 35 years and almost 59% by age 50 years. The incidence is even higher among African-American women, at 59% by age 35 years and more than 75% by age 50 years.

3. **What causes leiomyomas?**

   Leiomyomas are thought to arise from a somatic mutation of a monoclonal myometrial cell line. Possible factors responsible for initiating genetic changes include intrinsic abnormalities of the myometrium, congenitally increased estrogen receptors in the myometrium, hormonal changes, and ischemic injury at the time of menses.

4. **How does estrogen affect leiomyomas?**

   Leiomyomas contain both progesterone and estrogen receptors and are sensitive to estrogen levels. Factors that increase overall lifetime exposure to estrogen, such as obesity and early menarche, increase the incidence of these tumors.

5. **How common is malignancy in a leiomyoma?**

   Very rare. Genetic differences between leiomyomas and leiomyosarcomas indicate that these tumors most likely have distinct origins and that leiomyosarcomas do not result from malignant degeneration of leiomyomas. Malignancy should always be considered when leiomyomas increase in size after menopause.

6. **How are leiomyomas classified?**

   Leiomyomas are classified by their location (Fig. 5-1).
   - **Submucosal:** beneath the endometrium; distort the uterine cavity; can also become pedunculated and prolapse through the cervix
   - **Intramural:** within the myometrium
   - **Subserosal:** beneath the peritoneal surface of the uterus; can become pedunculated or even detach and obtain blood supply from another organ ("parasitic leiomyoma")
   - **Cervical:** within the cervix

7. **What symptoms are associated with leiomyomas?**

   Although leiomyomas are asymptomatic in approximately 50% of affected women, they can also cause significant morbidity and affect a woman's quality of life. The peak incidence of symptoms occurs among women in their 30s and 40s, and it is often related to the location and size of the leiomyomas. The most common symptoms overall are dysmenorrhea, abnormal uterine bleeding, and pressure. Submucosal leiomyomas are often associated with heavy menstrual bleeding. Intramural leiomyomas may be associated with dysmenorrhea or abnormal bleeding. Although leiomyomas in any location can cause pain through dysmenorrhea or degeneration, large leiomyomas can cause symptoms in adjacent organ systems (e.g., urinary frequency or constipation).

8. **How do leiomyomas cause abnormal uterine bleeding?**

   Several mechanisms are possible:
   - Increased surface area of the endometrium
   - Increased vascularity of the uterus
   - Ulceration of the overlying endometrium

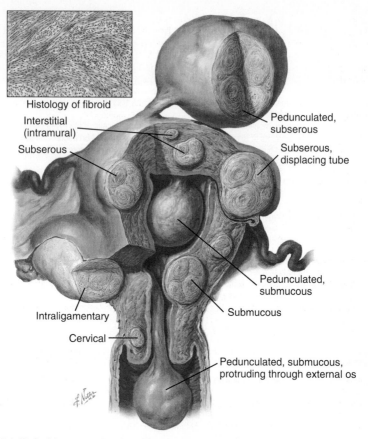

Histology of fibroid

Interstitial (intramural)

Subserous

Intraligamentary

Cervical

Pedunculated, subserous

Subserous, displacing tube

Pedunculated, submucous

Submucous

Pedunculated, submucous, protruding through external os

Figure 5-1. Uterine leiomyomata. *(From Smith RP: Netter's Obstetrics and Gynecology. 2nd ed. Philadelphia: Elsevier; 2015. Copyright 2015 Elsevier Inc. All rights reserved. www.netterimages.com.)*

- Distortion of the uterine wall that prevents contraction and subsequent closure of spiral arteries during menses
- Development of abnormal microvasculature, with stasis and changes in venous drainage

9. **Do leiomyomas affect fertility?**
   In general, leiomyomas are not thought to be a major cause of infertility. Although the American Society of Reproductive Medicine reports that these tumors may be associated in up to 5% to 10% of cases, this number falls to only 2% to 3% when all other causes of infertility are excluded. If leiomyomas do have an impact, it is thought to be through distortion of the uterine cavity that leads to recurrent miscarriage. Data from assisted reproduction technology (ART) suggest that submucosal and intramural leiomyomas that distort the uterine cavity should be removed.

10. **What effect do leiomyomas have on an ongoing pregnancy, and how does pregnancy affect these tumors?**
    Some studies have shown leiomyomas to be associated with an increased risk of preterm delivery, placenta previa, postpartum hemorrhage, and cesarean section.
    Degeneration manifesting with acute pain is the classically recognized complication during pregnancy. Its incidence is believed to be approximately 5%. Pregnancy also appears to have a variable and unpredictable effect on leiomyoma growth; the size of the tumors may increase, decrease, or remain the same.

11. **Can leiomyomas be treated with medication?**
Yes, although medical therapy directed at reducing abnormal uterine bleeding (progestin analogues, oral contraceptives, the levonorgestrel-releasing intrauterine device, or depot medroxyprogesterone acetate) does not directly affect the leiomyomas. Gonadotropin-releasing hormone (GnRH) agonists can reduce leiomyoma size by inducing a menopausal-like state of reduced estrogen levels; maximum reduction in tumor size (30% to 64%) occurs within 3 to 6 months. GnRH agonists have also been shown to improve preoperative and postoperative hemoglobin and hematocrit levels significantly. Use of these agents is generally considered to be a short-term solution because side effects can be severe, and drug cessation often results in a return of symptoms.

12. **What are the indications for surgical treatment?**
- Persistent abnormal bleeding unresponsive to medical therapy
- Excessive pain or pressure
- Cases in which fertility is believed to be affected
- Case in which tumor growth occurs after menopause (malignancy should also be considered)

13. **What surgical and nonmedical treatment options are available?**
- **Uterine artery embolization (UAE):** This procedure disrupts the blood supply to the uterus, which can decrease leiomyoma size and improve symptoms. Efficacy is limited when leiomyomas are large. Potential complications include premature ovarian failure, chronic vaginal discharge, and pelvic infection.
- **Hysteroscopic resection:** This procedure is appropriate for submucosal leiomyomas, and it can allow many patients to avoid hysterectomy.
- **Myomectomy:** This surgical removal of only the leiomyoma is most commonly offered to women who would like to preserve the ability to have children.
- **Hysterectomy:** The only definitive treatment, hysterectomy is appropriate for women who do not wish to have children. It can be performed by several different routes: vaginally, laparoscopically, by laparotomy, or with use of a robotic surgical system.

KEY POINTS: LEIOMYOMATOUS UTERUS

1. Fibroids are hormone-sensitive, fibromuscular benign tumors that are thought to originate from a monoclonal cell line.
2. Leiomyomas can cause abnormal uterine bleeding, dysmenorrhea, pelvic pressure, and even bladder and bowel symptoms.
3. Fibroids can be treated medically, surgically, or with uterine artery embolization.

BIBLIOGRAPHY

1. Aharoni A, Reiter A, Golan D, et al. Patterns of growth of uterine leiomyomas during pregnancy: a prospective longitudinal study. *Br J Obstet Gynaecol.* 1988;95:510–513.
2. Candiani GB, Fedele L, Parazzini F, Villa L. Risk of recurrence after myomectomy. *Br J Obstet Gynaecol.* 1991;98: 385–389.
3. Cook JD, Walker CL. Treatment strategies for uterine leiomyoma: the role of hormonal modulation. *Semin Reprod Med.* 2004;22:105–111.
4. Cramer SF, Patel A. The frequency of uterine leiomyomas. *Am J Clin Pathol.* 1990;94:435–438.
5. Day Baird D, Dunson DB, Hill MC, Cousins D, Schectman JM. High cumulative incidence of uterine leiomyoma in black and white women: ultrasound evidence. *Am J Obstet Gynecol.* 2003;188:100–107.
6. Evans P, Brunsell S. Uterine fibroid tumors: diagnosis and treatment. *Am Fam Physician.* 2007;75:1503–1507.
7. Fernandez H, Sefrioui O, Virelizier C, et al. Hysteroscopic resection of submucosal myomas in patients with infertility. *Hum Reprod.* 2001;16:1489–1492.
8. Friedman AJ, Haas ST. Should uterine size be an indication for surgical intervention in women with myomas? *Am J Obstet Gynecol.* 1993;168:751–755.
9. Gupta S, Jose J, Manyonda I. Clinical presentation of fibroids. *Best Pract Res Clin Obstet Gynaecol.* 2008;22:615–626.
10. Hurskainen R, Teperi J, Rissanen P, et al. Quality of life and cost effectiveness of levonorgestrel releasing intrauterine system versus hysterectomy for treatment of menorrhagia: a randomised trial. *Lancet.* 2001;35:273–277.
11. Kjerulff KH, Langenberg P, Seidman JD, Stolley PD, Guzinski GM. Uterine leiomyomas: racial differences in severity, symptoms and age at diagnosis. *J Reprod Med.* 1996;41:483–490.
12. Leibsohn S, d'Ablaing G, Mishell Jr DR. Leiomyosarcoma in a series of hysterectomies performed for presumed uterine leiomyomas. *Am J Obstet Gynecol.* 1990;162:968–974.
13. Lethaby A, Vollenhoven B, Sowter M. Pre-operative GnRH analogue therapy before hysterectomy or myomectomy for uterine fibroids. *Cochrane Database Syst Rev.* 2000;2. CD000547.

14. Marshall LM, Spiegelman D, Barbieri RL, et al. Variation in the incidence of uterine leiomyoma among premenopausal women by age and race. *Obstet Gynecol.* 1997;90:967–973.
15. Maruo T, Ohara N, Matsuo H, et al. Effects of levonorgestrel-releasing IUS and progesterone receptor modulator PRM CDB-2914 on uterine leiomyomas. *Contraception.* 2007;75:S99–S103.
16. Munro MG. *Abnormal Uterine Bleeding.* Cambridge: Cambridge University Press; 2010.
17. Parker WH. Etiology, symptomatology, and diagnosis of uterine myomas. *Fertil Steril.* 2007;87:725–736.
18. Practice Committee of the American Society for Reproductive Medicine. Myomas and reproductive function. *Fertil Steril.* 2004;82(Suppl. 1):S111–S116.
19. Qidwai GI, Caughey AB, Jacoby AF. Obstetric outcome in women with sonographically detected uterine leiomyomata. *Obstet Gynecol.* 2006;107:376–382.
20. Quade BJ, Wang TY, Sornberger K, Dal Cin P, Mutter GL, Morton CC. Molecular pathogenesis of uterine smooth muscle tumors from transcriptional profiling. *Genes Chromosomes Cancer.* 2004;40:97–108.
21. Sankaran S, Manyonda SI. Medical management of fibroids. *Best Pract Res Clin Obstet Gynaecol.* 2008;22:655–676.
22. Smith RP. Uterine leiomyomata. In: *Netter's Obstetrics and Gynecology.* 2nd ed. Philadelphia: Saunders; 2008:304.
23. Stenchever MA, Droegemueller W, Herbst AL, Mishell DR, eds. *Comprehensive Gynecology.* 4th ed. St. Louis: Mosby; 2001.
24. Stewart EA, Friedman AJ, Peck K, Nowak RA. Relative overexpression of collagen type I and collagen type III messenger ribonucleic acids by uterine leiomyomas during the proliferative phase of the menstrual cycle. *J Clin Endocrinol Metab.* 1994;79:900–906.
25. Walker CL, Stewart EA. Uterine fibroids: the elephant in the room. *Science.* 2005;308:1589–1592.
26. Wallach EE, Vlahos NF. Uterine myomas: an overview of development, clinical features, and management. *Obstet Gynecol.* 2004;104:393–406.

CHAPTER 6

ANOVULATION

Jacob Casey, MD, and Judy H. Chen, MD

1. **What is anovulation, and what is the general cause?**
   Anovulation is the absence of ovulation from the ovary. It is referred to as either primary (when the patient has no earlier history of normal ovulation) or secondary (when normal ovulation was previously present). Generally speaking, the cause of anovulation is dysfunction at any level of the hypothalamic-pituitary-ovarian (HPO) axis. Because the HPO axis involves a complex interaction of multiple organ systems, more precise causes are not always identifiable.

2. **What are primary disruptions of the HPO axis that cause anovulation?**
   - Hypothalamic dysfunction
   - Gonadal dysgenesis
   - Weight-related issues
   - Early-onset hypothyroidism

3. **What are common causes of secondary anovulation?**
   - Obesity
   - Hyperprolactinemia
   - Hypothyroidism or hyperthyroidism
   - Adrenal disorders
   - Stress
   - Pregnancy
   - Primary ovarian insufficiency (POI)
   - PCOS (polycystic ovarian syndrome)

4. **What are common symptoms of anovulation?**
   Amenorrhea, abnormal uterine bleeding, signs of androgen excess, and infertility are common symptoms.

5. **How does anovulation lead to abnormal uterine bleeding?**
   The absence of normal cycles leads to a state of unopposed estrogen, which destabilizes the endometrium and leads to irregular, noncyclic shedding.

6. **How does obesity cause anovulation?**
   Androgens are converted to estrogen in adipose tissue, a process that leads to an elevated estrogen-to-progesterone ratio. In turn, this change can suppress progesterone production and result in a state of unopposed estrogen. High levels of estrogen suppress gonadotropin-releasing hormone (GnRH) release from the hypothalamus; result is suppression of follicle-stimulating hormone (FSH). Numerous studies have shown that weight loss in an obese female patient with PCOS helps restore ovulation and subsequent normal menses. (For more detailed information on the normal menstrual cycle, see Chapter 1.)

7. **How does hyperprolactinemia affect the HPO axis?**
   Hyperprolactinemia decreases GnRH release through negative feedback on the hypothalamus.

8. **What are common causes of hyperprolactinemia?**
   - Prolactinoma
   - Breastfeeding
   - Hypothyroidism
   - Medications
   - Stress

9. **How is hyperprolactinemia treated?**
   Dopamine agonists are the mainstays of treatment.

Prolactinomas are benign and are the most common tumors of the pituitary gland. Treatment depends on size; microadenomas (<10 mm) that are asymptomatic can be followed with medical therapy and follow-up imaging. Macroadenomas (>10 mm) may require surgical intervention in addition to medical therapy.

10. **How does thyroid dysfunction cause anovulation?**
Hypothyroidism can lead to overproduction of thyroid-releasing hormone (TRH) and thyroid-stimulating hormone (TSH), as well as disrupting the release of GnRH. In experimental models, TRH is a stimulus for prolactin release, which, in turn, exerts negative feedback on GnRH and results in anovulation. However, hypothyroidism leads to menstrual irregularities more frequently than to anovulation.

Hyperthyroidism can increase the production of sex hormone–binding globulin (SHBG), the conversion of androgens to estrogens, and baseline levels of gonadotropins. This can result in menstrual irregularities and, less frequently, anovulation.

11. **How do adrenal disorders cause anovulation?**
In conditions such as congenital adrenal hyperplasia and Cushing syndrome, abnormal corticosteroid production leads to androgen excess. This condition disrupts the HPO axis and results in anovulation.

12. **What are some factors that affect GnRH release from the hypothalamus?**
   - Weight loss: Significant weight loss and loss of body fat in particular are associated with hypothalamic anovulation and amenorrhea. Extreme weight loss such as that associated with eating disorders can also be associated with other endocrine abnormalities. These conditions carry a mortality rate as high as 5% to 15%. Therefore, this condition requires careful assessment; patients require intensive psychotherapy for both mental and physical health.
   - Exercise: Increased opioid production from excess exercise, in combination with the loss of weight and body fat that accompany strenuous exercise, may inhibit ovulation through positive effects on norepinephrine or leptin inhibition on the release of GnRH.
   - Stress: Extreme stress may induce anovulation by the opioid pathways similar to those noted with exercise.

13. **What is the female athlete triad?**
The female athlete triad is a hypoestrogenic state consisting of insufficient caloric intake, amenorrhea, and decreased bone mineral density. Elevated cortisol centrally inhibits the release of gonadotropins, thus resulting in decreased estrogen production and suppression of ovulation.

14. **What is Kallmann syndrome?**
Kallmann syndrome is characterized by primary amenorrhea and anosmia. It results from failed neuronal migration of GnRH neurons and can be inherited in an X-linked or autosomal recessive pattern. Women with Kallmann syndrome have normal ovaries and can undergo successful ovulation induction (for more detailed information on ovulation induction, see Chapter 24.)

15. **What is POI?**
POI is a condition in which the resting pool of primordial follicles in a female patient is prematurely depleted before 40 years of age, with resulting early menopause. Although the exact mechanism of primordial follicle depletion is unknown, causes include genetic factors, chemotherapy, radiotherapy, and surgical intervention.

16. **What are dysgenetic gonads?**
The term *dysgenetic gonads* refers to limited gonadal development. This includes patients with abnormal karyotypes (e.g., 45 XO, phenotypic female patients with 46 XY karyotype), gonadal agenesis, or rudimentary gonads.

KEY POINTS: ANOVULATION

1. Anovulation commonly manifests as infrequent, irregular menses or amenorrhea.
2. Common causes of anovulation are pregnancy, thyroid disease, hyperprolactinemia, PCOS, and weight extremes.
3. Ovarian failure is normal at menopause (average age, 51 years) and is premature, referred to as Premature Ovarian Insufficiency, when it occurs before 40 years of age.

BIBLIOGRAPHY

1. American College of Obstetricians and Gynecologists. Management of Abnormal Uterine Bleeding Associated With Ovulatory Dysfunction. ACOG practice bulletin 136. Washington, DC: American College of Obstetricians and Gynecologists; 2013.
2. De Vos M, Devroey P, Fauser BC. Primary ovarian insufficiency. *Lancet.* 2010;376:911–921.
3. ESHRE/ASRM PCOS Consensus Workshop Group. Consensus on infertility treatment related to polycystic ovary syndrome. *Hum Reprod.* 2008;23:462–477.
4. Lash MM, Armstrong A. Impact of obesity on women's health. *Fertil Steril.* 2009;91:1712–1716.
5. Lentz GM, Lobo RA, Gershenson DM, Katz VL, eds. *Comprehensive Gynecology.* 6th ed. Philadelphia: Mosby; 2013.
6. Poppe K, Velkeniers B. Female infertility and the thyroid. *Best Pract Res Clin Endocrinol Metab.* 2004;18:153–165.
7. Practice Committee of the American Society for Reproductive Medicine. Practice guidelines: use of exogenous gonadotropins in anovulatory women. A technical bulletin. *Fertil Steril.* 2008;90:S7–S12.
8. Practice Committee of the American Society for Reproductive Medicine and the Practice Committee of the Society for Assisted Reproductive Technology. Criteria for number of embryos to transfer: a committee opinion. *Fertil Steril.* 2013;99:44–46.
9. Practice Committee of the American Society for Reproductive Medicine. Use of clomiphene citrate in infertility women: a committee opinion. *Fertil Steril.* 2013;100:341–348.
10. Speroff L, Fritz MA. *Clinical Gynecologic Endocrinology and Infertility.* 7th ed. Philadelphia: Lippincott Williams &Wilkins; 2005.
11. Unuane D, Tournaye H, Velkeniers B, Poppe K. Endocrine disorders and female infertility. *Best Pract Res Clin Endocrinol Metab.* 2011;25:861–873.

1. **With which aspects of sexuality should a gynecologist be familiar?**
   Gynecologists should be familiar with the physiology of sexual response and phases of the sexual response cycle. They should be able to obtain a thorough sexual history, which includes screening for sexual dysfunction, abuse, number of partners, use of barrier protection methods, sexually transmitted infection (STI) history, and current method of birth control. They should also be familiar with disorders of the genital tract that may hinder sexual responsiveness.

2. **What are the phases of the sexual response cycle?**
   Masters and Johnson originally described four physiologic stages of sexual response: excitement, plateau, orgasm, and resolution. Kaplan and colleagues subsequently modified these stages to desire, arousal, and orgasm.

3. **List the normal physiologic changes seen in desire and arousal.**
   - Increased blood flow to the labia and vagina
   - Lubrication of the genital tract (subepithelial transudate resulting from engorgement)
   - Clitoral engorgement and protrusion
   - Vaginal expansion
   - Breast enlargement
   - Nipple erection
     The dopamine system is thought to be responsible for sexual desire, and the noradrenergic system is thought to be responsible for sexual arousal.

4. **What characterizes orgasm in women?**
   Simultaneous rhythmic contractions of the orgasmic platform, uterus, and rectal sphincter occur at 0.8-second intervals and then diminish in intensity, duration, and regularity. Generalized myotonia occurs, as well as tachycardia, tachypnea, and an elevation in blood pressure. This response is not affected by hysterectomy, and it is possible for women to be multiorgasmic.
   Resolution of vasocongestion results in a return to normal anatomy and physiology.

5. **What is sexual dysfunction?**
   In general, sexual dysfunction is a heterogeneous group of disorders that hinder a person's ability to experience sexual pleasure. For women, this can encompass problems in the sexual response cycle (e.g., Kaplan's stages of desire, arousal, or orgasm), as well as pain, discomfort, or stress associated with sexual activity.

6. **What is the prevalence of sexual dysfunction?**
   The fifth edition of the *Diagnostic and Statistical Manual of Mental Disorders* (DSM-V) estimates the prevalence of female orgasmic problems to be greater than 40%, but not all women who report orgasmic problems report associated distress. In other words, some women with orgasmic problems still report high sexual satisfaction.

7. **What are the types of disorders seen in female sexual dysfunction?**
   The DSM-V describes the following types of sexual dysfunctions in women:
   - Female orgasmic disorder
   - Female sexual interest/arousal disorder
   - Genitopelvic pain/penetration disorder
   - Substance/medication-induced sexual dysfunction

8. **How does the DSM-V define the different sexual dysfunction disorders?**
   - **Female orgasmic disorder:** Marked delay, infrequency, reduction in intensity, or absence of orgasm that is distressing to the patient. It is critical in this diagnosis that this is *not* the result of relationship stressors that may cause these symptoms. The prevalence of this

condition varies widely depending on age, culture, and severity of symptoms. A medication review should be undertaken to ensure that this disorder is not medication induced (e.g., selective serotonin reuptake inhibitors [SSRIs] are known to cause difficulties with orgasm).

- **Female sexual interest/arousal disorder:** A persistent or recurrent deficiency or absence of sexual desire or receptivity to sexual activity that causes marked distress or interpersonal difficulty. Imbalanced sexual desire between partners is *not* sufficient to make the diagnosis. This was previously termed hypoactive sexual desire disorder but was broadened to female sexual interest/arousal disorder in the DSM-V. If this condition is secondary to a mood disorder or interpersonal issues, this diagnosis should not be made.
- **Genitopelvic pain/penetration disorder:** Persistent difficulty or pain with penetration during intercourse that may be associated with fear, anxiety, or tensing of the pelvic muscles during attempts at penetration. This disorder ranges from total inability to have vaginal penetration to minimal symptoms, but to fit the diagnosis the condition must be distressing to the patient. Approximately 15% of women in North America report recurrent pain during intercourse, and this complaint is a frequent cause for referral to specialists in sexual dysfunction.
- **Substance/medication-induced sexual dysfunction:** Any sexual dysfunction that has a temporal relationship or should be attributed to a substance or medication change.

These disorders must persist for approximately 6 months or more and must be present during almost all occasions of sexual activity. They should also not be attributable to a medical comorbidity (e.g., SSRI use, endometriosis) or personal issue (e.g., relationship problems, life stressors).

9. What is the etiology of sexual dysfunction?

Sexual dysfunction is multifactorial; causes can include abuse, psychologic factors, racial and religious influences, comorbid conditions (e.g., hypertension, dyslipidemia, spinal cord dysfunction, premature ovarian insufficiency), earlier surgical history, and medication history (e.g., SSRIs, antihypertensives, antihistamines, hormonal medications).

10. How is sexual dysfunction evaluated?

By systematically evaluating the causes of sexual dysfunction, gynecologists can offer targeted solutions that may resolve a frustrating issue. A complete sexual history should be obtained, including questions about sexual orientation, type and frequency of sexual activity, information on previous and current partners, and sexual satisfaction. A pelvic examination can be used to evaluate pelvic pain disorders. Based on the patient's history, further diagnostic studies (e.g., gonorrhea or *Chlamydia* cultures, ultrasound) may be indicated. Androgen levels should not be used to diagnose sexual dysfunction.

11. What are potential barriers to treatment?

- Reluctance to discuss this topic with health care providers
- Perception that few or no treatment options exist
- Inadequate provider training
- Inadequate time to obtain a complete sexual history
- Underestimation of the prevalence of sexual dysfunction

12. Does hysterectomy affect sexual function?

No. Hysterectomy does not affect sexual function or the ability to achieve orgasm.

13. What treatment options exist for female sexual dysfunction?

- **Dyspareunia:** Topical estrogens may improve symptoms, especially in postmenopausal women. If estrogen is contraindicated (e.g., a history of hormone-sensitive cancer), nonestrogen lubricants may be helpful. Systemic estrogen with or without progestin therapy has not been shown to improve sexual function.
- **Orgasmic disorders:** Studies on the benefit of sildenafil have been inconclusive.
- **Female sexual interest/arousal disorder:** Transdermal testosterone can be an effective short-term treatment; however, it should not be used for longer than 6 months. Treatment should also be balanced with the risks of androgen replacement therapy, which include hirsutism, acne, virilization, possible cardiovascular effects, and a potential increased risk of breast cancer.

The safety and efficacy of herbal supplements for treating female sexual dysfunction are unproven.

In many cases a multidisciplinary approach should be used, which may include a primary care physician, a gynecologist, a psychiatrist, a psychotherapist, a sex therapist, and a pelvic physical therapist. Partner and couples therapy may also be of benefit. Any identifiable underlying disorders should be treated; for example, a patient with dyspareunia that is thought to be secondary to endometriosis should have either laparoscopy or hormonal medication.

14. **What devices can be used to treat female sexual dysfunction?**
The Food and Drug Administration (FDA) has approved a battery-powered device that is applied to the clitoris to increase blood flow and engorgement. It has been shown to benefit patients with arousal and orgasm dysfunction.

KEY POINTS: FEMALE SEXUAL DYSFUNCTION

1. In general, sexual dysfunction is a heterogeneous group of disorders that hinder a person's ability to experience sexual pleasure.
2. Sexual dysfunction is multifactorial, and a multidisciplinary approach should be used for treatment.
3. A complete sexual history should include questions about sexual orientation, type and frequency of sexual activity, information on previous and current partners, and sexual satisfaction.

BIBLIOGRAPHY

1. American College of Obstetricians and Gynecologists. Female sexual dysfunction. ACOG practice bulletin number 119. *Obstet Gynecol.* 2011;117:996–1007.
2. American Psychiatric Association. *Diagnostic and Statistical Manual of Mental Disorders.* 5th ed. Washington, DC: American Psychiatric Association; 2013.
3. Basson R. Female sexual response: the role of drugs in the management of sexual dysfunction. *Obstet Gynecol.* 2001;98:350–353.
4. Basson R, Berman J, Burnett A, et al. Report of the International Consensus Development Conference on Female Sexual Dysfunction: definitions and classifications. *J Urol.* 2000;163:888–893.
5. Berman JR, Goldstein I. Female sexual dysfunction. *Urol Clin North Am.* 2001;28:405–416.
6. Kaplan H. *Disorders Of Sexual Desire And Other New Concepts And Techniques In Sex Therapy.* New York: Simon and Schuster; 1979.
7. Laumann EO, Paik A, Rosen RC. Sexual dysfunction in the US: prevalence and predictors. *JAMA.* 1999;281:537–554.
8. Masters W, Johnson V. *Human Sexual Response.* Boston: Little, Brown and Company; 1966.

CHAPTER 8

MENOPAUSE

Rachel Rosenheck, MD, and Judy H. Chen, MD

1. What are the differences between menopause and perimenopause?

Perimenopause is the period immediately before menopause and is characterized by irregular menstrual cycles and hormonal fluctuations. It is associated with hot flashes, vaginal dryness, sleep disturbances, and mood symptoms. The average age for perimenopause to start is 47.5 years, and an average of 4 years will pass before the final menstrual period.

Menopause is a retrospective diagnosis after a woman has experienced 12 months of amenorrhea without any other obvious pathologic or physiologic cause. It is a reflection of complete ovarian follicular depletion resulting in high follicle-stimulating hormone (FSH) concentrations and hypoestrogenemia. In the United States, the average age for menopause is 51.4 years. Menopause that occurs before the age of 40 years is called premature ovarian failure or primary ovarian insufficiency.

2. What causes menopause to occur? What endocrine changes are seen?

Menopause is caused by a gradual depletion of functioning ovarian follicles. Declining inhibin B levels from the granulosa cells lead to increased FSH production from the pituitary that accelerates the follicular phase of the menstrual cycle. High basal estradiol levels can be seen during menses, often in association with follicular cysts. As the granulosa cells gradually lose their ability to produce estradiol, FSH levels rise (as do luteinizing hormone [LH] levels, to a lesser extent). After menopause, androgen levels decline by 50%. The greater decline of estradiol, however, favors a higher androgen-to-estrogen ratio. This change can lead to signs of hirsutism and alopecia in some women. Estrogen production after menopause is principally in the form of estrone and results from aromatization of androstenedione in adipose tissues.

3. What are common symptoms of perimenopause and menopause?

Shorter follicular and luteal phases result in shortened, irregular menstrual cycles. Anovulation then occurs and results in "skipped" menstrual periods, oligomenorrhea, and eventually amenorrhea. Vasomotor symptoms, also known as hot flashes, occur in approximately 80% of women and can persist for 5 to 15 years after menopause. Over time, symptoms of urogenital atrophy can develop; these include dyspareunia, vulvar pruritus, and incontinence. Other associated symptoms are sleep and mood disturbances, as well as new-onset depression. Although not a symptom of menopause, accelerated bone loss also occurs.

4. What are the available treatments for menstrual irregularities associated with menopause?

In the absence of contraindications (e.g., tobacco use, hypertension, or vascular disease), irregular menstrual cycles can be treated with low-dose oral contraceptive pills. Another effective way to control irregular bleeding while reducing the risk of endometrial hyperplasia is monthly withdrawal bleeding induced by progestins. When patients do not experience bleeding after withdrawal of the progestin, hypoestrogenism is diagnosed, and estrogen replacement therapy can be considered. Another treatment option is continuous progestin use, but breakthrough bleeding is a common undesired side effect.

5. What is a hot flash?

A hot flash is a sudden sensation of warmth, often accompanied by a flushed sensation of the upper body and face that quickly becomes generalized. Typically lasting from 1 to 5 minutes, it is often associated with profuse perspiration. Palpitations or feelings of anxiety can also occur. Hot flashes result from alterations in the hypothalamic thermoregulatory center caused by fluctuations in steroid and peptide hormone levels.

6. How can vasomotor symptoms be treated?

For women with moderate to severe hot flashes, the most effective therapy is estrogen. This treatment can stop hot flashes completely in approximately 80% of women and reduce the frequency and severity of hot flashes in the remainder.

7. **What are the health risks and benefits of hormone therapy (HT) in perimenopausal and menopausal women?**
Aside from reducing vasomotor symptoms and improving urogenital atrophy, HT is associated with a 2% to 5% increase in bone mineral density (BMD) and a 25% to 50% decreased risk of vertebral and hip fractures. Observational studies found HT to be cardioprotective, but this finding was not replicated in randomized controlled trials. In 2002, a large, randomized controlled study showed an increased risk of stroke, thromboembolic events, and breast cancer in women who used HT. Reductions in colon cancer and fracture risk, however, were also seen. The absolute risks and benefits for any individual woman are small. Because of these findings, the long-term risks are considered to exceed the benefits of HT use in healthy postmenopausal women; this treatment should be reserved for symptomatic women and used for as short a duration as possible.

8. **What are the different types of estrogen preparations available for HT?**
Box 8-1 contains a list of currently available preparations for HT. All routes of administration appear to be equally effective for symptomatic relief, but their metabolic effects differ. Oral estrogen has a more favorable effect on lipid profiles, but it is associated with an increase in serum triglycerides and C-reactive protein. Use of transdermal or vaginal estrogen appears to have a higher risk of venous thromboembolism and stroke.

9. **What progestins are available for use in perimenopausal and menopausal women, and what is the key benefit of these hormones?**
Currently available progestins used for HT include medroxyprogesterone acetate, norethindrone, and micronized progesterone. Progestins reduce the risk of endometrial hyperplasia and endometrial cancer in women who receive estrogen therapy and must always be given in patients who still have a uterus.

10. **What are the contraindications to HT?**
HT is contraindicated in pregnancy, active thromboembolic disease, chronic liver impairment, undiagnosed genital bleeding, or estrogen-dependent neoplasms.

11. **What are selective estrogen receptor modulators (SERMs), and what are their indications?**
SERMs comprise a class of drugs that have differential estrogen agonistic and antagonistic properties in various tissues. They have no proven benefits in preventing cardiovascular disease and carry an increased risk of thrombotic events. Raloxifene is currently approved for the prevention and treatment of osteoporosis; it does not improve hot flashes or urogenital atrophy. The side effect profile of raloxifene is similar to that of tamoxifen, and it does not have established benefits in breast cancer therapy. Bazedoxifene is an SERM that has been marketed for the control of hot flashes.

12. **Does HT increase the risk of breast cancer?**
More than 50 epidemiologic studies and more than a half-dozen meta-analyses have tried to answer this question. With few exceptions, these studies were observational and subject to bias. In addition, the types of hormones used, their respective doses, and their duration of administration varied, as did the criteria for the diagnosis of breast cancer. The majority of meta-analyses did not find compelling evidence for an association between estrogen-only HT and breast cancer.
   The Women's Health Initiative Study was halted prematurely because of an increased relative hazard for breast cancer of 1.24 (or 8 in 10,000 women/year more breast cancers) after 5.6 years of follow-up in patients treated with combination estrogen-progestin versus placebo. Women in the estrogen-progestin arm of the study were also diagnosed with later stage cancer and more aggressive types of tumors.

13. **Define osteoporosis and how it is diagnosed.**
Osteoporosis is a progressive bone disease characterized by a decrease in bone mass and density that leads to an increase risk of fracture. BMD is best assessed by a dual-energy x-ray absorptiometry (DEXA) study. The World Health Organization (WHO) defines osteoporosis as a BMD that is greater than 2.5 SD below the young adult mean (called a T-score). Osteopenia is a BMD greater than 1.0 to less than 2.5 standard deviations (SD) below the young adult mean. A Z-score is the BMD of the patient compared with the expected mean at her own age, with greater than 1 SD below the mean considered abnormal.
   Although not diagnostic of osteoporosis, biochemical markers of bone remodeling exist and include serum markers of bone *formation* (osteocalcin, bone specific alkaline phosphatase, and procollagen extension peptides) and urinary markers of bone *resorption* (pyridinoline cross-linked peptides, N-telopeptides, hydroxyproline, and hydroxylysine).

Box 8-1. Currently Available Preparations for Hormone Therapy

17β-Estradiol
- Oral
  - Activella (with norethindrone acetate)
  - Estrace
  - Gynodiol
  - Ortho-Prefest (with norgestrel)
- Vaginal
  - Estrace cream
  - Estring (ring)
  - Vagifem (tablets)
- Transdermal
  - Alora
  - Climara
  - CombiPatch (with norethindrone acetate)
  - Esclim (stretchable)
  - Estraderm
  - FemPatch
  - Vivelle ("Dot" is smallest patch available)

Ethinyl Estradiol (EE)
- Estinyl (20- and 50-μg EE tablets)
- (5 μg EE/1 mg norethindrone acetate)

Conjugated Equine
- Premarin (PO, IV, vaginal)
- Premphase (with Provera, 5 mg × 14 days)
- Prempro (with 2.5 mg Provera QD)

Synthetic Conjugated
- Cenestin

Estropipate
- Ogen (PO and vaginal)
- Ortho-Est

Esterified
- Estratab
- Estratest (with 2.5 mg methyltestosterone)
- Menest

Other
- BiEst (estradiol and estriol)
- TriEst (estrone, estradiol, and estriol)
- Delestrogen (estradiol valerate IM)
- Estrocare (black cohosh extract)

IM, intramuscular; *IV,* intravenous; *PO,* oral; *QD,* daily.

14. **How common is osteoporosis, and why is it such a health concern?**
    More than 200 million people worldwide are estimated to have osteoporosis. Osteoporosis affects 25 million Americans and results in 1.5 million fractures annually in the United States, at an estimated cost of 10 billion dollars. The prevalence of postmenopausal osteoporosis is estimated at 11.5%, and 1 in 3 women older than 50 years of age will experience an osteoporotic fracture. Up to 25% of fractures (particularly of the hip) lead to death within 1 year, and another 25% of patients will remain bedridden. Spinal compression fractures lead to loss of height, pain, and the "dowager's hump."

15. **What are the types and causes of osteoporosis?**
    - **Primary osteoporosis** (type 1) is caused by estrogen deprivation, advancing age, excessive smoking and alcohol consumption, poor nutrition (particularly calcium, vitamin D, and protein),

Table 8-1. Major Studies Demonstrating Efficacy of Treatment Modalities for Osteoporosis

TREATMENT	STUDY	DOSE	STUDY TYPE	BMD			Fracture		
				VERTEBRAL	FEMUR		VERTEBRAL	FEMUR	NONVERTEBRAL
HRT	PEPI (1996)	0.625 mg	RCT (3 yr)	Inc 5.0%	Inc 1.7%		—	—	—
	Torgerson (2001)		Meta-analysis	—	—		—	—	Dec 27%
	WHI (2002)	0.625 mg RCT	—	—	—		Dec 33%	Dec 33%	Dec 24%
Bisphosphonates									
Alendronate	FIT (1996)	10 mg/day	RCT (3 yr)	—	—		Dec 55%	Dec 51%	—
	FOSIT (1999)	10 mg/day	RCT (1 yr)	Inc 4.9%	Inc 3%		—	—	Dec 47%
Risedronate	VERT (1999)	5 mg/day	RCT (3 yr)	Inc 5.4%	Inc 1.6%		Dec 41%	—	Dec 39%
SERMs									
Tamoxifen	NSABP PI (1998)	20 mg/day	RCT (5 yr)	—	—		Dec 26%	Dec 45%	—
Raloxifene	MORE (1999)	60 mg/day	RCT (3 yr)	Inc 2.6%	Inc 2.1%		Dec 30%	No change	No change
Calcitonin	PROOF (2000)	200 IU/day	RCT (5 yr)	Inc 1.5%	—		Dec 33%	—	—
Fluoride	Pak (1995)	25 mg bid	RCT (4 yr)	Inc 4%	—		Dec 68%	—	—
Vitamin D	Chapuy (1994)	800 IU/day	RCT (3 yr)	—	—		—	Dec 27%	Dec 28%

BMD, Bone mineral density; *Dec*, decrease; *FIT*, Fracture Intervention Trial; *FOSIT*, Fosamax Interventional Trial; *HRT*, hormone replacement therapy; *Inc*, increase; *MORE*, Multiple Outcomes of Raloxifene Evaluation; *NSABP*, National Surgical Adjuvant Breast and Bowel Project; *PEPI*, Postmenopausal Estrogen/Progestin Interventions Trial; *PROOF*, Prevent Recurrence of Osteoporotic Fractures Study; *RCT*, randomized controlled trial; *SERMs*, selective estrogen receptor modulators; *VERT*, Vertebral Efficacy with Risedronate Therapy; *WHI*, Women's Health Initiative.

inadequate weight-bearing exercise, and hereditary factors such as race (Asians and whites are at higher risk) and a slender body habitus.

- **Secondary osteoporosis** (type 2) can be caused by the following: endocrine abnormalities such as parathyroid, thyroid, and cortisol excess, diabetes, and hypogonadism; gastrointestinal abnormalities such as malabsorption and anorexia; and medications such as anticonvulsants, cyclosporine, glucocorticoids, gonadotropin-releasing hormone (GnRH) agonists, heparin, isoniazid, lithium, methotrexate, and thyroid hormone.

16. **How is osteoporosis treated?**

    Table 8-1 is an overview of efficacy studies of treatments for osteoporosis. Numerous treatment options are available. Weight-bearing exercise, smoking and alcohol cessation, calcium supplementation, and vitamin D supplementation can both prevent and treat osteoporosis. Medications in women diagnosed with osteoporosis include bisphosphonates (etidronate, alendronate, and risedronate), calcitonin, tibolone, and parathyroid hormone. HT offers protection against fractures at both the hip and spine, but it is not used for treatment of osteoporosis.

KEY POINTS: MENOPAUSE

1. The average age of menopause in the United States is 51 years.
2. Symptoms of menopause include hot flashes, vaginal atrophy, and sleep and mood disturbances.
3. Most expert groups agree that HT is indicated for the management of severe menopausal symptoms.
4. In women who still have a uterus and who receive estrogen replacement therapy, progesterone must be given to prevent endometrial hyperplasia and cancer.
5. Osteoporosis, defined as a T-score greater than or equal to 2.5 standard deviations below the mean for young controls, is commonly treated with calcium and vitamin D, bisphosphonates, or SERMs.

BIBLIOGRAPHY

1. Bush TL, Whiteman M, Flaws JA. Hormone replacement therapy and breast cancer: a qualitative review. *Obstet Gynecol.* 2001;98:498–508.
2. Chestnut 3rd CH, Silverman S, Andriano K, et al. A randomized trial of nasal spray salmon calcitonin in postmenopausal women with established osteoporosis: the Prevent Recurrence of Osteoporotic Fractures Study (PROOF). *Am J Med.* 2000;109:267–276.
3. Collaborative Group on Hormonal Factors in Breast Cancer. Breast cancer and hormone replacement therapy: collaborative reanalysis of data from 51 epidemiological studies of 52,705 women with breast cancer and 108,411 women without breast cancer. *Lancet.* 1997;350:1047–1059.
4. Effects of hormone therapy on bone mineral density. results from the Postmenopausal Estrogen/Progestin Interventions (PEPI) trial. *JAMA.* 1996;276:1389–1396.
5. Ettinger B, Black DM, Mitlak BH, et al. Reduction of vertebral fracture risk in postmenopausal women with osteoporosis treated with raloxifene: results from a 3 year randomized clinical trial. Multiple Outcomes of Raloxifene Evaluation (MORE) investigators. *JAMA.* 1999;282:637–645.
6. Grady D, Herrington D, Bittner V, et al. Cardiovascular disease outcomes during 6.8 years of hormone therapy: Heart and Estrogen/Progestin Replacement Study Follow-up (HERS II). *JAMA.* 2002;288:49–57.
7. Manson JE, Martin KA. Postmenopausal hormone replacement therapy. *N Engl J Med.* 2001;345:34–40.
8. Martin KA, Barbieri RL. Treatment of menopausal symptoms with hormone therapy. Uptodate. Available at www.uptodate.com. Accessed October 13, 2015.
9. National Osteoporosis Society. Hormone replacement therapy for the treatment and prevention of osteoporosis. National Osteoporosis Society Position Statement. December 2010 NOS 00190. Available at www.nos.org.uk/document.doc?id=823. Accessed October 13, 2015.
10. North American Menopause Society. A decision tree for the use of estrogen replacement therapy or hormone replacement therapy in postmenopausal women: consensus opinion. *Menopause.* 2000;7:76–86.
11. North American Menopause Society. The 2012 hormone therapy position statement of the North American Menopause Society. *Menopause.* 2012;19:257.
12. Shifren JL, Schiff I. Role of hormone therapy in the management of menopause. *Obstet Gynecol.* 2010;115:839.
13. Taffe JR, Dennerstein L. Menstrual patterns leading to the final menstrual period. *Menopause.* 2002;9:32.

CHAPTER 9

BENIGN LESIONS OF THE VULVA AND VAGINA

Susan Park, MD

1. What are the components of the vulva (Fig. 9-1)?
   - Labia majora
   - Labia minora
   - Mons pubis
   - Clitoris
   - Vestibule
   - Urethral meatus
   - Vaginal orifice
   - Hymenal ring
   - Bartholin glands
   - Skene ducts
   - Vestibulovaginal bulbs

2. What are the seven infections that can cause vulvar lesions?
   1. Chancroid *(Haemophilus ducreyi)*
   2. Syphilis *(Treponema pallidum)*
   3. Lymphogranuloma venereum (LGV; *Chlamydia trachomatis* serovar)
   4. Condylomata acuminata (human papillomavirus [HPV])
   5. Genital herpes
   6. Molluscum contagiosum
   7. Granuloma inguinale (donovanosis)

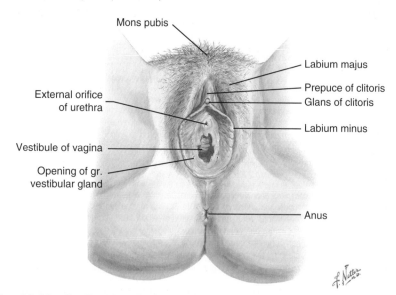

Figure 9-1. Vulva. *(From Netter's Atlas of Human Anatomy. 6th ed. Philadelphia: Elsevier; 2014:354. Copyright 2014 Elsevier Inc. All rights reserved. www.netterimages.com.)*

3. Describe the microbiologic and clinical features and treatment of chancroid (*Haemophilus ducreyi* infection).

Chancroid is caused by a nonmotile, anaerobic, gram-negative bacillus. It has an incubation period of 3 to 10 days. Diagnosis made by culture or polymerase chain reaction (PCR), or it is made clinically after exclusion of other potential causes. It manifests as small papules that evolve into pustules and then painful ulcers. Approximately 50% of patients will have tender inguinal adenopathy **(buboes).** Treatment options include azithromycin, erythromycin, ceftriaxone, or ciprofloxacin.

4. Describe the microbiologic and clinical features and treatment of syphilis (*Treponema pallidum* infection).

This infection with an anaerobic spirochete has an incubation period of 2 weeks. Diagnosis made by dark-field microscopy, rapid plasma reagin (RPR), and fluorescent treponemal antibody absorption (FTA-ABS) tests. Syphilis has three stages:
1. Primary syphilis: Painless ulcer with dull red base **(chancre)**, may go unnoticed. If untreated, it spontaneously heals in 3 to 8 weeks.
2. Secondary syphilis: Occurs 6 weeks to 6 months after primary infection. It has a variable presentation including diffuse macular, papular, pustular, or nodular rash, or pustular lesions (can involve palms or soles of feet), lymphadenopathy, alopecia, hepatitis, neurologic and ocular abnormalities, gastrointestinal abnormalities, renal abnormalities, musculoskeletal abnormalities, and vulvar **condyloma lata** (confluent gray masses with flat tops and broad bases on the periphery of the vulva).
3. Late (tertiary) syphilis: Occurs 4 to 20 years after primary infection. It manifests as **gummas** (can occur anywhere on the body including the vulva), aortitis, and neurologic abnormalities such as tabes dorsalis, optic atrophy, pupillary disturbances **(Argyll Robertson pupil)**, and general paresis.

   All stages can be treated with penicillin G. Doxycycline, tetracycline, or azithromycin may be considered as alternatives if a person is allergic to penicillin. In pregnancy, however, allergic patients must be desensitized and given penicillin G.

5. What is the Jarisch-Herxheimer reaction?

Acute fever with headache and myalgias may occur within hours of treatment. It is caused by release of large amounts of endotoxin from dying spirochetes and the subsequent inflammatory reaction.

6. Describe the clinical features and treatment of LGV.

LGV is a chronic infection of lymphatic tissue by *Chlamydia trachomatis*. It has an incubation period of 3 to 12 days and is found most frequently in tropical climates. Diagnosis made by serology, culture, immunofluorescence, or nucleic acid detection. LGV has primary and secondary stages:
- Primary stage: Manifests as small painful ulcers at inoculation sites, typically in the fourchette, but they can also occur on labia. The ulcers spontaneously heal within days.
- Secondary stage: Occurs 2 to 6 weeks later with painful inguinal masses resulting from lymphadenopathy. The "groove sign" (depressions between lymph nodes) is visible.

   Treatment is with doxycycline (first line) or erythromycin, along with aspiration of fluctuant lymph nodes if needed. LGV can cause fibrosis or elephantiasis if untreated.

7. Describe the clinical features and treatment of condyloma acuminatum (HPV infection).

HPV is a double-stranded DNA virus. It has an incubation period of 3 weeks to 8 months. Infection manifests as irregular, fleshy or pink-colored lesions anywhere on the vulva, perineum, or perianal region. Many treatment options exist: trichloroacetic acid, podophyllin, topical imiquimod, cryotherapy, laser surgery, or excision. Most can be prevented by the quadrivalent or nonvalent HPV vaccine.

8. Describe the clinical features and treatment of genital herpes.

It is caused by infection with herpes simplex virus or HSV (serotypes 1 and 2). Both serotypes can infect oral and genital tissues, although HSV 1 is more often associated with oral lesions and HSV 2 is more often associated with genital lesions. The incubation period is 2 to 10 days. Diagnosis made by viral culture, serology, immunofluorescence, PCR, or **Tzanck smear** (scraping of ulcer shows multinucleated giant cells). Presentation ranges from asymptomatic to painful vesicular lesions and ulcers with or without dysuria, fever, and lymphadenopathy. Prodromal symptoms (paresthesias, vulvar tenderness, and pruritus) can occur. Treatment options include acyclovir, valacyclovir, and famciclovir. Patients who experience frequent outbreaks should be offered suppression therapy.

9. Describe the clinical features and treatment of molluscum contagiosum.
   This is caused by a double-stranded DNA poxvirus and has an incubation period of 2 to 7 weeks. It manifests as painless, umbilicated lesions 1 to 5 mm in diameter. Treatment is rarely needed, but options include trichloroacetic acid, imiquimod, or Monsel solution (ferric subsulfate).

10. Describe the clinical features and treatment of granuloma inguinale (*Calymmatobacterium granulomatis* infection; also known as donovanosis).
    This is caused by a nonmotile, gram-negative bacillus. It has an incubation period of 1 to 12 weeks. Diagnosis made by **Wright** or **Giemsa stain** (will show **Donovan bodies**). It manifests as painless nodules that progress to locally destructive, painless ulcers with a beefy red appearance (highly vascular). No regional lymphadenopathy occurs. Treatment is with doxycycline, azithromycin, erythromycin, ciprofloxacin, or trimethoprim-sulfamethoxazole.

11. What are the three vulvar dermatoses, also known as the "three lichens"?
    1. Lichen sclerosis: Most common in postmenopausal patients. It is characterized by epithelial thinning (parchment-like tissue), with fibrosis and agglutination of the labia. It can cause introital stenosis, dyspareunia, and intense pruritus. It is associated with increased risk for squamous cell carcinoma. Diagnosis is confirmed by biopsy. Treatment is with topical corticosteroids.
    2. Lichen planus: A papulosquamous, chronic, inflammatory dermatosis of unknown origin. Vaginal involvement is common. Lesions are painful, usually violaceous, and frequently have white striae **(Wickham striae)** either at the margins of lesions or on the oral mucosa. It can cause dysuria and dyspareunia, and loss of normal vulvar architecture may be extreme. Diagnosis is confirmed by biopsy. Treatment is with topical corticosteroids.
    3. Lichen simplex chronicus: Pruritus leads to hyperplastic, leathery epithelium from chronic scratching. Diagnosis is confirmed by biopsy. Treatment is with topical corticosteroids.

12. What is hidradenitis suppurativa?
    A chronic follicular occlusive disease in which obstruction of apocrine glands leads to draining sinuses, abscess formation, and scarring. It can occur anywhere along the "milk line" from the vulva to the axilla. Treatment can be complex and may require topical antibiotics, systemic antibiotics, meticulous hygiene, wardrobe modifications, oral contraceptives, or surgical resection. It is associated with increased risk for squamous cell carcinoma, and recurrence is very common.

13. Describe the benign pigmented lesions of the vulva.
    - Melanocytic nevi: Usually asymptomatic, varying in color and size (from 1 to 2 mm to 1 to 2 cm). Diagnosis is confirmed by biopsy.
    - Acanthosis nigricans: Poorly defined, velvety hyperpigmentation can affect labiocrural folds (areas where the labia majora and the inner thighs meet) in addition to the axillae, nipples, and umbilical area.
    - Vitiligo: Depigmentation of an otherwise normal area of skin. It is usually well-defined and symmetric.

14. What are the common cystic lesions of the vulva and vagina?
    - Cysts of epidermal origin: These include sebaceous cysts, epidermal inclusion cysts, hidradenoma, syringoma, and **Gartner duct cysts** (arise from vestigial remnants of the vaginal portion of the wolffian ducts).
    - Duct cysts: **Bartholin gland cysts** and **Bartholin abscesses** (Fig. 9-2) are found at the 4 and 8-o'clock positions of the vestibule. Treatment is with incision and drainage from the mucosal (not cutaneous) side, followed by Word catheter placement to promote a fistulous tract to prevent recurrence. Refractory cases can be treated with marsupialization or gland excision.
    - Cysts of urethral and paraurethral origin: These include **Skene duct cysts** and urethral or suburethral diverticula.

15. What are the benign solid tumors of the vulva and vagina?
    - Epithelial squamous tumors: seborrheic keratosis, fibroepithelial polyp, vestibular papillomatosis
    - Epithelial glandular tumors: hidradenoma, syringoma, fibroadenomas
    - Mesenchymal origin: angiomas, angiokeratomas, leiomyomas, lipomas, neurofibroma
    - Urethral origin: caruncle

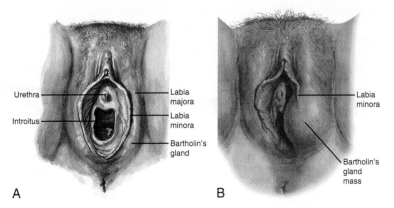

Figure 9-2. Normal Bartholin gland location **(A, left)** and enlargement of the Bartholin gland possibly due to abscess, enlarged cyst, or tumor **(B, right)**. *(From Roberts JR, ed. Roberts and Hedges' Clinical Procedures in Emergency Medicine. 6th ed. Philadelphia: Saunders; 2014:740.)*

16. **What is extramammary Paget disease of the vulva?**
    Extramammary Paget disease is intraepithelial neoplasia causing severe pruritus. It can occur in the groin, vulvar, or perianal areas and appears well demarcated and eczematoid. Diagnosis is made by biopsy. Treatment is with excision, and recurrence is high. Up to 25% to 35% of cases are associated with an underlying or in situ adenocarcinoma, and patients should be evaluated for synchronous neoplasms elsewhere in the body.

17. **What are the developmental abnormalities of the vagina, and how are they treated?**
    - Imperforate hymen: usually recognized after puberty when retention of menses leads to **hematocolpos.** Inspection of the introitus often reveals a bulging mass, and hematocolpos can be confirmed with ultrasound. Treatment is with hymenotomy.
    - Longitudinal vaginal septum: may be partial or complete; usually associated with uterine anomalies (e.g., septum or didelphys). Treatment is with excision, although it is not necessary if the condition is asymptomatic.
    - Transverse vaginal septum: failure of normal fusion and canalization of the urogenital sinus and müllerian ducts that divides the vagina into upper and lower compartments. A fenestration is often present, and pregnancy can occur, but repair (resection) is required to allow for vaginal delivery. Repair is also necessary if menstrual flow is obstructed.

KEY POINTS: BENIGN LESIONS OF THE VULVA AND VAGINA

1. The ulcer of primary syphilis is usually single and painless, whereas the ulcer of herpes is more often multiple and painful.
2. The warty lesions of HPV are treated with destructive agents, such as TCA, cryotherapy, and laser.
3. Vulvar epithelial disorders differ in that lichen sclerosis is a butterfly distribution of thin epithelium, lichen simplex is local and thick, and lichen planus is inflammatory.

BIBLIOGRAPHY

1. Berek J. *Berek and Novak's Gynecology.* 14th ed. Philadelphia: Lippincott Williams & Wilkins; 2007.
2. Edwards L. New concepts in vulvodynia. *Am J Obstet Gynecol.* 2003;189:S24–S30.
3. Foster DC. Vulvar disease. *Obstet Gynecol.* 2002;100:145–163. 2002.
4. Lentz GM. *Comprehensive Gynecology.* 6th ed. Philadelphia: Mosby; 2012.
5. Maldonado V. Benign vulvar tumors. *Best Pract Res Clin Obstet Gynaecol.* 2014;28:1088–1097.
6. Workowski KA, Berman S. Centers for Disease Control and Prevention. Sexually transmitted diseases treatment guidelines, 2010. *MMWR Recomm Rep.* 2010;59:1–110.

CHAPTER 10

LOWER GENITAL TRACT INFECTIONS

Manpreet Singh, MD

1. **What are the characteristics of normal vaginal fluid?**
   Normal vaginal fluid is white and generally not malodorous, with a pH of approximately 4.5. Microscopically, it contains squamous epithelial cells and bacteria but no white or red blood cells. The principal organisms of normal flora are lactobacilli (also called Döderlein bacilli), which are aerobic gram-variable rods. The vagina also contains gram-negative bacteria and anaerobes. Infectious organisms (e.g., *Trichomonas, Neisseria gonorrhoeae* [gonococcus], *Chlamydia*) or alterations in the normal flora (e.g., bacterial vaginosis, candidiasis) can cause vaginitis.

2. **What are the most common forms of vaginitis, and what are their symptoms?**
   Vaginitis is characterized by one or more of the following symptoms: increased vaginal discharge, malodorous discharge, vaginal or vulvar pruritus, dyspareunia, vaginal or vulvar burning, vulvar edema, and erythema. The characteristics of the symptoms and the gross description of the discharge are not sufficient to establish the diagnosis.
   - **Candidiasis** is caused by an overgrowth of *Candida* species.
   - **Bacterial vaginosis** is caused by an imbalance in the normal flora, with an increase in anaerobic bacteria.
   - **Trichomoniasis** is caused by the parasite *Trichomonas vaginalis*. It is a sexually transmitted infection (STI).
   - **Atrophic vaginitis** is irritation and inflammation secondary to atrophy of the vaginal epithelium.

3. **What are the diagnostic tests for vaginitis?**
   The various causes of vaginitis are most easily distinguished by performing four simple tests:
   1. Examination of the vulva, vagina, vaginal discharge, and cervix
   2. Determination of vaginal fluid pH
   3. Microscopic evaluation of vaginal fluid that has been mixed with saline and potassium hydroxide (KOH)
   4. The "whiff test," which is performed by mixing a sample of vaginal fluid with KOH and assessing for an amide odor (Table 10-1)

4. **What are the characteristics of vulvovaginal candidiasis?**
   Candida species cause vulvar and vaginal itching and burning, dysuria, dyspareunia, and abnormal vaginal discharge. The most common species isolated is *Candida albicans*. Other species include *Candida glabrata* and *Candida tropicalis*. Vulvovaginal candidiasis has a distinct thick, white, "cottage cheese" appearance on gross examination. Diagnosis is made by the appearance of budding hyphae (*C. albicans, C. tropicalis*) or spores (*C. glabrata*) seen in a KOH preparation under medium power, a test that is approximately 80% sensitive. Treatment is with either a single dose of an oral agent such as fluconazole or a short course (1 to 7 days) of a vaginal preparation (e.g., miconazole, clotrimazole, tioconazole).

5. **How is recurrent vulvovaginal candidiasis treated?**
   The diagnosis of recurrent candidiasis is made when a patient has four or more infections unrelated to antibiotic use in a single year. Predisposing conditions include pregnancy, diabetes, and human immunodeficiency virus (HIV) infection. Because different forms of vaginitis have similar symptoms, a patient's history alone or a pattern of self-treatment with over-the-counter antifungal agents is insufficient to establish this diagnosis. Treatment is aimed at eradicating the yeast systemically through long courses of oral antifungals. Topical treatment with agents such as boric acid and gentian violet may be effective in some cases.

Table 10-1. Distinguishing Characteristics of the Common Forms of Vaginitis

FEATURES	PHYSIOLOGIC DISCHARGE	BACTERIAL VAGINOSIS	TRICHOMONIASIS	CANDIDIASIS	GONOCOCCAL OR CHLAMYDIAL VAGINITIS
Color	White	Gray	Grayish yellow	White	Greenish yellow
Consistency	Nonhomogenous	Homogenous	Purulent	Thick, curdlike ("cottage cheese")	Mucopurulent or purulent
pH	<4.5	>4.5	>4.5	<4.5	N/A
Microscopic findings	Squamous epithelial cells, lactobacilli, few WBCs	Rare WBCs, ↑bacteria, "clue" cells	Motile trichomonads, WBCs	Pseudohyphae, yeast buds, WBCs	>10 WBCs/HPF
Vulva characteristics	Normal	Normal	Edematous, erythematous	Erythematous	Normal or erythematous
Vaginal mucosa	Normal	Normal	Normal	Erythematous	Normal
Cervix	Normal	Normal	Petechiae ("strawberry" cervix)	May have patches of discharge	Friable, erythematous, purulence visible at os
Amine odor	Absent	Present	Present	Absent	Absent

HPF, High-power field; *WBCs,* white blood cells.

6. What are the characteristics of bacterial vaginosis?

Bacterial vaginosis occurs as a result of an alteration in the normal vaginal flora, with overgrowth of anaerobic bacteria (*Gardnerella vaginalis, Mycoplasma hominis, Ureaplasma urealyticum, Peptostreptococcus, Mobiluncus, Prevotella,* and *Bacteroides*). This disorder can be precipitated by elevated vaginal pH from antibiotics or douching. Symptoms include pruritus and odor, especially after intercourse. A thin, white-gray discharge is often seen on physical examination. A common method of diagnosis is the **Amsel criteria** (see later). Other methods include assessing a Gram stain (uses **Hay/Ison** or **Nugent criteria**), employing a DNA probe–based test, or using a rapid proline aminopeptidase test card.

7. What are the Amsel criteria?
1. Thin, white, homogeneous discharge
2. Clue cells on microscopy: vaginal epithelial cells with spherical bacteria obscuring the usually sharp border
3. Vaginal fluid pH >4.5
4. Release of a fishy, amide odor on adding 10% KOH solution ("whiff test")

Three of the four criteria must be met for a diagnosis of bacterial vaginosis.

8. How is bacterial vaginosis treated?

It can be treated with either oral or topical medications. Oral medications include metronidazole, tinidazole, and clindamycin; vaginal preparations exist for both metronidazole and clindamycin. In general, bacterial vaginosis is not considered to be sexually transmitted, and partners do not require cotreatment.

9. What are the characteristics of trichomoniasis?

Trichomoniasis is an STI caused by *T. vaginalis,* a unicellular protozoan parasite. It causes pruritus and increased discharge, often copious. Trichomonads are tear-shaped or ovoid, mobile, and flagellated. They are usually identified by their motility and their visible flagella, and they can be identified under a microscope. Although a positive "whiff test" is generally specific for bacterial vaginosis, it can also occur in trichomoniasis. Treatment with a single oral dose of metronidazole or tinidazole is highly effective, but resistant cases requiring a longer course of therapy do exist.

10. What are the characteristics of atrophic vaginitis?

Atrophic vaginitis comprises irritation and inflammation secondary to atrophy of the vaginal epithelium, usually associated with the hypoestrogenic states of menopause or breastfeeding. It is not an infection and does not require antibiotics. Treatment is with either vaginal or oral estrogen.

11. What are the most common STIs that affect the lower genital tract and their causative organisms?
- Syphilis: *Treponema pallidum*
- Gonorrhea: *N. gonorrhoeae*
- *Chlamydia* infection: *C. trachomatis*
- Trichomoniasis: *T. vaginalis*
- Genital herpes: herpes simplex virus (HSV)

12. Why is screening for STIs important?

Many STIs can be asymptomatic at some stage of the disease; screening benefits the person screened and can help prevent the spread of the disease. No ironclad rules exist for selection of candidates for screening and for choice of STIs in screening. Various criteria can be applied using demographics and risk-scoring systems, or the criteria can be based on the site of care. However, any system other than universal screening misses some individual persons perceived to be at low risk. The U.S. Preventive Services Task Force (USPSTF) recommends screening for *Chlamydia* infection and for gonorrhea for all sexually active women younger than 25 years of age, even if they are not engaging in high-risk sexual behaviors.

13. What are two of the most important principles in managing and controlling STIs?
1. Education on safe sexual practices
2. Treatment of all sexual contacts

14. What are the clinical features of syphilis, and how is it treated?

Syphilis is spread by sexual contact and progresses through well-described stages.

- In the **primary stage**, an initial ulcer appears at the point of infection and is usually visible on the vulva. In contrast to genital herpes, the ulcer is painless.
- The **secondary stage** follows 4 to 10 weeks after the primary infection and involves systemic symptoms (e.g., fever, weight loss, hair loss, headache). Patients usually have a characteristic maculopapular rash on the palms and soles of the feet.
- In the **latent stage**, patients have serologic proof of infection without symptoms of disease. These patients are at risk for **tertiary syphilis**, which affects multiple organ systems: cardiovascular system (e.g., aortitis), skin (e.g., chronic gummas), and central nervous system (e.g., dementia, tabes dorsalis, **Argyll Robertson pupil**, seizures, meningitis).

Syphilis is diagnosed by visualization of the organism using dark-field microscopy or through serologic testing with either the fluorescent-labeled *Treponema* antibody test (**FTA-ABS**) or *Treponema pallidum* particle agglutination assay (**TPPA**).

Screening is performed using nontreponemal tests, either the rapid plasma reagin (**RPR**) or the Venereal Disease Research Laboratories (**VDRL**) test. If results of either of these tests are positive, a confirmatory test is required. False-positive screening test results can be caused by some viral infections (e.g., varicella, measles) and other disease processes (e.g., tuberculosis [TB], lymphoma).

Treatment depends on the stage of the disease, a patient's allergy status, and whether a patient is pregnant. In general, intramuscular penicillin is the antibiotic of choice. Doxycycline, tetracycline, or azithromycin may be considered as alternatives except in pregnancy. Physicians should be aware of the **Jarisch-Herxheimer reaction**, which is caused by the release of inflammatory cytokines on death of the bacteria. This reaction can cause fever, chills, rigors, hypotension, tachycardia, vasodilation, and myalgia.

15. What are the characteristics of *Chlamydia* infection?
    Chlamydia infection is caused by *C. trachomatis* and produces mucopurulent discharge, although the infection is often asymptomatic. *C. trachomatis* can be cultured, or the diagnosis made by identifying *Chlamydia* mRNA with a genetic probe. Treatment is with doxycycline, azithromycin, or one of several quinolones. Undiagnosed infection can cause infertility and chronic pelvic pain. *Chlamydia* can also infect the upper genital tract and cause pelvic inflammatory disease (PID).

16. What causes genital herpes?
    Herpes infection is caused by one of two herpes simplex viruses, HSV-1 and HSV-2. HSV-1 more commonly causes perioral infection ("cold sores"), and HSV-2 is more commonly isolated in genital infections. As with other herpes viruses (e.g., herpes zoster), infection with HSV is chronic. The virus becomes dormant after the initial outbreak, but it can always reactivate and cause subsequent outbreaks.

17. How does genital herpes manifest?
    Herpes typically causes small vesicular eruptions—which may or may not be clustered—that rapidly progress to shallow, painful ulcers. Lesions can occur anywhere on the labia, vaginal epithelium, cervix, or perineum. Inguinal adenopathy can be present, as well as vaginal discharge. However, the most common complaint is pain. Systemic symptoms (e.g., fever and malaise) may also be present. Although rare, urinary retention requiring bladder catheterization can result from involvement of the sacral portions of the spinal cord. Asymptomatic infection is also possible; herpes antibodies can be isolated from women with no known history of infection.

18. Does a difference exist between a primary and a recurrent herpes outbreak?
    Yes. A primary herpes outbreak is typically more severe and longer in duration (12 to 21 days). Recurrent outbreaks generally manifest with relatively mild symptoms and last 2 to 5 days. The frequency of recurrence is quite variable; some women experience only a single outbreak, and others may have several recurrences each year.

19. When is genital herpes contagious?
    The virus can be shed and transmitted at any time, during both symptomatic and asymptomatic periods. Spread is through direct contact, although healed ulcers are no longer considered infectious. Patients are also contagious in the days just before an outbreak. During this time, they may or may not experience prodromal symptoms such as tingling or burning in the affected region.

20. How is genital herpes treated?
    HSV infection cannot be cured, but the symptoms and duration of primary and recurrent outbreaks can be reduced with antiviral agents. Several agents are effective and include acyclovir, valacyclovir, and famciclovir. Initial treatment is for 7 to 10 days, and treatment for 2 to 5 days is indicated for recurrences.

21. **Does HSV suppression have a role?**

Suppression therapy with antivirals is effective in reducing the frequency of recurrences. The decision to use suppressive therapy is up to the patient. In general, suppression is recommended for women who have more than two or three outbreaks a year.

22. **Does HSV infection have any other sequelae?**

Primary HSV infection during pregnancy is potentially very serious. Transmission to the newborn can occur if a woman has an active herpes outbreak or prodrome at the time of vaginal delivery. Although the rate of neonatal infection is greatest for women experiencing an initial outbreak, it can occur even during a secondary outbreak. For this reason, women with prodromal symptoms or active lesions at the time of labor should be delivered by cesarean section. To prevent recurrences around the time of delivery and avoid cesarean section, the American Congress of Obstetricians and Gynecologists (ACOG) recommends that suppressive antiviral therapy be given in the last 4 weeks of pregnancy to all women with a history of recurrent genital HSV.

Although rare, other potential sequelae include ocular infections (e.g., conjunctivitis or herpetic keratoconjunctivitis with dendritic corneal ulcers), skin infections (e.g., eczema herpeticum, herpetic whitlow, herpes gladiatorum), visceral infections, and central nervous system complications (e.g., aseptic meningitis, myelitis, encephalitis).

23. **What is a Bartholin cyst, and what causes it?**

A Bartholin cyst is a noninfectious dilation of the Bartholin gland, which is located at the 4-o'clock and 8-o'clock positions of the labia minora. These glands are mucin secreting and provide vaginal lubrication through the Bartholin duct, which can become obstructed by infection, inflammation, or physical blockage (e.g., mucus plug). Obstruction causes the gland to dilate and eventually fill with fluid; this condition is referred to as a Bartholin cyst, which can be asymptomatic or cause discomfort.

24. **Can Bartholin cysts become infected?**

Most Bartholin cysts are sterile and contain only the mucinous material produced by the gland. However, secondary infection can occur. In these cases the cyst becomes filled with purulent material and is termed a Bartholin abscess. These infections are usually polymicrobial, but *N. gonorrhoeae* can sometimes be isolated.

25. **How is a Bartholin cyst or abscess treated?**

Although treatment is not required for asymptomatic cases, three options are available for symptomatic women: incision and drainage, marsupialization, and excision. Most cases respond to incision, drainage, and placement of a Word catheter. The incision should be approximately 5 mm long and made on the mucosal surface. The Word catheter keeps the cyst walls from reapproximating and allows for continued drainage; the goal is for the catheter to stay in place for 4 to 6 weeks to allow for epithelialization. Wound care generally involves intercourse abstinence, sitz baths, and antibiotics for surrounding cellulitis or signs of infection.

In the case of recurrence, the cyst wall can be opened and the edges sutured to leave an open space. This procedure is called marsupialization. Another option is excision of the entire gland and duct, although this procedure involves significant dissection and requires regional or general anesthesia.

26. **Can Bartholin cysts be malignant?**

Most Bartholin cysts are benign and do not need routine biopsy or excision. However, a new cyst in a woman older than 40 years of age should be examined for possible malignancy.

KEY POINTS: LOWER GENITAL TRACT INFECTIONS

1. Trichomoniasis and candidiasis are diagnosed by visualizing the organisms on microscopy of vaginal discharge.
2. The presence of bacterial vaginosis is suggested by the "whiff test" and the appearance of "clue cells."
3. Syphilis has several stages: primary (vulvar lesion), secondary (systemic rash), latent, and tertiary (systemic effects).
4. Primary herpes outbreaks are typically more severe and longer in duration than recurrences.

BIBLIOGRAPHY

1. Arduino PG, Porter SR. Oral and perioral herpes simplex virus type 1 (HSV-1) infection: review of its management. *Oral Dis*. 2006;12:254–270.
2. Baldwin HE. STD update: screening and therapeutic options. *Inter J Fertil Womens Med*. 2001;46:79–88.
3. Brocklehurst P, Gordon A, Heatley E, Milan SJ. Antibiotics for treating bacterial vaginosis in pregnancy. *Cochrane Database Syst Rev*. 2013;1. CD000262.
4. Centers for Disease Control and Prevention. Tracking the hidden epidemics 2000: trends in STDs in the United States. Available at http://www.cdc.gov/std/trends2000/trends2000.pdf. Accessed October 15, 2015.
5. Forna F, Gülmezoglu AM. Interventions for treating trichomoniasis in women. *Cochrane Database Syst Rev*. 2003;2. CD000218.
6. Islam A, Safdar A, Malik A. Bacterial vaginosis. *J Pak Med Assoc*. 2009;59:601–604.
7. Kimberlin DW, Rouse DJ. Clinical practice: genital herpes. *N Engl J Med*. 2004;350:1970–1977.
8. Kushnir VA, Mosquera C. Novel technique for management of Bartholin gland cysts and abscesses. *J Emerg Med*. 2009;36:388–390.
9. Morris M, Nicoll A, Simms I, et al. Bacterial vaginosis: a public health review. *Br J Obstet Gynaecol*. 2001;108:439–450.
10. Ormrod D, Scott LJ, Perry CM. Valaciclovir: a review of its long-term utility in the management of genital herpes simplex virus and cytomegalovirus infections. *Drugs*. 2000;59:839–863.
11. U.S. Preventive Services Task Force recommendations for STI screening. Available at http://www.uspreventiveservicestaskforce.org/Page/Name/uspstf-recommendations-for-sti-screening. Accessed October 15, 2015.
12. Wechter ME, Wu JM, Marzano D, Haefner H. Management of Bartholin duct cysts and abscesses: a systematic review. *Obstet Gynecol Surv*. 2009;64:395–404.
13. Workowski KA, Berman S. Centers for Disease Control and Prevention. Sexually transmitted diseases treatment guidelines, 2010. *MMWR Recomm Rep*. 2010;59:1–110. x.

CHAPTER 11

PELVIC INFLAMMATORY DISEASE

Mary Anne M. Baquing, MD

1. **What is pelvic inflammatory disease (PID)?**

   PID is a clinical syndrome that comprises a spectrum of inflammatory diseases of the upper female genital tract: endometritis (infection of endometrium), salpingitis (infection of the fallopian tubes), tubo-ovarian abscess, and pelvic peritonitis. It is caused by ascending infection from the vagina to the upper genital organs.

2. **What causes PID?**

   Most cases are polymicrobial. Previously, the most common pathogens were thought to be the sexually transmitted organisms *Neisseria gonorrhoeae* and *Chlamydia trachomatis*. More recent studies have shown that other organisms in the vaginal flora may also play a crucial role in the development of PID. These other organisms include enteric gram-negative rods and anaerobes such as *Mycoplasma genitalium*, *Ureaplasma urealyticum*, and *Gardnerella vaginalis*. Less than half of PID cases have cervical infection with gonorrhea or *Chlamydia*, likely from the active screening and treatment of sexually active women. Cervical or uterine instrumentation may increase the risk of PID.

3. **What are the incidence and prevalence of PID?**

   PID is estimated to occur in more than 750,000 women in the United States every year. These estimates are limited by the poor sensitivity of clinical diagnostic criteria and the lack of national surveillance.

4. **What are risk factors for PID?**
   - Young age: higher risk of acquiring sexually transmitted infections (STIs)
   - History of PID: damaged fallopian tubes are at higher risk for reinfection
   - History of gonorrhea or *Chlamydia* infection
   - High-risk sexual behaviors: multiple partners, male partners with gonorrhea or *Chlamydia* infection
   - Bacterial vaginosis
   - Socioeconomic status: related to health care access

5. **Are intrauterine devices (IUDs) associated with PID?**

   The risk of developing PID after IUD insertion is highest within the first 3 weeks. Historically, the IUD would be removed at the time of PID diagnosis. More recent studies, however, do not support this practice; patients respond just as well to treatment with the IUD in place.

6. **What are the clinical symptoms of PID?**

   Variable. PID may be asymptomatic, or it can manifest with moderate or even severe symptoms (also known as acute PID). In patients with symptoms, the most common are lower abdominal pain, cramping, postcoital bleeding, abnormal discharge, fever, nausea, and vomiting. Subclinical PID is more frequent and leads to misdiagnosis and mistreatment.

7. **What are the physical examination findings associated with PID?**

   During a pelvic examination, the classic sign of PID is cervical motion tenderness or the "chandelier sign." This is characterized by severe tenderness or an accompanying reaction to the pain the patient feels on manipulation of the cervix. Other physical examination findings include adnexal tenderness, right upper quadrant (RUQ) tenderness (associated with **Fitz-Hugh-Curtis syndrome**), and mucopurulent discharge on speculum examination.

8. **What are the diagnostic criteria for PID?**

   The Centers for Disease Control and Prevention (CDC) recommend treatment in sexually active patients if one of the following are met in the absence of any other explanation:
   - Uterine tenderness
   - Adnexal tenderness (bilateral or unilateral)

- Cervical motion tenderness ("chandelier sign")
  These additional findings support PID diagnosis but are not required:
- Fever higher than 38.3° C
- Abnormal discharge or friable cervix
- White blood cells (WBCs) on saline microscopy (the absence of WBCs makes the diagnosis less likely)
- Cervical infection with gonorrhea or *Chlamydia*
- Leukocytosis
- Elevated erythrocyte sedimentation rate
- Elevated C-reactive protein
- Imaging suggestive of a tubo-ovarian abscess or pyosalpinx
- Endometrial biopsy showing endometritis
- Laparoscopic findings consistent with PID

9. **What options exist for outpatient treatment of PID?**
   The following regimens are recommended by the CDC for treatment of PID in the outpatient setting:
   - Ceftriaxone 250 mg intramuscularly (IM) in a single dose AND doxycycline 100 mg orally twice a day for 14 days
   - Cefoxitin 2 g IM AND probenecid 1 g orally in a single dose AND doxycycline 100 mg orally twice a day for 14 days
   - Other parenteral third-generation cephalosporin AND doxycycline 100 mg orally twice a day for 14 days
   - Consider adding metronidazole to any of the foregoing regimens, especially in patients with bacterial vaginosis.

10. **How should patients who receive outpatient treatment be followed?**
    Patients should be reexamined within 72 hours of treatment. If they do not show significant clinical improvement, they need to be admitted for parenteral treatment.

11. **What are the criteria for inpatient treatment of PID?**
    - Failed outpatient treatment
    - Inability to tolerate or be compliant with an outpatient oral regimen
    - Pregnancy
    - Presence of tubo-ovarian abscess
    - Inability to exclude surgical emergencies such as appendicitis or ectopic pregnancy
    - Severe illness (vomiting, high fever)

12. **What are the recommended inpatient treatment options for PID?**
    The CDC recommends the following parenteral regimens:
    - Cefotetan 2 g intravenously (IV) every 12 hours *OR* cefoxitin 2 g IV every 6 hours AND doxycycline 100 mg orally or IV every 12 hours
    - Clindamycin 900 mg IV every 8 hours AND gentamicin loading dose of 2 mg/kg followed by maintenance dose 1.5 mg/kg every 8 hours (A single daily gentamicin dosing of 3 to 5 mg/kg may be considered.)
    - Alternative regimen: ampicillin/sulbactam 3 g IV every 6 hours AND doxycycline 100 mg orally or IV every 12 hours
    - If a tubo-ovarian abscess is present, clindamycin or metronidazole should be added to provide improved anaerobic coverage.

13. **What other considerations should be made when treating women for PID?**
    Women diagnosed with PID should be offered testing for all other STIs. Those who test positive for gonorrhea or *Chlamydia* infection during evaluation should be retested 3 to 6 months after treatment because of high rates of reinfection.

14. **How should sexual partners of women diagnosed with PID be managed?**
    Men who have had sexual contact within 60 days of a women diagnosed with PID should be tested for STIs and empirically treated for both *Chlamydia* infection and gonorrhea.

15. **What are the potential long-term consequences of PID?**
    - Infertility
    - Tubo-ovarian abscess
    - Increased risk of ectopic pregnancy
    - Chronic pelvic pain

KEY POINTS: PELVIC INFLAMMATORY DISEASE

1. PID is diagnosed by any of the following findings on physical examination: uterine tenderness, adnexal tenderness, or cervical motion tenderness.
2. The CDC recommends different oral and parenteral regimens for the treatment of PID.
3. Women in whom outpatient therapy fails or who are poor candidates for it should be hospitalized.
4. Long-term sequelae of PID include infertility, tubo-ovarian abscesses, chronic pelvic pain, and ectopic pregnancy.

BIBLIOGRAPHY

1. Centers for Disease Control and Prevention. *U.S. Selected practice recommendations for contraceptive use, 2013: Adapted from the World Health Organization Selected Practice Recommendations for Contraceptive Use.* 2nd ed. MMWR Recomm Rep; 2013. 62.
2. Centers for Disease Control and Prevention. Sexually transmitted diseases treatment guidelines, 2015. *MMWR Recomm Rep.* 2015;64:1–137. Available at http://www.cdc.gov/std/tg2015/default.htm. Accessed October 15, 2015.
3. Hoffman B, Schorge J, Schaffer J, et al., eds. *Williams Gynecology.* 2nd ed. New York: McGraw-Hill; 2012.
4. Wiesenfeld HC, Hillier SL, Meyn LA, et al. Subclinical pelvic inflammatory disease and infertility. *Obstet Gynecol.* 2012;120:37–43.
5. Wiesenfeld HC, Hillier SL, Meyn L, et al. *Mycoplasma genitalium: is it a pathogen in acute pelvic inflammatory disease (PID)?.* Vienna, Austria: Presented at the STI and AIDS World Congress; 2013 (Joint Meeting of the 20th ISSTDR and 14th IUSTI Meeting), July 14-27, 2013.

CHAPTER 12

ECTOPIC PREGNANCY

Ryan Pedigo, MD

1. **What is an ectopic pregnancy?**

   An ectopic pregnancy occurs when an embryo implants itself outside the uterine cavity, usually inside the fallopian tube.

2. **Is ectopic pregnancy a serious condition?**

   Yes. Although mortality has declined considerably because of early detection, advances in resuscitation, and definitive management, hemorrhagic shock from a ruptured ectopic pregnancy remains the most common cause of pregnancy-related maternal death in the first trimester. The overall death rate is approximately 1 death per 2000 ectopic pregnancies.

3. **What is the epidemiology of ectopic pregnancy?**

   The incidence of ectopic pregnancy is estimated to be 1% to 2% of all pregnancies. The incidence has increased over the past few decades secondary to (1) increased risk factors for salpingitis (e.g., *Chlamydia trachomatis* or *Neisseria gonorrhoeae* infection), (2) increased detection of unruptured ectopic pregnancies by using more advanced diagnostic strategies, and (3) assisted reproductive technology (ART). Patients in the first trimester of pregnancy who present to an emergency department with vaginal bleeding, abdominal pain, or both have approximately a 10% chance of having an ectopic pregnancy.

4. **What are the risk factors for ectopic pregnancy?**

   Anything that may impede embryo movement from the fallopian tube to the uterus confers an increased risk. Keep in mind that because ectopic pregnancy is so common, half of all women who are diagnosed have no risk factors.

   • Salpingitis from sexually-transmitted infections is the major contributing factor, with an odds ratio (OR) of 3.5. The increased incidence of ectopic pregnancy in patients with a history of salpingitis results from inflammation and morphologic changes that occur in the fallopian tube after infection.

   • A history of tubal surgical intervention also increases risk (OR, 3.5), but this is mainly attributable to the underlying cause of the surgical procedure (e.g., salpingitis with a tubo-ovarian abscess, previous ectopic pregnancy).

   • Smoking causes ciliary dysmotility in the fallopian tubes and predisposes to ectopic pregnancy in a direct dose-response relationship (OR, 2, which rises to 4 if a patient smokes more than one pack/day).

   • A history of an earlier ectopic pregnancy carries a very large risk; approximately 25% of subsequent pregnancies will also be ectopic.

   • Women who have been exposed to diethylstilbestrol (DES) in utero have a 5% risk of ectopic pregnancy; this risk rises to 13% if abnormalities are seen on a hysterosalpingogram.

   • Although it is very rare for a patient with an intrauterine device (IUD) to become pregnant, the risk of an ectopic pregnancy is high if it happens.

5. **Where do ectopic pregnancies implant, if not inside the uterus?**

   Almost all ectopic pregnancies implant in the fallopian tube (97.7%) (Fig. 12-1). Most tubal pregnancies implant in the ampullary portion of the tube (>80%), but they can also implant in the isthmus (12%) and fimbrial region (5%). Ectopic pregnancies that do not occur in the fallopian tube are rare (2.3%), and they are interstitial (also referred to as "cornual"), cervical, or abdominal pregnancies. The risk of hemorrhagic shock and death from an interstitial or abdominal pregnancy is five times greater compared with a tubal pregnancy.

6. **What is a heterotopic pregnancy, and what is the incidence?**

   A heterotopic pregnancy is defined as the coexistence of an intrauterine pregnancy (IUP) and an ectopic pregnancy. Previous estimates for heterotopic pregnancy were 1 in 30,000, but it is likely as common as 1 in 4000 (albeit still very rare). Heterotopic pregnancy should always be seriously considered in women undergoing ART; depending on the technique used, the risk of an associated heterotopic pregnancy can be as high as 1 in 100.

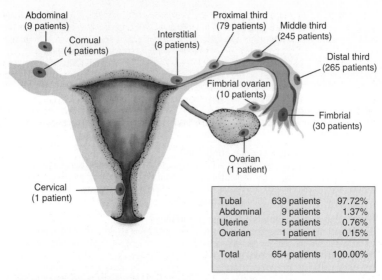

Figure 12-1. Locations of implantation in ectopic pregnancy. *(From Lentz GM, Lobo RA, Gershenson DM, et al, eds. Comprehensive Gynecology. 6th ed. Philadelphia: Mosby; 2012.)*

7. **What are the most common symptoms of an ectopic pregnancy?**
An ectopic pregnancy should be considered in any pregnant patient who has abdominal pain or vaginal bleeding. All women of reproductive age who present with these complaints should receive a pregnancy test. Because a standard urine pregnancy test can detect human chorionic gonadotropin (hCG) levels as low as 20 mIU/mL, a negative result almost always rules out the diagnosis. In a patient with a positive pregnancy test result, additional evaluation is necessary.

8. **How is an ectopic pregnancy diagnosed?**
Evaluation begins with a urine pregnancy test; if the result is negative, an ectopic pregnancy is excluded. If the urine pregnancy test result is positive and the patient stable, serologic testing and ultrasonography should be performed.
The following tests should always be ordered:
1. Serum quantitative hCG (discussed later in question 9).
2. Blood type and antibody screen; women with vaginal bleeding who are Rh negative require anti-D immunoglobulin (RhoGAM) to prevent isoimmunization and hemolytic disease of the newborn in subsequent pregnancies.
3. Hemoglobin level; keep in mind that this can be normal in the early stages of acute blood loss. Significant anemia is cause for concern.
A transvaginal ultrasound (TVUS) scan should be performed to attempt to locate the pregnancy. Four general categories of results are seen:
1. Nondiagnostic: Normal anatomy is present, but no IUP is identified.
2. Suggestive of ectopic pregnancy: An adnexal mass is present, and no IUP is seen.
3. Diagnostic of an ectopic pregnancy: A gestational sac with a yolk sac or embryo is seen outside the uterine cavity.
4. Diagnostic of an IUP: A gestational sac with a yolk sac or embryo is seen inside the uterine cavity. If a pregnant patient has not undergone ART, the diagnosis of ectopic pregnancy is essentially excluded in the presence of an IUP.

9. **In patients without an IUP on TVUS, how does the quantitative hCG determination help?**
If no IUP is visualized on TVUS, a quantitative hCG determination can guide management. A single level guides interpretation of ultrasound results on that day, and serial levels can be used to guide prognosis and management in the outpatient setting. Evidence of an IUP (i.e., a gestational sac) should

be seen with TVUS when the hCG level reaches approximately 1500 mIU/mL, and an IUP is virtually always seen when hCG exceeds 2500 mIU/mL. Traditionally, a quantitative hCG level of 1500 mIU/mL has been called the **discriminatory zone** because this is the level at which one expects to visualize an IUP if the pregnancy is normal. However, more recent data support a higher threshold, with 99% of gestational sacs visible with TVUS when the hCG level reaches 3500 mIU/mL. Absence of an IUP on TVUS with an hCG greater than the discriminatory zone is highly suggestive of an abnormal pregnancy (either an ectopic pregnancy or a nonviable intrauterine gestation). If a patient without an IUP on ultrasound has an hCG level lower than the discriminatory zone and is stable, she can be followed with a repeat hCG level in 48 hours. These patients should be instructed to seek emergency medical care if they have worsening abdominal pain, lightheadedness or syncope (concerning for blood loss), or other concerns.

The discriminatory zone for transabdominal ultrasound is much higher (6000 mIU/mL) because it is much more difficult to visualize an early IUP with this method. However, some providers prefer to perform a transabdominal ultrasound scan first because visualization of an IUP eliminates the need for a subsequent TVUS (Tables 12-1 and 12-2).

Table 12-1. Normal Intrauterine Pregnancy

GESTATIONAL AGE	STRUCTURES
4-5 weeks from LMP	Eccentrically placed small gestational sac
5 weeks from LMP	Double decidua sign (two echogenic rings surrounded by intrauterine fluid collection); can be mistaken for pseudo-sac
5.5 weeks from LMP	Diagnostic findings start here: Yolk sac visualized within gestational sac
6 weeks from LMP	Embryonic pole
6.5 weeks from LMP	Fetal cardiac activity present

LMP, Last menstrual period.

Table 12-2. Ectopic Pregnancy

Extrauterine pregnancy	Yolk sac or fetal pole (100% positive predictive value for ectopic pregnancy) is diagnostic
Ring sign	Adnexal mass with hyperechoic ring surrounding gestational sac
Nonhomogenous mass (not ovarian)	Positive predictive value for ectopic pregnancy is 80% to 90%

10. **How are serial quantitative hCG measurements useful?**
In patients who have an hCG lower than the discriminatory zone and who are stable for discharge, serial hCG levels can guide outpatient management (Fig. 12-2). In early pregnancy (before 6 to 7 weeks of gestation), hCG normally doubles every 48 hours and should increase by *at least* 66%. If the level does not rise significantly or declines, a nonviable pregnancy (either ectopic or spontaneous abortion) is highly likely. If the level rises to greater than the discriminatory zone and no IUP is identified, suspicion of an ectopic pregnancy should increase.

11. **Can other blood tests predict the viability of a pregnancy?**
Progesterone levels can potentially be used to predict pregnancy viability, although most hospitals cannot readily perform this test and produce a result within the same patient visit. In one large series, all women in the first trimester of pregnancy who had a serum progesterone level lower than 5 ng/mL had an abnormal pregnancy (ectopic or nonviable IUP), and almost all women (97%) with a progesterone level higher than 25 ng/mL were eventually diagnosed with a viable IUP. This is test is not currently considered part of the standard workup for ectopic pregnancy.

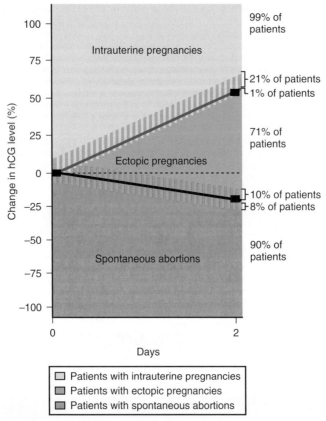

Figure 12-2. Change in human chorionic gonadotropin (hCG) level over 48 hours (2 days) in intrauterine pregnancies, ectopic pregnancies, and spontaneous abortions. *(From Lentz GM, Lobo RA, Gershenson DM, et al, eds. Comprehensive Gynecology. 6th ed. Philadelphia: Mosby; 2012.)*

12. What is the role of dilation and curettage (D&C) in the diagnosis of an ectopic pregnancy?

When a patient has a nondiagnostic TVUS and the hCG level is greater than the discriminatory zone, D&C can be considered for both diagnostic and therapeutic purposes. However, this option is reserved for undesired pregnancies. If chorionic villi are identified by histologic examination of the tissue obtained during the procedure, a nonviable IUP was present, and the patient is considered to have received definitive treatment (i.e., therapeutic abortion). If chorionic villi are not identified, the diagnosis of an ectopic pregnancy is presumed. A D&C can also be considered in patients with an abnormally low rate of rise in hCG because this indicates an abnormal pregnancy.

13. How is an ectopic pregnancy managed medically, and who is eligible?

Medical management of an ectopic pregnancy is achieved with methotrexate (MTX), a folic acid antagonist. In properly selected patients, outcomes are comparable to those of surgical intervention. Before the patient receives MTX, the following laboratory tests should be ordered: complete blood count (CBC), chemistry panel, liver function tests (LFTs), quantitative hCG, blood type, and antibody screen. Absolute contraindications to MTX are breastfeeding, immunodeficiency, blood dyscrasias, active pulmonary disease, any renal or hepatic dysfunction, alcoholism, or active peptic ulcer disease.

The ideal patient for MTX therapy (1) is asymptomatic or minimally symptomatic with an unruptured tubal ectopic pregnancy, (2) is reliable for follow-up, and (3) has an hCG level higher than

5000 mIU/mL. No fetal cardiac activity should be present, and the size of the ectopic mass should be relatively small (e.g., <3 to 4 cm). An hCG level lower than 5000 mIU/mL raises the risk of treatment failure by 5.5 times.

Intramuscular MTX is the most common route of administration, and both single- and multiple-dose protocols exist. Single-dose MTX is more than 90% effective, has fewer side effects, and does not require folinic acid rescue therapy. Common side effects (seen in 30% of patients) include severe pelvic pain (usually days 3 to 7 after initiating therapy), stomatitis, and conjunctivitis. However, more rare and severe reactions (e.g., hepatotoxicity, pulmonary toxicity, myelosuppression, nephrotoxicity) are possible.

The day MTX is given is considered day 1, and hCG levels should fall by at least 15% between days 4 and 7 (it is not unusual for hCG levels to rise on days 1 to 3). If a 15% decline is not achieved, an additional dose of MTX per week can be given to a maximum of three additional doses until the hCG falls by 15%. After three additional doses have been given, a lack of decline is considered treatment failure, and surgical treatment should be performed.

14. **What does surgical management of an ectopic pregnancy involve, and who is eligible?**
Indications for surgical management include hemodynamic instability, suspicion of rupture, contraindications to MTX, or treatment failure. The most common procedure is laparoscopy with salpingostomy or salpingectomy. In a salpingostomy, the fallopian tube is incised, the ectopic pregnancy is removed, and the tube is left to heal by secondary intention. This method preserves future fertility through that fallopian tube, but it does carry the risk of leaving some trophoblastic tissue in the fallopian tube (termed a persistent ectopic pregnancy). Patients should be followed with weekly hCG levels until these levels are undetectable. A salpingectomy is removal of the fallopian tube with the ectopic pregnancy; although it does not preserve future fertility on that side, it has an extremely low risk of persistent ectopic pregnancy.

KEY POINTS: ECTOPIC PREGNANCY

1. Ectopic pregnancy is the most common cause of maternal pregnancy-related death in the first trimester.
2. The most significant risk factor for ectopic pregnancy is a history of salpingitis resulting from sexually-transmitted infections such as *Chlamydia* infection or gonorrhea.
3. The most common symptoms of an ectopic pregnancy are abdominal pain and vaginal bleeding.
4. A quantitative hCG of more than 1500 mIU/mL with no evidence of an IUP visualized on TVUS is concerning for an ectopic pregnancy.
5. The management of an ectopic pregnancy can be either medical or surgical, depending on the patient's preference and the clinical characteristics.
6. Consider heterotopic pregnancy in any patient who has recently undergone ART.

BIBLIOGRAPHY

1. American College of Obstetricians and Gynecologists. Medical management of ectopic pregnancy. ACOG practice bulletin no. 94. *Obstet Gynecol.* 2008;111:1479–1485.
2. Barnhart K. Ectopic pregnancy. *N Engl J Med.* 2009;361:379–387.
3. Connolly A, Ryan DH, Stuebe AM, Wolfe HM. Reevaluation of the discriminatory and threshold levels of Serum β-hCG in early pregnancy. *Obstet Gynecol.* 2013;121:65–70.
4. Lobo RA. Ectopic pregnancy. In: Lentz GM, Lobo RA, Gershenson DM, et al., eds. *Comprehensive Gynecology.* 6th ed. Philadelphia: Mosby; 2013.
5. Murray H, Baadkah H, Bardell T, Tulandi T. Diagnosis and treatment of ectopic pregnancy. *CMAJ.* 2005;173:905–912.
6. Stovall TG, Ling FW, Carson SA, Buster JE. Serum progesterone and uterine curettage in differential diagnosis of ectopic pregnancy. *Fertil Steril.* 1992;57:456–457.

CHAPTER 13

INDUCED ABORTION

Lirona Katzir, MD

1. **What percentage of pregnancies is unintended?**
   Approximately 51% of pregnancies are unintended. Of these, 20% are unwanted, and 31% are mistimed.

2. **What percentage of pregnancies ends in abortion?**
   Approximately 20% of all pregnancies end in abortion; among unintended pregnancies, this rises to 4 out of every 10.

3. **What are the major methods used to terminate a pregnancy?**
   - Medical abortion
   - Surgical abortion: either dilation and curettage (D&C) or dilation and evacuation (D&E)
   - Labor induction

4. **At what gestational age are abortions most often performed?**
   Almost 90% of abortions occur in the first trimester; 30% of all abortions occur at 6 weeks or earlier, and less than 1% of abortions are performed after 20 weeks.

5. **What workup is needed before offering or performing an abortion?**
   - A complete history and physical examination
   - Ultrasound scan to confirm pregnancy and determine gestational age
   - Hemoglobin or hematocrit if anemia is suspected
   - Rh testing; if a woman is Rh negative, RhD immunoglobulin should be administered at the time of the procedure

6. **How does gestational age affect the type of abortion that can be offered?**
   - Less than 9 weeks: Medical or surgical options can be offered based on the patient's preference. Evidence-based medical regimens are most effective for pregnancies of less than 49 days.
   - 9 to 13 weeks: Both medical and surgical options can still be offered, although medical abortions at this gestational age are typically done in an inpatient setting.
   - More than 13 weeks: Surgical abortion or labor induction can be offered.

7. **What are the major differences between medical and surgical abortions in the first trimester?**
   Table 13-1 provides a comparison of medical and surgical abortions.

8. **What percentage of abortions is completed medically?**
   Fifteen percent to 20% of all abortions are completed medically.

9. **What medications are used for medical abortions? How do they work?**
   - **Mifepristone (RU-486):** a progesterone antagonist that causes decidual necrosis of the uterine lining, softening of the cervix, and increased contractility of the uterus. It is most commonly used in combination with a prostaglandin.
   - **Misoprostol:** a prostaglandin that is used off-label for medical abortion and labor induction. It can be administered orally, buccally, or vaginally, and it is most effective when combined with mifepristone.
   - **Methotrexate:** a folate antimetabolite that interferes with DNA synthesis and the implantation process. Before mifepristone became available, it was used in combination with misoprostol. At present, this regimen is rarely used.

10. **What are the most common regimens used for medical abortions? How do their success rates differ?**
    Regimens approved by the Food and Drug Administration (FDA) are based on the original regimen registered in France in the 1980s. More recent evidence-based regimens have proved to be superior in terms of cost, safety, efficacy, and incidence of adverse effects (Table 13-2). Misoprostol-only

Table 13-1. Major Differences Between Medical And Surgical Abortions in the First Trimester

MEDICAL ABORTION	SURGICAL ABORTION
Usually avoids an invasive procedure	Involves an invasive procedure
Usually avoids anesthesia and requires only oral pain medication	May require sedation or local anesthesia
Can be completed in the privacy of a home	Completed in the clinic, office, or operating room
May take days to weeks to complete	Generally completed at the time of the procedure
Higher rates of cramping; bleeding not commonly perceived as "light"	Bleeding commonly perceived as "light"
Generally a multistep procedure, requiring at least two visits	Generally a single-step process, requiring only one visit
Follow-up required to ensure that the abortion is completed	Most cases do not require follow-up
Success rates ~95%	Success rates ~99%

Table 13-2. Food and Drug Administration–Approved Regimen Versus Evidence-Based Regimens for Induced Abortion

FDA-APPROVED REGIMEN	EVIDENCE-BASED REGIMENS
Gestations up to 49 days	Gestations up to 63 days
Regimen: Mifepristone 600 mg orally followed by misoprostol 400 µg orally 48 hours later	Regimens: Mifepristone 200 mg orally followed by misoprostol 800 µg vaginally, buccally, or sublingually 24-48 hours later (Alternatively, misoprostol can be can administered vaginally 6-8 hours after mifepristone)
Timing between mifepristone and misoprostol administration cannot be varied	More flexibility in timing between mifepristone and misoprostol ($<$6 hours up to 48 hours depending on route)
Must return to the office or clinic for misoprostol administration	Can self-administer misoprostol in the privacy of a home
Greater time to expulsion	Less time to expulsion
More expensive	Lower cost
Efficacy: 92% (rates are higher at earlier gestations)	Efficacy: 95%-99%

regimens are only 84% to 85% effective and have a significantly higher incidence of adverse effects compared with combined regimens.

11. **What are the major side effects of the medications used for medical abortions?**
Bleeding and cramping are the most common side effects experienced by women undergoing a medical abortion. Other common side effects include nausea (20% to 60%), vomiting (5% to 40%), headaches (10% to 40%), diarrhea (1% to 35%), dizziness (10% to 40%), and thermoregulatory effects (10% to 60%) such as warmth, hot flushes, fever, or chills.

12. **What are the major complications of medical abortion?**
Major complications are hemorrhage requiring emergency D&C, incomplete abortion requiring further management, and postabortal infections. Depending on the regimen used, less than 5% of patients will require a D&C. Overall, the rate of complications is less than 1%.

13. **What are contraindications to medical abortion?**
    - Allergy or intolerance to mifepristone or misoprostol
    - Suspected or confirmed ectopic pregnancy
    - Severe anemia, known coagulopathy, or anticoagulant therapy
    - Severe liver, renal, cardiovascular, or respiratory disease
    - Patients who are unreliable or unable to be contacted for follow-up

14. **What are the different techniques used to perform a surgical abortion?**
    - Less than 13 weeks: A D&C can be performed in the office with a mechanical vacuum aspirator (MVA), or a suction D&C can be performed in a procedure room with an electric vacuum aspiration system (EVA). Specimens should always be inspected for villi.
    - More than 13 weeks: In the second trimester, D&Cs and D&Es are typically performed in an operating or procedure room with either anesthesia or analgesia and sedation. After 14 weeks of gestation, D&Es are the standard procedure and may require cervical preparation.
    - Prophylactic antibiotics are recommended during surgical abortions to prevent infection.

15. **What are the major complications of surgical abortions?**
    Surgical abortions are extremely safe, with very low complication rates. Rare complications include uterine perforation (0.5%), hemorrhage (0.1% to 0.7%), postabortal infection (0.1% to 4%), incomplete abortion (<1%), and cervical laceration (3%). Abortions are safest early in pregnancy; although the risk is very low, mortality increases with each week of gestation.

16. **What is the preferred method of second trimester termination?**
    The patient's preference, the provider's comfort, cost, safety, indication, and logistics should all be taken into consideration when determining the method of pregnancy termination in the second trimester. Compared with labor induction, D&Es by experienced providers are associated with lower complication rates (4% versus 29%). The most common complication of second trimester labor induction is retained placenta (20%), which can increase the risk of postabortal hemorrhage and the need for a D&C.

17. **How is a second trimester surgical termination performed?**
    Depending on gestational age, cervical preparation may be required. This can be accomplished with cervical ripening agents (typically misoprostol) or osmotic dilators before the procedure. Once anesthesia or adequate sedation is achieved, further cervical dilation may be needed. When sufficient dilation is achieved, amniotic fluid is aspirated, and the uterine cavity is evacuated with the use of grasping forceps.

18. **Is induced fetal demise necessary before second trimester abortions?**
    No. Although no evidence exists to recommend for or against routine induced fetal demise before an abortion, it is a commonly employed technique. It can be done by intraamniotic or intrafetal injection with digoxin, transection of the umbilical cord, or fetal intracardiac injection of potassium chloride. In cases of abortion by labor induction after 20 weeks of gestation, induced fetal demise may be preferred for the patient's comfort and to avoid transient fetal survival.

19. **When is labor induction performed, and what methods are used?**
    Labor induction is an alternative to a surgical abortion. It is often preferred in cases with fetal anomalies to provide an intact fetus for autopsy. It can be performed with mifepristone, cervical ripening agents such as misoprostol, or mechanical dilation. Intravenous oxytocin may be used with later gestations.

20. **How soon after an abortion can birth control be initiated?**
    Oral contraceptives, the transdermal patch, the vaginal ring, and subdermal implants can be initiated on the same day as the administration of misoprostol or the surgical procedure. Intrauterine devices can be placed immediately following surgical abortion or as early as 1 week following a completed medical abortion.

21. **What was the impact of the 1973 U.S. Supreme Court decision in Roe v. Wade?**
    - Roe v. Wade legalized abortion across the United States.
    - Before Roe v. Wade, illegal abortions accounted for 17% of maternal deaths. This rate has dramatically decreased to approximately 0.6 deaths per 100,000 procedures.

KEY POINTS: INDUCED ABORTION

1. More than 50% of pregnancies are unintended.
2. Pregnancies can be terminated medically or surgically.
3. Most complications are related to incomplete abortion, hemorrhage, and infection.
4. Abortions are now among the safest procedures for women in the Unites States.

BIBLIOGRAPHY

1. American College of Obstetricians and Gynecologists. Second trimester abortion. ACOG practice bulletin no. 135. *Obstet Gynecol.* 2013;121:1394–1406.
2. American College of Obstetricians and Gynecologists. Medical management of first trimester abortion. ACOG practice bulletin no. 143. *Obstet Gyecol.* 2014;123:676–692.
3. Borgatta L, Kapp N. Society of Family Planning. Clinical guidelines: labor induction abortion in the second trimester. *Contraception.* 2011;84:4–18.
4. Guttmacher Institute. *Fact sheet: facts on induced abortion worldwide;* 2012. Available at http://www.guttmacher.org/pubs/fb_IAW.html. Accessed October 22, 2015.
5. Guttmacher Institute. *Fact sheet: induced abortion in the United States;* 2014. Available at http://www.guttmacher.org/pubs/fb_induced_abortion.html. Accessed October 22, 2015.
6. Sawaya GF, Grady D, Kerlikowske K, Grimes DA. Antibiotics at the time of induced abortion: the case for universal prophylaxis based on a meta-analysis. *Obstet Gynecol.* 1996;87:884.

CHAPTER 14

CONTRACEPTION

Elena Martinez, MD

1. **What methods of contraception are currently available to women in the United States?**
   - Abstinence, withdrawal, and fertility awareness
   - Permanent sterilization (tubal ligation, tubal occlusion, vasectomy)
   - Hormonal
     - Oral contraceptive pills (OCPs; combination estradiol and progestin or progestin only)
     - Injectable progestin (depot medroxyprogesterone acetate)
     - Subdermal implant (etonogestrel implant)
     - Vaginal ring (etonogestrel and ethinyl estradiol)
     - Transdermal patch (norelgestromin and ethinyl estradiol)
   - Intrauterine device (IUD)
     - Levonorgestrel IUD
     - Copper IUD
   - Barrier methods
     - Condoms
     - Diaphragm
     - Cervical cap
     - Contraceptive sponge
   - Spermicides
   - Emergency contraception (oral levonorgestrel, ulipristal acetate, high-dose oral contraceptives, or copper IUD)

2. **What percentage of women will have an unintended pregnancy in the first year of using contraception, and what percentage of women will continue to use contraception after 1 year?**
   This depends on the method used (Table 14-1).

Table 14-1. Percentage of Women in the United States Who Experience an Unintended Pregnancy During the First Year of Typical Use and the First Year of Perfect Use of Contraception and the Percentage Continuing Use at the End of the First Year

METHOD COLUMN (1)	Percentage of Women Experiencing an Unintended Pregnancy Within the First Year of Use (%)		PERCENTAGE OF WOMEN CONTINUING USE AT 1 YEAR (%)* COLUMN (4)
	TYPICAL USE† COLUMN (2)	PERFECT USE‡ COLUMN (3)	
No method§	85	85	—
Spermicides¶¶	28	18	42
Fertility awareness–based methods	24	—	47
Standard Days method¶	—	5	—
TwoDay method¶	—	4	—
Ovulation method¶	—	3	—
Symptothermal method¶	—	0.4	—
Withdrawal	22	4	46

Table 14-1. Percentage of Women in the United States Who Experience an Unintended Pregnancy During the First Year of Typical Use and the First Year of Perfect Use of Contraception and the Percentage Continuing Use at the End of the First Year *(Continued)*

METHOD COLUMN (1)	Percentage of Women Experiencing an Unintended Pregnancy Within the First Year of Use (%)		PERCENTAGE OF WOMEN CONTINUING USE AT 1 YEAR (%)* COLUMN (4)
	TYPICAL USE† COLUMN (2)	PERFECT USE‡ COLUMN (3)	
Sponge	—	—	36
Parous women	24	20	—
Nulliparous women	12	9	—
Condom#			
Female	21	5	41
Male	18	2	43
Diaphragm**	12	6	57
Combined pill and progestin-only pill	9	0.3	67
Evra patch	9	0.3	67
NuvaRing	9	0.3	67
Depo-Provera (depot medroxyprogesterone acetate)	6	0.2	56
IUCs			
ParaGard (copper T)	0.8	0.6	78
Mirena (LNG)	0.2	0.2	80
Implanon	0.05	0.05	84
Female sterilization	0.5	0.5	100
Male sterilization	0.15	0.1	100
LAM is an effective, temporary method of contraception.††			

IUC, Intrauterine contraceptive; *LAM,* lactational amenorrhea method; *LNG,* levonorgestrel.

*Among couples attempting to avoid pregnancy, the percentage of couples who continue to use a method for 1 year.

†Among typical couples who initiate use of a method (not necessarily for the first time), the percentage of couples who experience an accidental pregnancy during the first year if they do not stop use for any other reason. Estimates of the probability of pregnancy during the first year of typical use for spermicides and the diaphragm are taken from the 1995 National Survey of Family Growth (NSFG) corrected for underreporting of abortion; estimates for fertility awareness–based methods, withdrawal, the male condom, the oral contraceptive pill, and Depo-Provera are taken from the 1995 and 2002 NSFG corrected for underreporting of abortion.

‡Among couples who initiate use of a method (not necessarily for the first time) and who use it perfectly (both consistently and correctly), the percentage of couples who experience an accidental pregnancy during the first year if they do not stop use for any other reason.

§The percentages of becoming pregnant in columns (2) and (3) are based on data from populations where contraception is not used and from women who cease using contraception to become pregnant. Among such populations, approximately 89% of women become pregnant within 1 year. This estimate was lowered slightly (to 85%) to represent the percentage of women who would become pregnant within 1 year among women now relying on reversible methods of contraception if they abandoned contraception altogether.

¶¶Foams, creams, gels, vaginal suppositories, and vaginal film.

¶The ovulation and TwoDay methods are based on evaluation of cervical mucus. The Standard Days method avoids intercourse on cycle days 8 through 19. The symptothermal method is a double-check method based on evaluation of cervical mucus to determine the first fertile day and evaluation of cervical mucus and temperature to determine the last fertile day.

#Without spermicides.

**With spermicidal cream or jelly.

††However, to maintain effective protection against pregnancy, another method of contraception must be used as soon as menstruation resumes, the frequency or duration of breastfeeding is reduced, bottle feedings are introduced, or the baby reaches 6 months of age.

Modified from Trussell J. Contraceptive failure in the United States. *Contraception.* 2011;83:397-404.

3. **What is the most commonly used contraceptive in the United States?**
   The OCP. First approved for use in 1960, OCPs have evolved into a safe and popular option. This is likely because of their relative safety profile for the average user, the flexibility to start, stop, or manipulate regimens, and their multiple noncontraceptive benefits.

4. **How do OCPs work?**
   OCPs work through progestin- and estrogen-mediated effects.
   - Progestins
     - Suppress both luteinizing hormone (LH) and follicle stimulating hormone (FSH), thus preventing ovulation
     - Thicken cervical mucus and hamper sperm transport
     - Induce endometrial gland atrophy and decrease the likelihood of embryo implantation
     - May alter secretions and motility of the fallopian tubes, thereby interfering with fertilization
   - Estrogen
     - Suppresses both LH and FSH, although to a lesser effect than progestins
     - Potentiates the antigonadotropin effects of progestins, thus enhancing their effects
     - Importantly, stabilizes the endometrium and prevents irregular shedding

5. **What are the noncontraceptive benefits of OCPs?**
   - Decreases in menstrual flow, anemia, primary dysmenorrhea, risk of symptomatic pelvic inflammatory disease, risk of ectopic pregnancy, and incidence of benign breast disease (fibroadenomas, fibrocystic changes)
   - Reduced risk of ovarian and endometrial cancer
   - Improvement in hirsutism and acne

6. **What is the primary risk associated with combination OCPs?**
   Venous thromboembolism (VTE) is the most common, serious side effect of estrogen-containing hormonal contraception. The highest risk is thought to occur during the first year of use, and an increased risk persists until discontinuation. However, the absolute risk is low.

7. **What are other risks associated with OCPs?**
   Stroke and myocardial infarction, although the absolute risk is still very low.

8. **What are some common therapeutic uses of OCPs?**
   - **Menstrual disorders:** Primary dysmenorrhea in most women can be successfully treated with OCPs. OCPs can also be used to treat both heavy bleeding and intermenstrual bleeding, and high doses (three or four pills a day) of combination formulations can effectively suppress acute episodes of bleeding. Once the bleeding has stopped, the regimen can be tapered and then stopped to allow for withdrawal bleeding.
   - **Endometriosis:** A Cochrane Collaboration review supported the use of OCPs for long-term treatment.
   - **Hyperandrogenism:** OCPs suppress ovarian, adrenal, and peripheral androgen metabolism. The estrogen component of OCPs also increases sex hormone–binding globulin levels and inhibits 5α-reductase in the skin, thus resulting in lower levels of dihydrotestosterone. For more information on this topic, see Chapter 26.
   - **Hypoestrogenic states:** OCPs have been used in women with hypothalamic amenorrhea as a method of hormone replacement therapy. OCP use in the perimenopausal period can prevent pregnancy, regulate uterine bleeding, and treat vasomotor and vaginal dryness symptoms. Estrogen replacement in the form of OCPs can also benefit patients who are amenorrheic after radiation therapy, chemotherapy, or bilateral oophorectomy.
   - **Menstrual migraines:** Likely triggered by changes in estrogen levels immediately before menses, these headaches occur immediately before the onset of menses and not at any other time during the cycle. Continuous OCP dosing, with no withdrawal, is most effective at prevention.

9. **What is the association of OCPs with cancer?**
   - **Ovarian cancer:** Users of OCPs are less likely to develop epithelial ovarian cancer, with the risk decreasing by 40% with as little as 3 to 6 months of OCP use. The protective effect persists for at least 15 years after OCP discontinuation.
   - **Endometrial cancer:** OCP users are 50% less likely to develop endometrial cancer, with the risk reduced by 20% with 1 year of use, 40% with 2 years of use, and 60% with 4 or more years of use. This reduction in risk also persists for at least 15 years after discontinuation.

- **Breast cancer:** In the past, concern existed that OCPs were an independent risk factor for developing breast cancer. However, the 2002 Women's CARE Study by the National Institute of Child Health and Human Development established that current or former OCP use was not associated with an increased risk of breast cancer.
- **Cervical cancer:** Although a 2014 quantitative review of the link between OCPs and cervical cancer showed that long-term (>5 year), current, or recent OCP use is related to a nearly twofold increased risk of cervical cancer, this risk levels off after stopping OCP use and approaches baseline within 10 years.

10. **What are contraindications to OCP use?**
    - Known presence or history of VTE or pulmonary embolism
    - History of stroke, coronary artery disease, or ischemic heart disease
    - Diabetes with microvascular complications (neuropathy, retinopathy) or duration of more than 20 years
    - History of estrogen-dependent cancer
    - Migraines with focal neurologic symptoms (aura)
    - Age older than 35 years in the setting of smoking more than 20 cigarettes a day
    - Poorly controlled hypertension (blood pressure >160/100 mm Hg) or in the setting of vascular disease
    - Active liver disease
    - Major surgical procedure with prolonged immobilization
    - Personal history of acquired or inherited thrombophilia

11. **What are the other forms of hormonal contraception?**
    - **Depot medroxyprogesterone acetate:** This is given as an intramuscular injection of 150 mg every 12 weeks. Amenorrhea is common after 1 year of use (50%), and headaches are the most common nonmenstrual side effects. Although transient bone mineral density (BMD) loss may occur, it is comparable to loss seen with lactation and reverses on discontinuation. Neither the World Health Organization (WHO) nor the American College of Obstetricians and Gynecologists (ACOG) recommends restricting its use or performing BMD testing in women who use it.
    - **Etonogestrel subdermal implant:** A single rod containing 68 mg of etonogestrel is placed in the subcutaneous tissue of the upper arm in the supracondylar area. Lasting up to 3 years, this method carries the lowest failure rate for any contraceptive at 0.05 pregnancies in the first year of use. Common side effects include irregular bleeding, amenorrhea, gastrointestinal difficulties, headaches, acne, breast tenderness, and weight gain; the continuance rate for this method, however, is 84% at 1 year.
    - **Etonogestrel and ethinyl estradiol vaginal ring:** A flexible vaginal ring that delivers 120 µg/day of etonogestrel and 15 µg/day of ethinyl estradiol remains in place for 3 weeks, followed by a ring-free week. Common side effects include headache, vaginitis, leucorrhea, and ring slippage. The continuation rate at 1 year is 68%.
    - **Norelgestromin and ethinyl estradiol transdermal patch:** One patch containing 6 mg norelgestromin and 0.75 mg ethinyl estradiol is applied once a week for 3 consecutive weeks, followed by a patch-free week. The most common side effects are headache and nausea. Conflicting evidence exists regarding a potential increase in VTE risk (compared with OCPs) with this method.

12. **What is the effect of hormonal contraception on an unsuspected pregnancy?**
    The use of any hormonal method of contraception early in an unsuspected pregnancy has not been shown to increase the risk of congenital anomalies or early pregnancy loss.

13. **What is emergency contraception and how does it work?**
    Emergency contraception is intended for use after unprotected intercourse to prevent pregnancy. It works by inhibiting or delaying ovulation, and it may also impair endometrial receptivity to implantation. Other possible mechanisms include interference with corpus luteum function, thickening of cervical mucus, and alterations in tubal transport of sperm, egg, or embryo. *It does not interrupt or harm an already established pregnancy.*

14. **What are the forms of emergency contraception?**
    - **Levonorgestrel pill (1.5 mg):** 89% effective if taken within 72 hours of unprotected intercourse, can be taken up to 120 hours with less efficacy. Slightly less effective in women with a BMI >25-30. Side effects are minimal and mostly include nausea and vomiting. Available without a prescription.

- **Ulipristal acetate pill (30 mg):** This is 89% effective when taken up to 120 hours after unprotected intercourse and is slightly less effective in women with a body mass index (BMI) greater than 35. Side effects include headache, nausea, and abdominal pain. It is available by prescription only.
- **High-dose combination OCPs (Yuzpe method):** 100 µg of ethinyl estradiol and 0.5 to .075 mg of levonorgestrel are divided into two doses and taken 12 hours apart. This is 74% effective if taken by 72 hours after unprotected intercourse. Major side effects include headache, nausea, and vomiting.
- **Copper IUD:** This can be inserted up to 7 days after ovulation to prevent pregnancy and is 99.9% effective.

15. **How does an IUD prevent pregnancy?**
An IUD induces a local inflammatory reaction that renders the uterus an unfavorable environment for pregnancy. This reaction also alters sperm motility or integrity and tubal fluids, thus interfering with ova and sperm transport and interaction. IUDs are appropriate for use in both nulliparous and adolescent women, and insertion can be performed at any point in the menstrual cycle as long as a diagnosis of pregnancy is excluded.

16. **What are the different types of IUD?**
    - **Copper IUD:** This releases copper ions that enhance the inflammatory response and reach concentrations that are toxic for spermatozoa. The continuation rate is 78% at 1 year, and the failure rate is 0.6%. The most common side effects are dysmenorrhea and heavy bleeding, seen in approximately 10% of women.
    - **Levonorgestrel IUD:** This provides additional protection by inducing endometrial gland atrophy and thickening cervical mucous. The continuation rate is 80% at 1 year, and the failure rate is 0.2%. The most common side effects are breakthrough bleeding and amenorrhea. Systemic side effects can also occur and include headaches, nausea, breast tenderness, and ovarian cysts.

17. **What are contraindications to IUD insertion?**
    - Confirmed or suspected pregnancy
    - Known or suspected pelvic malignant disease
    - Undiagnosed vaginal bleeding
    - Acute or chronic pelvic infection
    - Hyperbilirubinemia secondary to Wilson disease (for copper-containing devices only)

18. **What are the major risks associated with IUD use?**
    - Displacement of the device that leads to difficult removal
    - Uterine perforation
    - Pelvic infection
    The IUD itself does not cause pelvic infection. In general, it is believed that the risk of pelvic inflammatory disease is greater with an IUD in place when a woman has a sexually transmitted infection. A WHO multicenter review estimated the overall risk of pelvic inflammatory disease to be concentrated in the first 20 days after insertion, when the risk was sixfold higher, than at later times. The ACOG supports the practice of screening asymptomatic women at the time of IUD insertion and treating for infection in the case of a positive result, without the need to remove the IUD.

19. **What are barrier methods of contraception?**
Barrier methods of contraception provide a physical barrier that prevents sperm and ovum interaction, and some forms also use a spermicidal chemical to help decreasing the odds of pregnancy. Barrier methods include male and female condoms, diaphragms, cervical caps, and sponges. Benefits include protection against some sexually transmitted infections (depending on the barrier method used), provision of immediate protection without much advance planning, easy access, and the absence of systemic side effects. Disadvantages comparatively higher failure rates, discomfort with placement or use, and possible allergic reactions.

20. **What are the forms of permanent sterilization?**
    - **Tubal ligation:** In this surgical procedure, the fallopian tubes are cut, thermally damaged, removed, or otherwise destroyed. It can be performed with regional anesthesia if it is performed within the first few days post partum; otherwise, general anesthesia is used. Less than 1% of women will become pregnant in the first year. The risk of failure varies by the method used and the age of the patient.
    - **Tubal occlusion:** First approved in the United States in 2002, this is performed using hysteroscopy and does not necessarily require general anesthesia; inert microinserts designed to initiate

localized tissue ingrowth are placed into the proximal portion of the fallopian tubes. A hysterosalpingogram (HSG) is then performed 3 months after the procedure to ensure that complete occlusion has occurred. Benefits include avoiding the need for an abdominal incision and general anesthesia, and this method may be a viable option for women who are not good surgical candidates.

- **Vasectomy:** Interruption of the vas deferens to prevent sperm from entering the ejaculate is typically performed as an outpatient procedure using local anesthesia. Pregnancy rates are reported to be 0% to 2%. Associated risks are minor but can rarely include hematoma, infection, hydrocele, granuloma formation, and chronic pain syndrome.

In the United States, permanent female sterilization is the most common method of contraception used by couples who are more than 30 years old.

21. **What is fertility awareness?**

Two types of fertility awareness are used. First, assuming a cycle length of 28 days, ovulation should occur on or near cycle day 14. Abstinence between days 8 and 19 will most likely avoid pregnancy. Second, physiologic changes in cervical mucus and basal body temperature are observable during the time surrounding ovulation and can be used to time abstinence.

KEY POINTS: CONTRACEPTION

1. Combination OCPs work by inhibiting ovulation through suppression of LH and FSH, thus creating a decidualized endometrium, thickening cervical mucus, and decreasing tubal motility.
2. Venous thromboembolic events are the most common serious side effects of OCPs.
3. OCPs have multiple secondary benefits and are commonly used to treat many different medical conditions.
4. Emergency contraception is available over the counter, by prescription, and by a medical provider. It is most effective when used within 72 to 120 hours of unprotected intercourse.
5. Long-acting reversible contraceptives (IUDs, implant) are recommended for women who desire effective long-term contraception that is completely reversible.

BIBLIOGRAPHY

1. American College of Obstetricians and Gynecologists. Sterilization. ACOG technical bulletin no. 222. Washington, DC: American College of Obstetricians and Gynecologists; 1996.
2. American College of Obstetricians and Gynecologists. Emergency contraception. ACOG technical bulletin no. 25. Washington, DC: American College of Obstetricians and Gynecologists; 2001.
3. American College of Obstetricians and Gynecologists. Long-acting reversible contraception: implants and intrauterine devices. ACOG practice bulletin no. 121. *Obstet Gynecol.* 2011;118:184–196.
4. Andersson K, Odlind V, Rybo G. Levonorgestrel-releasing and copper-releasing (Nova T) IUDs during five years of use: a randomized comparative trial. *Contraception.* 1994;49:56–72.
5. Barnhart KB, Dayal M. Contraception. In: Rakel RE, Bope ET, eds. *Conn's Current Therapy 2002.* Philadelphia: Saunders; 2002:1103–1111.
6. Burkman RT. Transdermal hormonal contraception: benefits and risks. *Am J Obstet Gynecol.* 2007;197:134–136.
7. Dayal MB, Barnhart KB. Noncontraceptive benefits and therapeutic uses of the oral contraceptive pill. *Semin Reprod Med.* 2001;19:295–303.
8. Dean EL, Grimes DA. Intrauterine devices for adolescents: a systematic review. *Contraception.* 2009;79:418–423.
9. Forste RR, Tanfer K, Tedrow L. Sterilization among currently married men in the United States, 1991. *Fam Plann Perspect.* 1995;(2):100–107.
10. Gemzell-Danielsson K. Mechanism of action of emergency contraception. *Contraception.* 2010;82:404–409.
11. Grimes DA. Intrauterine device and upper genital tract infection. *Lancet.* 2000;356:1013–1019.
12. Grimes DA, Jones LB, Lopez LM, Schultz KF. Oral contraceptives for functional ovarian cysts. *Cochrane Database Syst Rev.* 2014;4. CD006134.
13. Gillium LA, Mamidipudi SK, Johnston SC. Ischemic stroke risk with oral contraceptives. *JAMA.* 2000;284:72–78.
14. Hubacher D. Copper intrauterine device use by nulliparous women: review of side effects. *Contraception.* 2007;75(Suppl 6):8–11.
15. Iyer V, Farquahr C, Jepson R. Oral contraceptive pills for heavy menstrual bleeding. *Cochrane Database Syst Rev.* 1999;2. CD000154.
16. Kaunitz AM, Arias R, McClung M. Bone density recovery after depot medroxyprogesterone acetate injectable contraception use. *Contraception.* 2008;77:67–76.
17. Kerin JK, Munday DN, Ritossa MG, Pesce A, Rosen D. Essure hysteroscopic sterilization: results based on utilizing a new coil catheter delivery system. *J Am Assoc Gynecol Laparosc.* 2004;11:388–393.

18. La Vecchia C, Boccia S. Oral contraceptives, human papillomavirus and cervical cancer. *Eur J Cancer Prev.* 2014;23:110–112.
19. Marchbanks PA, McDonald JA, Wilson HG, et al. Oral contraceptives and the risk of breast cancer. *N Engl J Med.* 2002;346:2025–2032.
20. Mohllajee AP, Curtis KM, Peterson HB. Does insertion and use of an intrauterine device increase the risk of pelvic inflammatory disease among women with sexually transmitted infection? A systematic review. *Contraception.* 2006;73:145–153.
21. Moreno V, Bosch FX, Muñoz N, et al. Effect of oral contraceptives on risk of cervical cancer in women with human papillomavirus infection: the IARC multicentric case-control study. *Lancet.* 2002;359:1085–1092.
22. Ortiz ME, Croxatto HB. Copper T intrauterine device and levonorgestrel intrauterine system: biological bases of their mechanism of action. *Contraception.* 2007;75:S16–S30.
23. Roumen F. Review of the combined contraceptive vaginal ring, NuvaRing. *Ther Clin Risk Manag.* 2008;4:441–451.
24. Schlesselman JJ. Net effect of oral contraceptive use on the risk of cancer in women in the United States. *Obstet Gynecol.* 1995;85:793–801.
25. Schwingl PJ, Guess HA. Safety and effectiveness of vasectomy. *Fertil Steril.* 2000;3:923–936.
26. Schwingl PJ, Ory HW, Visness CW. Estimates of the risk of cardiovascular death attributable to low-dose oral contraceptives in the United States. *Am J Obstet Gynecol.* 1999;180:242–249.
27. Steen R, Shapiro K. Intrauterine contraceptive devices and risk of pelvic inflammatory disease: standard of care in high STI prevalence settings. *Reprod Health Matters.* 2004;12:136–143.
28. Speroff L. Oral contraceptives and breast cancer risk: summary and application of data. *Int J Fertil.* 2000;45(Suppl 2): 113–120.
29. Trussel J. Contraceptive failure in the United States. *Contraception.* 2011;83:397–404.
30. U.S. Department of Health and Human Services. National Center for Health Statistics. Fertility, family planning, and reproductive health of U.S. women: data from the 2002 National Survey of Family Growth. Vital and Health Statistics. *Series 23, no.* 2005;25. Available at www.cdc.gov/nchs/data/series/sr_23/sr23_025.pdf. Accessed October 22, 2015.
31. Vandenbrouke JP, Rosing J, Bloemenkamp KWM, et al. Oral contraceptives and the risk of venous thrombosis. *N Engl J Med.* 2001;334:1527–1535.
32. Westhoff C. Emergency contraception. *N Engl J Med.* 2003;349:1830–1835.
33. Workowski KA, Berman S. Centers for Disease Control and Prevention. STD treatment guidelines. *MMWR Recomm Rep.* 2010;59:1–110.

CHAPTER 15

BENIGN ADNEXAL MASSES

Carrie E. Jung, MD

1. **How are adnexal masses diagnosed, and why do they need to be evaluated?**
   Adnexal masses are generally detected at the time of an abdominal or pelvic examination or by imaging performed for other indications. Ultrasound is used to confirm any palpable pelvic mass. Although most adnexal masses are physiologic or benign neoplasms, a physician must consider an extensive differential diagnosis that includes malignancy. Ovarian cancer is the second most common malignant disease of the female genital tract and the leading cause of death from gynecologic neoplasm in the United States. This high mortality reflects late diagnosis—patients usually do not become symptomatic until the disease is widespread.

2. **What is the differential diagnosis for an adnexal mass?**
   Table 15-1 provides differential diagnoses for benign and malignant adnexal masses.

Table 15-1. Differential Diagnosis of Adnexal Masses

BENIGN	MALIGNANT
Physiologic (Functional) Ovarian Cysts	**Ovarian Malignancies**
Follicular cyst	Epithelial cell
Corpus luteum cyst	Sex cord stromal cell
Theca lutein cyst	Germ cell
Nonfunctional Ovarian Cysts	**Fallopian Tube Cancer**
Endometrioma	
Polycystic ovaries	**Nongynecologic Cancers**
	Gastrointestinal tumors
Benign Ovarian Neoplasms	Lymphoma
Mature cystic teratoma	Other metastases
Fibroma, adenofibroma, cystadenofibroma	
Serous cystadenoma, mucinous cystadenoma	
Brenner tumor	
Fallopian Tube Origin	
Ectopic pregnancy	
Paratubal cyst	
Hydrosalpinx, hematosalpinx	
Tubo-ovarian abscess	
Nonadnexal	
Diverticulitis	
Appendiceal abscess	
Pelvic kidney	
Leiomyomas	

3. **What patient-related characteristics should be considered when evaluating an adnexal mass?**
   A patient's age and menstrual status are the most important characteristics to consider when creating a differential diagnosis. Adnexal masses in women who are menstruating regularly are frequently physiologic (follicular cysts, corpus luteum, theca lutein cysts). Most malignant adnexal masses occur in women older than 45 years of age, with the exception of germ cell and sex cord stromal tumors, which occur in younger women at the same frequency as in postmenopausal women.

Other factors to consider are the patient's symptoms (e.g., weight loss, abdominal distention, and pulmonary, gastrointestinal, or genitourinary complaints are more likely associated with malignancy), parity (nulliparity is associated with an increased risk for ovarian malignancy), and family history of gynecologic or breast cancers.

4. **What characteristics help differentiate between benign and malignant adnexal masses?**
Table 15-2 summarizes the basic differences between benign and malignant masses. The following are additional points to consider:
- Very large masses tend to be of borderline (low-grade) malignant potential.
- Mucinous tumors are capable of reaching very large sizes (up to 40 pounds!).
- Malignant lesions are more likely to have areas of necrosis and hemorrhage compared with benign masses. Hemorrhagic corpus luteum cysts and endometriomas are exceptions to this rule.
- The presence of ascites usually indicates a malignant process.

Table 15-2. Basic Differences Between Benign and Malignant Masses

CHARACTERISTIC	BENIGN	MALIGNANT
Size	Usually <10 cm	Usually >10 cm
Number	Unilocular ("simple cyst")	Multilocular ("complex cyst")
Borders	Smooth, regular, well-defined	Irregular borders with nodularity, excrescences, studding, papillary projections
Laterality	Unilateral	Bilateral
Mobility	Mobile	Fixed or adherent to other structures
Growth rate	Slowly enlarging	Rapidly enlarging

5. **How do follicular cysts form, and what physical characteristics do they have?**
Follicular cysts result from failed rupture of a dominant follicle or failed atresia of secondary follicles. They are simple cysts that average approximately 2 cm in size, although they can vary from a few millimeters to 10 cm. They are thin walled and filled with clear, straw-colored fluid. If rupture occurs, they can cause pain and intraperitoneal hemorrhage (albeit rarely).

6. **How should benign-appearing cysts be managed?**
In menstruating women, cysts that have a benign appearance on ultrasound examination and are smaller than 10 cm can be observed. Almost all physiologic cysts resolve spontaneously. Suppression with oral contraceptives to prevent additional cysts may be helpful.

7. **What is polycystic ovarian syndrome (PCOS), and what characteristics do patients with this syndrome possess?**
The definition of PCOS is somewhat controversial. The National Institutes of Health (NIH) uses the working definition of "ovulatory dysfunction with evidence of hyperandrogenism, clinically or by laboratory means, without other causes of hyperandrogenism identified."
Ovulatory dysfunction manifests clinically either as abnormal menstrual cycles (usually oligomenorrhea or amenorrhea) or, with more subtlety, as infertility. Obesity and insulin resistance can also occur, although they are not required for diagnosis. See Chapter 26 for additional information.

8. **How are the follicular cysts associated with PCOS different from other follicular cysts?**
The follicular cysts in PCOS are usually bilateral and more numerous, but smaller, than other physiologic follicular cysts (<12 mm in diameter). When a state of anovulation persists for a prolonged period of time numerous small follicles form, producing the classic "beads on a string" or "pearl necklace" appearance on ultrasound examination. However, multiple cysts visible on ultrasound scans are not required for the diagnosis of PCOS, nor can ultrasound findings alone be used for diagnosis.

9. **What are endometriomas?**
   Endometriomas (also known as "chocolate cysts" because of the color of the cyst fluid) are endometrial implants on the ovary. If symptomatic, they can cause chronic pelvic pain, dysmenorrhea, dyspareunia, or infertility. See Chapter 4 for additional information.

10. **How are endometriomas managed?**
    Because endometriomas often appear as complex adnexal masses on ultrasound examination, surgical management is usually chosen to rule out malignancy. At the time of surgical intervention, the endometrioma should be resected, along with any implants suggestive of endometriosis. If residual disease is suspected, medical management with leuprolide (a gonadotropin-releasing hormone agonist), continuous oral contraceptives, or depot medroxyprogesterone acetate can be done postoperatively. See Chapter 4 for additional information on the treatment of endometriosis.

11. **Why do theca lutein cysts develop, and how are they managed?**
    Theca lutein cysts can develop with prolonged or excessive ovarian stimulation by either exogenous or endogenous gonadotropins. They are seen in association with molar pregnancies, choriocarcinomas, and multiple gestations, as well as with the use of ovulation induction agents. Gonadotropins cause luteinization of mature, immature, and atretic follicles, thus resulting in bilateral ovarian enlargement. Theca lutein cysts resolve spontaneously and are usually managed expectantly.

12. **What are benign cystic teratomas?**
    Benign cystic teratomas (also known as "dermoid cysts") are ovarian neoplasms that contain mature tissue of ectodermal, mesodermal, or endodermal origin. The most common elements are ectodermal derivatives such as skin, hair follicles, teeth, bone, and sebaceous or sweat glands. Rarely, they can even have functional thyroid tissue and lead to hyperthyroidism ("struma ovarii").

13. **What is the most frequent complication associated with benign cystic teratomas?**
    Ovarian torsion is the most common complication of dermoid cysts and causes severe, acute abdominal pain. If the cyst ruptures, chemical peritonitis can result from spillage of cholesterol-laden debris and cyst fluid. Although they can reach very large dimensions, benign cystic teratomas rarely rupture.

14. **How are patients with ovarian torsion managed?**
    Ovarian torsion is a *gynecologic emergency* and requires prompt surgical management. Most cases of torsion can be managed with laparoscopy. In young women for whom fertility and preservation of ovarian function are important issues, conservative treatment with untwisting of the adnexa and ovarian cystectomy is preferred. However, this mode of surgical management requires prompt diagnosis and intervention to avoid strangulation and necrosis of twisted tissue. If strangulation and necrosis do occur, adnexectomy should be performed. Ovarian torsion occurs most often in children and young women.

15. **What laboratory tests are useful when evaluating an adnexal mass?**
    - Complete blood count with differential to rule out infection
    - β-Human chorionic gonadotropin (β-hCG) to rule out pregnancy or ectopic pregnancy
    - Gonorrhea and Chlamydia testing should be performed when tubo-ovarian abscess or pelvic inflammatory disease is suspected.
    - Tumor markers
      - *CA-125* (cancer antigen 125) is commonly elevated in epithelial ovarian cancer.
      - *HE-4* (human epididymis protein 4) is elevated in epithelial ovarian cancer and is used in combination with CA-125.
      - α-*Fetoprotein* is elevated in germ cell tumors (endodermal sinus tumors, embryonal cell cancer, mixed germ cell malignant tumors).
      - β-*hCG* is unusually elevated in molar pregnancy and choriocarcinoma.
      - *Lactate dehydrogenase* is elevated with dysgerminomas.

16. **What is CA-125, and in which patients should it be tested?**
    CA-125 levels are most useful in evaluating postmenopausal women with adnexal masses. The CA-125 antigen is expressed by epithelial ovarian tumors and is markedly elevated with epithelial ovarian malignant diseases. However, it can also be elevated with a variety of other conditions such as endometriosis, uterine leiomyomas, pregnancy, pelvic infections, and menstruation. Because these conditions are more likely to occur in menstruating women, CA-125 levels are less specific for ovarian cancer in the premenopausal age group.

17. What is the ROMA score?

The ROMA (Risk of Ovarian Malignancy Algorithm) score is calculated using a combination of a patient's CA-125 and HE-4 results. It is used to assess risk for epithelial ovarian cancer and has a higher sensitivity than either serum marker used alone. Different cutoffs are used, based on a patient's menopausal status. Although the ROMA score is most useful in postmenopausal women, it has a high negative predictive value (≈97%) for epithelial ovarian cancer and for tumors of low malignant potential in both premenopausal and postmenopausal women.

18. At what size do all adnexal masses warrant surgical exploration?

Because functional cysts rarely exceed 7 to 8 cm, any patient with an adnexal mass larger than 10 cm requires surgical exploration. In addition size, ultrasound characteristics that help differentiate between benign and malignant masses should also be considered when determining whether surgical intervention is indicated.

KEY POINTS: BENIGN ADNEXAL MASSES

1. When evaluating adnexal masses it is important to consider age, menstrual status, associated symptoms, and family history.
2. The most common neoplasm in young women is a benign teratoma.
3. In menstruating women, cysts smaller than 10 cm with benign features on ultrasound examination can be observed.
4. Ovarian torsion is a gynecologic emergency and requires prompt surgical management.

BIBLIOGRAPHY

1. American College of Obstetricians and Gynecologists. Medical management of endometriosis. ACOG practice bulletin no. 11. Washington, DC: American College of Obstetricians and Gynecologists; 1995.
2. DiSaia P, Creasman W. *Clinical Gynecologic Oncology*. 5th ed. St. Louis: Mosby; 1997:253–281.
3. Goldstein S. Postmenopausal adnexal cysts: how clinical management has evolved. *Am J Obstet Gynecol.* 1996;175:1498–1502.
4. Lewis V. Polycystic ovary syndrome: a diagnostic challenge. *Obstet Gynecol Clin North Am.* 2001;28:1–20.
5. Mishell DR, Stenchever MA, Droegemueller W, Herbst AL. *Comprehensive Gynecology*. 8th ed. St. Louis: Mosby; 1997:905–912.
6. Pfeifer S, Gosman G. Evaluation of adnexal masses in adolescents. *Pediatr Clin North Am.* 1999;46:573–592.
7. Speroff L, Glass RH, Kase NG. *Clinical Gynecologic Endocrinology and Infertility*. 6th ed. Baltimore: Lippincott Williams & Wilkins; 1999:493–511.
8. Modesitt S. Risk of malignancy in unilocular ovarian cystic tumors less than 10 centimeters in diameter. *Obstet Gynecol.* 2003;102:594–599.
9. American College of Obstetricians and Gynecologists. *Management of adnexal masses. ACOG practice bulletin no. 83*. Washington, DC: American College of Obstetricians and Gynecologists; 2007.
10. Moore RG, Miller MC, Disilvestro P, et al. Evaluation of the diagnostic accuracy of the risk of ovarian malignancy algorithm in women with a pelvic mass. *Obstet Gynecol.* 2011;118:280–288.
11. Lobo RA. Endometriosis. In: Lentz GM, Lobo RA, Gershenson DM, Katz VL, eds. *Comprehensive Gynecology*. 6th ed. Philadelphia: Mosby; 2013:433–452.

CHAPTER 16

ACUTE AND CHRONIC PELVIC PAIN

Judy H. Chen, MD

1. **What are the most common causes of acute pain related to the reproductive organs?**
   - **Mittelschmerz:** A dull pressure or aching sensation occurs in the middle of the menstrual cycle in either the right or left lower quadrant. It is secondary to ovulation, distention of the ovarian capsule, or mild bleeding associated with the process of ovulation.
   - **Functional ovarian cysts:** Cysts may be follicular or luteal in origin. Symptoms include an aching sensation in the right or left lower quadrant, and an enlarged, cystic ovary is seen on ultrasound examination. The clinical course is variable—spontaneous resolution, torsion with pain, rupture with pain, and rupture with hemorrhage are all possible.
   - **Intrauterine pregnancy:** This can cause abdominal pain through stretching of the visceral peritoneum, uterine contractions, stretching of the ovarian capsule from the corpus luteum, rupture of the corpus luteum, and threatened miscarriage.
   - **Ectopic pregnancy** (Fig. 16-1): This can cause pain before and after rupture secondary to stretching of the fallopian tube or hemoperitoneum. For more information on ectopic pregnancy, see Chapter 12.
   - **Pelvic infections:** Common causes are gonorrhea, *Chlamydia*, and anaerobic gram-negative species.
   - **Ovarian torsion** (Fig. 16-2): This may involve a normal or cystic ovary, tube, or uterine mass. Symptoms may be constant or intermittent and include nausea, vomiting, diaphoresis, and severe pelvic pain. For more information on ovarian torsion, see Chapter 15.
   - **Dysmenorrhea:** Lower abdominal or pelvic pain is associated with the immediate premenstrual and menstrual phase.

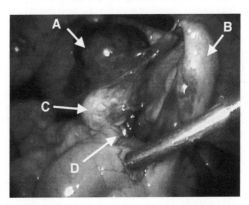

Figure 16-1. Laparoscopic view of an ectopic pregnancy *(A)* in the distal ampulla. Also evident are the proximal portion of the tube *(B)*, an ovary *(C)*, and bowel adhered to the ovary *(D)*.

2. **How are the individual pelvic organs innervated?**
   The pelvic organs receive their innervation from the autonomic nervous system, which comprises both sympathetic and parasympathetic fibers. Most afferent stimuli are transmitted by sympathetic nerves through cell bodies that lie in the thoracolumbar distribution. Parasympathetic nerve fibers are also involved in the transition of painful stimuli. Organs that are müllerian in embryonic origin—the uterus, fallopian tubes, and upper vagina—transmit impulses through sympathetic fibers into the spinal cord

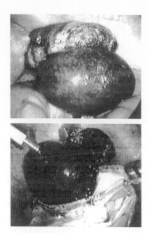

Figure 16-2. Ovarian torsion. Note the large, swollen ovary with a bluish hue resulting from venous obstruction.

at the level of T10 to T12 and L1. Impulses from the uterus travel through the uterosacral ligaments to the uterine inferior plexus. From the uterus, they join other pelvic afferents to form the hypogastric plexus at the level of the rectum and vagina. Impulses from the upper vagina, cervix, and lower uterine segment travel through the parasympathetic system to the sacral roots S2 to S4.

The ovaries and distal fallopian tubes derive their nerve supply independently and enter the spinal cord at T9 and T10. Stimulation from the kidneys, ureters, bowel, and skin dermatomes terminate on T11 and T12. The bladder, rectum, perineum, and anus are derived from the urogenital sinus and are innervated by both sympathetic and parasympathetic systems. Fibers from the perineum and anus combine to form branches of the pudendal nerve, eventually terminating in sacral roots S2 and S4.

3. **What is the major difference between acute pelvic pain and chronic pelvic pain (CPP)?**
   Acute pain is of short duration, typically of less than 6 months, typically of less than 6 months, and is generally associated with tissue damage appropriate to the degree of symptoms. CPP often has an indefinite beginning. It is occasionally derived from unresolved acute pain, but is more frequently neuropathic.

4. **What is the definition of CPP?**
   CPP is nonspecific pelvic pain of more than 6 months' duration that may or may not be relieved by analgesics (narcotics or nonsteroidal antiinflammatory drugs [NSAIDs]).

5. **How common is CPP?**
   CPP is the most common indication for referral to women's health services and comprises approximately 20% of all outpatient appointments. Approximately 1 billion dollars are spent annually on outpatient management alone. Ten percent to 35% of laparoscopies and 12% of hysterectomies are estimated to be performed for this indication.

6. **What is the differential diagnosis of CPP?**
   Table 16-1 provides differential diagnoses for CPP.

7. **What are the most common causes of chronic pain related to the reproductive organs?**
   - **Endometriosis** is the presence of endometrial glands and stroma at sites other than the uterine cavity. Endometriotic implants can cause bleeding and the formation of pelvic adhesions. Approximately 25% to 40% of patients with CPP will have evidence of endometriosis at the time of laparoscopy. Pain associated with endometriosis is characteristically present several days before menstruation and ends soon after onset. However, it may evolve to remain present throughout the menstrual cycle. For more information on endometriosis, see Chapter 4.
   - **Adenomyosis** is the presence of endometrial glands within the myometrium. Associated pain typically begins a week before menses and continues until the last day of the cycle. The uterus is usually enlarged. Magnetic resonance imaging may be helpful to differentiate adenomyomas (leiomyomas with endometrial glands) from normal leiomyomas. For more information on adenomyosis, see Chapter 4.

Table 16-1. Causes of Chronic Pelvic Pain

GYNECOLOGIC	UROLOGIC	GASTROINTESTINAL	MUSCULOSKELETAL
PID	IC/BPS	Irritable bowel syndrome	Psoas muscle pain
Endometriosis	Bladder spasms	IBD	Stress fracture of pelvis
Adenomyosis	Nephrolithiasis	Constipation	Abdominal wall pain
Pelvic adhesions	Recurrent UTIs	Diverticulosis or diverticulitis	Lower back pain
Adnexal neoplasms	Perinephric	Malabsorption syndromes	Malignant diseases
Uterine neoplasms	abscesses	Malignant diseases	
Vulvar pain disorders	Malignant		
Chronic vaginitis	diseases		
Primary dysmenorrhea			
Pelvic congestion			
syndrome			
Malignant diseases			

IBD, Inflammatory bowel disease; *IC/BPS*, interstitial cystitis/bladder pain syndrome; *PID*, pelvic inflammatory disease; *UTI*, urinary tract infection.

- **Pelvic adhesions** (Fig. 16-3): These adhesions occur after trauma to the visceral or parietal peritoneum from surgical intervention, endometriosis, or infection. Surgical procedures account for approximately 70% of all adhesions. Associated pain is presumed to arise from either stretching of visceral nociceptors or abnormal regeneration of injured nerve endings.
- **Uterine neoplasms:** Both benign and malignant tumors can cause pain secondary to torsion, necrosis, stretching of the visceral peritoneum of the uterus, or compression of surrounding intraabdominal structures. Abnormal or heavy vaginal bleeding is often present. For more information on leiomyomas, see Chapter 5. For more information on uterine cancer, see Chapter 30.
- **Adnexal neoplasms** can cause pain through hemorrhage, necrosis, torsion, rupture, or large size. Associated symptoms may include abdominal distention, nausea, vomiting, anorexia, or unilateral lower extremity edema. For more information on adnexal masses, see Chapters 15 and 31

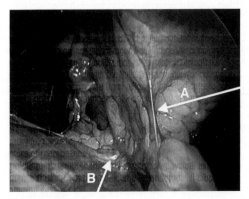

Figure 16-3. Dense adhesions between the bowel and anterior abdominal wall *(A)* and between the anterior uterus and anterior abdominal wall *(B)*.

8. What are the causes of vaginal pain?
   - Sexually transmitted infections
   - Vaginitis
   - Vulvodynia

   Although rare, endometriosis can manifest within the cervical ectropion, vaginal mucosa, or vestibule.

9. Which diseases of the urinary tract cause pelvic pain?
   - **Urinary tract infection (UTI), cystitis, and pyelonephritis** may manifest with lower abdominal pain, flank pain, dysuria, hematuria, and urinary frequency. Urinalysis often demonstrates leukocyte esterase and white blood cells on microscopy; nitrites are highly specific for UTI but are not sensitive (e.g., a positive result highly suggests UTI, but a negative result does not rule it out). Treatment includes appropriate antibiotic coverage for common uropathogens (almost always *Escherichia coli,* but occasionally other organisms). In the case of pyelonephritis, patients may also be febrile and have costovertebral angle tenderness on exam.
   - **Ureteral obstruction** can occur secondary to a stone, tumor, or adhesions. It can cause severe pain beginning in the flank and radiating into the groin and occasionally to the ipsilateral labia. While asymptomatic in the beginning, associated symptoms often include tachycardia, diaphoresis, nausea, vomiting, urinary frequency, and hematuria. Flank tenderness may be present on physical examination.
   - **Perinephric abscess** is usually unilateral. Symptoms include flank tenderness and recurrent fevers. Bacterial agents range from staphylococci to *E. coli.*
   - **Interstitial cystitis/bladder pain syndrome (IC/BPS):** Symptoms of frequency, urgency, and dysuria last for more than 6 weeks without evidence of infection or another identifiable cause.

10. What are the most common gastrointestinal causes of pelvic and lower abdominal pain?
    - **Irritable bowel syndrome** is an abdominal pain syndrome associated with altered bowel habits (e.g., diarrhea, constipation, bloating), possibly secondary to changes in gastrointestinal motility. Other potential causative factors include abnormal inflammatory responses and bacterial flora.
    - **Inflammatory bowel disease (IBD)** encompasses a range of diagnoses from Crohn disease to ulcerative colitis. Common presenting symptoms include lower abdominal pain, diarrhea, constipation, hematochezia, melena, and dyschezia.
    - **Diverticulitis** is most commonly seen in perimenopausal or postmenopausal women. Pain may be acute or severe with a history of chronic flares, and it may manifest with peritonitis similar to ovarian torsion or pelvic inflammatory disease.
    - **Appendicitis** occurs most frequently between the ages of 10 and 19 years. Pain is secondary to luminal distention and necrosis, and symptoms vary depending on the anatomic location of the appendix and the status of the infection.
    - **Bowel obstruction** has many possible causes. In developed nations, most cases are secondary to postoperative adhesions. Other causes include neoplasms, hernias, foreign bodies, gallstones, parasites, enteritis, or trauma. Presenting symptoms include abdominal pain and distention, vomiting, constipation, and lack of flatus.
    - **Hernias** occur when a fascial defect in the abdominal wall allows intraabdominal contents to pass through it. The most common forms of hernia are direct and indirect inguinal hernias, femoral hernias, incisional hernias, and umbilical hernias. Pain can occur if the intraperitoneal contents become trapped and their vascular supply is compromised.

11. How should CPP be evaluated?
    Evaluation should begin with a thorough history and detailed review of systems, followed by a physical examination. Positive findings can then direct subsequent steps. Helpful diagnostic tools include a complete blood count, metabolic panels, urine analysis, stool studies, and pelvic ultrasound scan or other imaging modalities.

12. How can CPP be treated?
    Treatment depends on the suspected cause. Greatest success rates are seen with a multidisciplinary approach incorporating the skills of gynecologists, physical therapists, and psychiatrists. The following list of options is not exhaustive:
    - Conservative methods: lifestyle modifications, counseling or support, cognitive-behavioral therapy (CBT)
    - Pelvic floor physical therapy
    - Analgesics:
      - Antiinflammatory: acetaminophen, NSAIDS
      - Opioids (not recommended for long-term management because of tolerance development)
      - Topical: lidocaine patch, capsaicin
    - Neuromodulating agents: gabapentin, pregabalin
    - Anxiolytics: diazepam, clonazepam

- Antidepressants: tricyclic antidepressants, monoamine oxidase inhibitors, serotonin-norepinephrine reuptake inhibitors
- Trigger point injections
- Surgical interventions: excisional procedures versus neuroablation
- Alternative therapies: acupuncture, meditation, herbal therapy

13. **What psychiatric considerations should be made for patients with CPP?**
Chronic pain often involves changes in the modulation of a stimulus ("peripheral sensitization," primarily through inflammatory pathways) or the patient's perception of a stimulus ("central sensitization," through sustained neurotransmitter response in the central nervous system). Mood and anxiety often influence pain intensity through central sensitization, and it is therefore important to address emotional contributions to chronic pain

KEY POINTS: ACUTE AND CHRONIC PELVIC PAIN

1. Not all pelvic pain is gynecologic in origin.
2. When evaluating pelvic pain, pregnancy should always be excluded.
3. CPP is defined as nonspecific pelvic pain of more than 6 months' duration. It is the most common indication for referral to women's health services, and the differential diagnosis is extensive.
4. Pain from pelvic organs may be referred to the dermatomes at the spinal cord level from which they are innervated.

BIBLIOGRAPHY

1. Baranowski AP. Chronic pelvic pain. *Best Pract Res Clin Gastroenterol.* 2009;23:593–610.
2. Buckius MT, McGrath B, Monk J, Grim R, Bell T, Ahuja V. Changing epidemiology of acute appendicitis in the United States: study period 1993-2008. *J Surg Res.* 2012;175:185–190.
3. Goodwin TM, Montoro MN, Muderspach L, Paulson R, Roy S. *Management of Common Problems in Obstetrics and Gynecology.* 5th ed. Oxford: Wiley-Blackwell; 2010:256.
4. Latthe P, Latthe M, Say L, Gulmezoglu M, Khan KS. WHO systematic review of prevalence of chronic pelvic pain: a neglected reproductive health morbidity. *BMC Public Health.* 2006;6:177.
5. Pezzone MA, Liang R, Fraser MO. A model of neural cross-talk and irritation in the pelvis: implications for the overlap of chronic pelvic pain disorders. *Gastroenterology.* 2005;128:1953–1964.
6. Vercellini P, Barbara G, Abbiati A, Somigliana E, Vigano P, Fedele L. Repetitive surgery for recurrent symptomatic endometriosis: what to do? *Eur J Obstet Gynecol Reprod Biol.* 2009;146:15–20.

CHAPTER 17

URINARY INCONTINENCE

Erin Mellano, MD, and Cecilia K. Wieslander, MD

1. **What is urinary incontinence (UI)?**

   UI is the involuntary loss of urine. Prevalence increases with age, and bothersome UI is estimated to affect between 20% and 40% of women older than 50 years of age. UI-related costs to society are estimated at between $20 and 30 billion a year.

2. **What are the types of UI?**
   - **Stress UI (SUI):** involuntary loss of urine with effort, exertion, sneezing, or coughing
   - **Urgency UI (UUI):** involuntary loss of urine associated with urgency
   - **Mixed UI:** involuntary loss of urine associated with urgency and also with effort or physical exertion or on sneezing or coughing
   - **UI associated with chronic urinary retention** (previously called overflow incontinence): involuntary loss of urine after overdistention of the bladder
   - **Nocturnal enuresis:** involuntary urinary loss of urine that occurs during sleep
   - **Continuous loss of urine:** continuous, involuntary loss of urine without preceding sensation or Valsalva event

3. **What is SUI?**

   SUI is the loss of urine resulting from increased intraabdominal pressure. It affects 10% to 20% of women. Risk factors include pregnancy and vaginal delivery, any chronic increase in intraabdominal pressure (obesity, chronic cough, or chronic constipation), and genetically inherited factors.

   The causes of SUI are generally multifactorial, but to some degree they are attributable to urethral hypermobility, impaired urethral sphincteric function, or a combination of the two. Urethral hypermobility is the most common cause of SUI. Normally, the urethra and bladder are supported by the pelvic floor musculature, and during episodes of increased intraabdominal pressure, the pelvic floor muscles contract and prevent loss of urine. In women with urethral hypermobility, descent of the proximal urethra and bladder neck occurs such that these structures are no longer compressed against the vagina during increased intraabdominal pressure, and leakage of urine results.

   Impaired urethral sphincteric function, often referred to as intrinsic sphincter deficiency (ISD), results from a weakness of the urethra sphincter muscle. Isolated ISD is most notable in women with nonmobile urethras who leak urine readily with minimal exertion. Common causes include advanced age, earlier urethral surgical procedures, and radiation treatment (Table 17-1).

4. **What is UUI?**

   UUI is the loss of urine resulting from detrusor overactivity (DO) leading to bladder contraction and loss of urine. This condition is often associated with overactive bladder (OAB) syndrome—urinary urgency, usually accompanied by frequency and nocturia, with or without UUI, in the absence of infection or other obvious disorder. The etiology of DO is generally divided into idiopathic and neurogenic, and most cases have no known cause (Table 17-1).

5. **What is UI associated with chronic urinary retention?**

   Loss of urine after overdistention of the bladder. This may result from weakening of the detrusor muscle from neuropathy (secondary to diabetes or neurologic disease), from obstruction caused by severe pelvic organ prolapse, or from postsurgical obstruction.

6. **What is continuous UI?**

   Continuous loss of urine, such as that caused by genitourinary fistulae. These fistulae may be congenital or secondary to obstetric trauma, pelvic surgery, or radiation.

7. **What are the physical examination findings associated with UI?**

   The primary purpose of the physical examination is to exclude other confounding or contributing factors to UI. These factors may include distorted anatomy, urethral diverticula, or genitourinary fistula.

Some women confuse vaginal discharge with urine. In SUI, it is not uncommon to see some degree of pelvic organ relaxation. Anterior vaginal wall prolapse, or a cystocele, is often associated with SUI; however, it does not cause UI. A cotton swab urethral mobility test (Q-tip test), defined as a 30-degree or greater movement of the urethra from the horizontal when the patient is supine and straining, may be performed. A neurologic examination is essential.

8. **What laboratory tests are helpful in evaluating UI?**
   All patients who complain of UI should have a **postvoid residual (PVR)** determination. This can be done, after a patient voids, by either an ultrasound scan of the bladder or catheterization. A patient with a PVR of 100 to 200 mL or greater may have an underlying neurologic disorder. This test is important because an elevated PVR is a relative contraindication to surgical treatment of SUI and to anticholinergic medications for OAB; either of these treatments can worsen the preexisting retention.

   Because an underlying urinary tract infection may contribute to voiding dysfunction, urinalysis and urine culture should be performed on all patients presenting for UI. Additional laboratory testing is not necessary unless one suspects a medical cause, such as diabetes or other systemic disorders.

9. **Which tests are *most* helpful in differentiating between SUI and UUI?**
   A simple **cystometrogram** involves placing a small catheter in the bladder and filling the bladder with fluid. This test measures the bladder capacity and bladder storage pressure, and it assesses for DO and urethral incontinence with a full bladder. **Normal bladder capacity is between 300 and 500 mL.** Patients with UUI secondary to DO often have reduced capacity and demonstrate involuntary bladder contractions (pressure increases above baseline). SUI can be demonstrated by loss of urine once the catheter is removed and the patient coughs or strains with a full bladder.

10. **Which tests are *less* helpful in differentiating between SUI and UUI?**
    The **Q-tip test** assesses urethral mobility by placing a sterile cotton swab through the urethra to the bladder neck to evaluate the movement of the urethra. A positive test result, indicating increased urethral mobility, is found when the cotton swab changes angle by more than 30 degrees with a Valsalva maneuver. Although this test may be helpful in assessing for urethral hypermobility, not all patients with SUI have urethral hypermobility—and women without UI may have a positive test result.

11. **What is multichannel urodynamics, and what are the indications for this test?**
    Multichannel urodynamics allows for the measurement of bladder filling pressures, capacity, compliance, DO, and voiding pressure. This test is indicated in complicated cases such as in women with recurrent UI after an earlier surgical procedure, painful UI, hematuria, recurrent urinary tract infections, a history of earlier or current pelvic irradiation, a history of radical pelvic surgical procedures, insensible urine loss, or suspected neurologic bladder dysfunction.

12. **Which nonsurgical treatments are available for SUI?**
    No good pharmacologic treatments are available for SUI. Pelvic floor muscle exercise (Kegel exercise) with or without biofeedback or electrical stimulation is an effective method for improving SUI. Behavioral modification (fluid intake reduction, scheduled voids, changing medications) can be helpful. Intravaginal incontinence dish pessary devices may help some women (Fig. 17-1). Vaginal estrogen may have some limited benefit in postmenopausal women, and α-adrenergic agonists may be useful for mild SUI caused by ISD.

13. **Which nonsurgical treatments are available for UUI?**
    Behavioral modifications and pelvic floor muscle exercises can be very effective in improving UUI symptoms. These modifications involve the following: avoidance of caffeine, alcohol, diuretics, citrus, and spicy foods (a "bladder diet"); decrease in fluid intake; management of medical conditions; change of medications; weight loss; and urge suppression techniques.

    Bladder contractions are caused by stimulation of the parasympathetic nervous system, mainly accomplished through the release of acetylcholine. In patients with DO, anticholinergic medications are often successful in controlling UI. These medications include oxybutynin, tolterodine, darifenacin, trospium chloride, fesoterodine, and imipramine. Some of the most common bothersome side effects of these medications include dry eyes, dry mouth, and constipation. Newer agents, such as mirabegron (a β_3 agonist that causes detrusor relaxation), have been developed to bypass some of the poorly

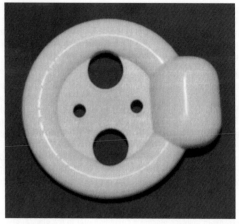

Figure 17-1. Incontinence ring pessary. *(From Lentz GM, Lobo RA, Gershenson DM, et al, eds.* Comprehensive Gynecology. *6th ed. Philadelphia: Mosby; 2012:475-502.)*

tolerated anticholinergic side effects. Imipramine is also advantageous in treating mixed UI because of its combined α-adrenergic and anticholinergic properties.

For women who do not tolerate oral pharmacotherapy, intradetrusor injections of botulinum toxin A can be offered. Intravesical botulinum toxin A administered by a physician is approved by the Food and Drug Administration and lasts for 6 to 9 months. This treatment eliminates the need for daily medication and avoids anticholinergic side effects. The primary risks include a 3% to 10% risk of urinary retention, which requires clean-intermittent catheterization and raises the risk of urinary tract infection.

Transcutaneous nerve stimulation, such as percutaneous posterior tibial nerve stimulation, has been shown to improve UUI symptoms without any significant side effects.

14. **Which surgical options exist for SUI?**
    Surgical management of SUI can be divided into (1) procedures to restore anatomic support to the proximal urethra and urethrovesical junction and (2) procedures designed to compensate for a poorly functioning urethral sphincter. Despite controversy surrounding transvaginal mesh, a midurethral mesh sling is still considered the "gold standard" for SUI. When artificial mesh is not desirable, slings made from autologous fascia can be performed. Autologous fascial slings can be placed at the bladder neck ("pubovaginal slings") or at the midurethra.

    Techniques to resuspend the urethrovesical angle vary based on surgical approach. For abdominal approaches, options include the Burch colposuspension (Fig. 17-2) and the Marshall-Marchetti-Krantz procedure. The Burch colposuspension is performed either laparoscopically or through an open incision, and it uses suture to attach the periurethral vaginal tissue to the Cooper ligament. Older transvaginal suspension procedures such as the Pereyra, Raz, and Stamey procedures are rarely used.

    Midurethral slings are also first-line options in patients with ISD. Another treatment is transurethral or periurethral injection of a bulking agent (e.g., collagen, calcium hydroxylapatite, pyrolytic carbon-coated beads, polytetrafluoroethylene, and polydimethylsiloxane). Transurethral injections are not permanent, however, and they often need to be repeated.

15. **What are the success rates of surgical treatment?**
    The midurethral mesh sling is the most effective surgical procedure for SUI, with a subjective cure rate of 78% to 88%. Long-term follow-up studies show that retropubic midurethral slings have a higher efficacy rate than transobturator slings or Burch colposuspensions. Retropubic midurethral slings have an efficacy comparable to that of pubovaginal slings, but patients with pubovaginal slings have an increased incidence of lower urinary tract symptoms (OAB syndrome and UUI).

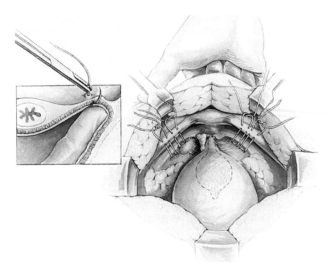

Figure 17-2. Burch colposuspension. *(From Walters MD, Karram MM, eds.* Urogynecology and Reconstructive Pelvic Surgery. *4th ed. Philadelphia: Saunders; 2015:253-261.)*

Long-term follow-up after Burch procedures show a success rates of 55% to 70%. However, the lack of standardized definitions of success used across different studies makes it difficult to make direct comparisons in meta-analyses.

The success rate of transurethral or periurethral bulking depends on the material used and on the underlying severity of UI.

16. Which surgical options exist for UUI resulting from DO?
Implantable sacral root neuromodulation is an effective treatment for refractory UUI. It involves stimulation of the pelvic plexus and pudendal nerves that innervate the bladder, pelvic floor muscles, and rectum, but the exact mechanism of action is uncertain.

Table 17-1. Differential Diagnosis and Treatment of Urinary Incontinence

CRITERIA	URGENCY URINARY INCONTINENCE	STRESS URINARY INCONTINENCE	INTRINSIC SPHINCTER DEFICIENCY
Basic pathologic feature	Irritable detrusor muscle	Loss of support to UVJ	Weakness of urethral sphincter
Symptoms	Urge incontinence, frequency, urgency, nocturia	Loss of urine with cough, laugh, sneeze, or activity	Severe loss of urine with cough, laugh, sneeze, or activity
Physical examination	Can be normal	Positive cough stress test Pelvic organ relaxation may be seen	Positive cough stress test
Q-tip test	Can be normal	Hypermobility of UVJ	Variable; UVJ can be hypermobile or fixed
Findings on cystometrogram	Involuntary detrusor contractions	Leak point pressure >60 cm of water	Leak point pressure <60 cm of water

Table 17-1. Differential Diagnosis and Treatment of Urinary Incontinence *(Continued)*

CRITERIA	URGENCY URINARY INCONTINENCE	STRESS URINARY INCONTINENCE	INTRINSIC SPHINCTER DEFICIENCY
Nonsurgical treatment	Behavioral changes: Pelvic floor muscle exercises Urge suppression techniques Oral pharmacotherapy Intravesical injection of botulinum toxin A Percutaneous tibial nerve stimulation	Behavioral changes Pelvic floor muscle exercise Intravaginal pessary device	Behavioral changes Pelvic floor muscle exercise Intravaginal pessary device
Surgical treatment	Sacral root neuromodulation	Slings: Retropubic midurethral mesh Transobturator mesh Pubovaginal fascial Midurethral fascial Transabdominal colposuspension (Burch colposuspension) Transvaginal needle suspension (Pereyra, Raz, Stamey)	Slings: Retropubic midurethral mesh Transobturator mesh Pubovaginal fascial Midurethral fascial Urethral bulking agents

UVJ, Urethrovesical junction.

KEY POINTS: URINARY INCONTINENCE

1. The two most common causes of UI are stress and DO.
2. SUI can result from urethral hypermobility or ISD of the urethra.
3. To guide treatment, it is vital to differentiate SUI from UUI.
4. Diagnostic tests for UI include the cough stress test, the cystometrogram, postvoid residual assessment, and multichannel urodynamics.
5. Treatment for SUI includes pelvic floor muscle exercises, medications to increase sphincter tone, pessaries, and surgical intervention.
6. UUI can be treated with behavioral modification, pelvic floor muscle exercises, medications, and nerve stimulation.

BIBLIOGRAPHY

1. American Urogynecologic Society and American College of Obstetricians and Gynecologists. Committee opinion: evaluation of uncomplicated stress urinary incontinence in women before surgical treatment. *Female Pelvic Med Reconstr Surg.* 2014;20:248–251.
2. Haylen BT, de Ridder D, Freeman RM, et al. An International Urogynecological Association (IUGA)/International Continence Society (ICS) joint report on the terminology for female pelvic floor dysfunction. *Neurourol Urodyn.* 2010;29:4–20.
3. Moore CK, Rackley RR. Surgical management of detrusor compliance abnormalities. In: Walters MD, Karram MM, eds. *Urogynecology and Reconstructive Pelvic Surgery.* 4th ed. Philadelphia: Saunders; 2015:555–565.
4. Nilsson CG, Palva K, Aarnio R, et al. Seventeen years' follow-up of the tension-free vaginal tape procedure for female stress urinary incontinence. *Int Urogynecol J.* 2013;24:1265–1269.
5. Norton P, Brubaker L. Urinary incontinence in women. *Lancet.* 2006;367:57–67.
6. Novara G, Artibani W, Barber MD, et al. Updated systematic review and meta-analysis of the comparative data on colposuspensions, pubovaginal slings, and midurethral tables in the surgical treatment of female stress urinary incontinence. *Eur Urol.* 2010;58:218–238.
7. Walters MD, Karram MM. Synthetic midurethral slings for stress urinary incontinence. In: Walters MD, Karram MM, eds. *Urogynecology and Reconstructive Pelvic Surgery.* 4th ed. Philadelphia: Saunders; 2015:272–294.

CHAPTER 18

PELVIC ORGAN PROLAPSE

Zaid Q. Chaudhry, MD, and Cecilia K. Wieslander, MD

1. **What is the pelvic floor?**
   The pelvic floor is composed of the levator muscle complex and the coccygeus muscle. This complex consists of three muscles: iliococcygeus, pubococcygeus, and puborectalis. These muscles are tonically contracted and provide support for the pelvic organs.

2. **How is the vagina supported in the pelvis?**
   Normal support can be described using a three-level system:
   - **Level 1:** apical support provided by the *uterosacral* and *cardinal ligaments.* This level helps maintain vaginal length and the horizontal axis of the upper vagina. Failure at this level can lead to uterovaginal or vaginal vault prolapse.
   - **Level 2:** midvaginal support. The connective tissue that supports this level attaches to the *arcus tendineus fascia pelvis* and the medial aspect of the levator muscles. Defects in this level lead to anterior or posterior vaginal wall prolapse.
   - **Level 3:** distal vaginal support. The *perineal body, perineal membrane*, and *endopelvic fascia* provide support at this level. Defects can lead to perineal descent or a rectocele (prolapse of the distal portion of the posterior vaginal wall).

3. **What is the endopelvic fascia?**
   Classically, the endopelvic fascia was thought to be a discrete layer between the bladder and the vagina as well as between the vagina and the rectum. However, histologic examination has shown that this is not true fascia; instead of being composed of organized collagen, it contains loosely arranged collagen, elastin, and adipose tissue.

4. **What is pelvic organ prolapse (POP)?**
   POP is the descent of the anterior vaginal wall, posterior vaginal wall, uterus, or apex of the vagina as a result of weakening of the pelvic floor musculature and connective tissue. It is generally described by the site of prolapse (i.e., anterior vaginal wall prolapse, posterior vaginal wall prolapse, or apical prolapse). Older terms include cystocele, rectocele, and enterocele (Table 18-1).

Table 18-1. Common Terminology Used in Pelvic Organ Prolapse

DEFECT LOCATION	CLINICAL CORRELATION(S)
Anterior vaginal wall	Cystocele
Apical	Enterocele Uterine prolapse
Posterior vaginal wall	Enterocele Rectocele

5. **What are the symptoms associated with POP?**
   Although some women may not have any symptoms, common complaints include feeling a vaginal "bulge" or pelvic pressure. Symptoms are generally worse with gravity (e.g., after long periods of standing or exercise), and they may be more prominent at times of abdominal straining (e.g., defecation). In advanced stages, women may need to reduce the prolapse manually (also known as "splinting") to void or defecate. Severe prolapse can also become raw and ulcerated from contact with clothing.

6. **What is procidentia?**
   This term is used to indicate that the entire uterus has prolapsed outside the introitus.

7. **How common is POP?**
   The prevalence of symptomatic prolapse is 3% to 8%. When both symptomatic prolapse and asymptomatic prolapse are combined, this incidence rises to more than 40%. In general, 10% to 20% of women will seek care for POP in their lifetime.

8. **What are the risk factors for POP?**
   POP is multifactorial; risk factors can be divided into predisposing, inciting, promoting, or decompensating events (Table 18-2). The most significant risk factor is a history of vaginal birth.

Table 18-2. Risk Factors for Pelvic Organ Prolapse

PREDISPOSING	INCITING	PROMOTING	DECOMPENSATING
Genetics	Pregnancy	Obesity	Age
Race	Vaginal birth	Smoking	Menopause
Gender	Prior hysterectomy	Pulmonary disease	Medications
	Myopathy	Constipation	
	Neuropathy		

9. **How is POP evaluated?**
   A pelvic examination is required to evaluate POP properly. If findings are not consistent with the presenting complaints, the examination should be repeated with the patient standing up.

10. **How is POP measured?**
    A standardized system known as the POP-Q (POP quantification) is used. It involves measurement of nine points and is highly reproducible. After all measurements have been obtained, a patient can be assigned to a stage ranging from 0 to 4. It is important for all points except total vaginal length to be measured with the patient straining or performing a Valsalva-type maneuver (Fig. 18-1).

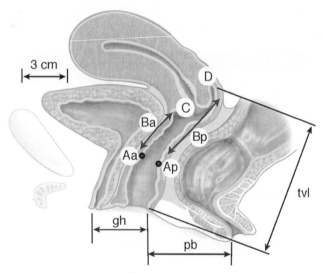

Figure 18-1. Six sites (points Aa, Ap, Ba, Bp, C, and D), genital hiatus (gh), perineal body (pb), and total vaginal length (tvl) used for pelvic organ support quantitation. *(From Walters MD, Karram MM, eds.* Urogynecology and Reconstructive Pelvic Surgery. *4th ed. Philadelphia: Saunders; 2015.)*

11. **Is treatment always necessary?**
    No. For the majority of women, symptoms generally stay the same without treatment. Ten percent of women will have worsening of their symptoms, and 3% will experience spontaneous improvement.

12. **What are nonsurgical options to manage POP?**
    Several options are available. The first is expectant management; POP is not life-threatening. Other options are pelvic floor exercises, weight loss, avoidance of heavy lifting, minimizing constipation or straining, and the use of pessaries. Pelvic floor exercises consist of contracting the pubococcygeus muscles several times a day, and they can be done under the supervision of a physical therapist.

13. **What are pessaries?**
    Pessaries are objects placed in the vagina to support the vaginal walls. They are generally made of silicone, and they come in an assortment of shapes and sizes. These devices are categorized as either supportive or space filling. Ring, Gellhorn, and donut pessaries are among the most commonly used pessaries (Fig. 18-2). All pessaries should be fitted by a health care provider with special training. Complications are rare, but they include urethral obstruction and vaginal wall erosions. Women occasionally complain of an increase in vaginal discharge. Some women may not be able to retain a pessary because of their vaginal anatomy.

14. **What types of surgical procedures are performed for POP?**
    Procedures can be performed transvaginally or transabdominally, and they can either restore or obliterate the vaginal canal. Selection is based on the patient's preference, the surgeon's preference, and the patient's age and comorbidities (Table 18-3).

15. **What types of grafts are used in POP repair, and what are their potential complications?**
    Grafts are exogenous materials used to reinforce repair at the time of surgical treatment. They are either synthetic or biologic (usually from a porcine source). Known complications are dyspareunia and mesh exposure, which may require a subsequent surgical procedure to remove the graft.

16. **What is the role of a hysterectomy in POP repair?**
    Hysterectomy has traditionally been performed when repairing apical prolapse, although the uterus can be left in place. A hysterectomy on its own does not correct prolapse.

17. **What is a colpocleisis, and when is it indicated?**
    A colpocleisis is a surgical procedure that completely closes the vaginal canal. It is reserved for patients with significant prolapse who no longer desire vaginal intercourse. A colpocleisis can be partial (also known as a LeFort colpocleisis) and leave the uterus in place or total (the uterus is removed or already absent). The benefits of this procedure are that it is extremely successful and can be done quickly with local or regional anesthesia.

KEY POINTS: PELVIC ORGAN PROLAPSE

1. The pelvic floor is composed of the levator muscle complex and the coccygeus muscle. This complex consists of three muscles: iliococcygeus, pubococcygeus, and puborectalis.
2. The causes of POP are multifactorial. The most significant risk factor is history of a vaginal birth.
3. The POP-Q is a standardized system to quantify POP.
4. POP is not life-threatening, and surgical treatment is not mandatory.

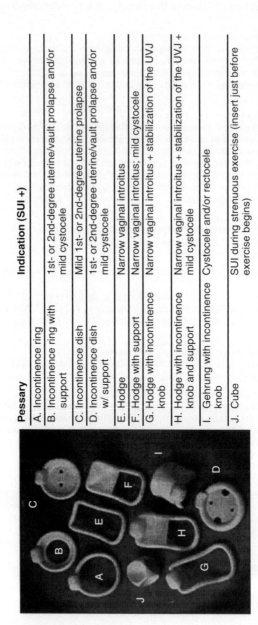

Pessary	Indication (SUI +)
A. Incontinence ring	
B. Incontinence ring with support	1st- or 2nd-degree uterine/vault prolapse and/or mild cystocele
C. Incontinence dish	Mild 1st- or 2nd-degree uterine prolapse
D. Incontinence dish w/ support	1st- or 2nd-degree uterine/vault prolapse and/or mild cystocele
E. Hodge	Narrow vaginal introitus
F. Hodge with support	Narrow vaginal introitus; mild cystocele
G. Hodge with incontinence knob	Narrow vaginal introitus + stabilization of the UVJ
H. Hodge with incontinence knob and support	Narrow vaginal introitus + stabilization of the UVJ + mild cystocele
I. Gehrung with incontinence knob	Cystocele and/or rectocele
J. Cube	SUI during strenuous exercise (insert just before exercise begins)

Figure 18-2. Pessary types and indications. *SUI,* Stress urinary incontinence; *UVJ,* ureterovesicular junction. *(From Walters MD, Karram MM, eds. Urogynecology and Reconstructive Pelvic Surgery. 4th ed. Philadelphia: Saunders; 2015.)*

Table 18-3. Surgical Treatment for Pelvic Organ Prolapse

TYPE OF PROLAPSE	SURGICAL OPTIONS
Anterior vaginal wall	Anterior colporrhaphy ("anterior repair") Paravaginal defect repair

Apical	Transvaginal:
	    Uterosacral ligament suspension
	    Sacrospinous ligament fixation
	    McCall culdoplasty
	    Colpocleisis*
	Transabdominal:
	    Sacrocolpopexy (via laparotomy or laparoscopy)

Posterior vaginal wall	Posterior colporrhaphy ("posterior repair") Site-specific repair

*Obliterates the vaginal canal

BIBLIOGRAPHY

1. American College of Obstetricians and Gynecologists. Pelvic organ prolapse. ACOG practice bulletin no. 85. *Obstet Gynecol.* 2007;110:717–729.
2. Bradley CS, Zimmerman MB, Qi Y, Nygaard IE. Natural history of pelvic organ prolapse in postmenopausal women. *Obstet Gynecol.* 2007;109:848–854.
3. Bump RC, Mattiasson A, Bø K, et al. The standardization of terminology of female pelvic organ prolapse and pelvic floor dysfunction. *Am J Obstet Gynecol.* 1996;175:10–17.
4. Culligan PJ. Nonsurgical management of pelvic organ prolapse. *Obstet Gynecol.* 2012;119:852–860.
5. DeLancey JO. Anatomy and biomechanics of genital prolapse. *Clin Obstet Gynecol.* 1993;36:897–909.
6. Haylen BT, de Ridder D, Freeman RM, et al. An International Urogynecological Association (IUGA)/International Continence Society (ICS) joint report on the terminology for female pelvic floor dysfunction. *Neurourol Urodyn.* 2010;29:4–20.
7. Khan AA, Eilber KS, Clemens JQ, et al. Trends in management of pelvic organ prolapse among female Medicare beneficiaries. *Am J Obstet Gynecol.* 2015;212:463. e1-e8.
8. Richter HE, Burgio KL. Stress urinary incontinence and pelvic organs prolapse: nonsurgical management. In: Walters MD, Karram MM, eds. *Urogynecology and Reconstructive Pelvic Surgery.* 4th ed. Philadelphia: Saunders; 2015:249.
9. Sung VW, Hampton S. Epidemiology and psychosocial impact of female pelvic floor disorders. In: Walters MD, Karram MM, eds. *Urogynecology and Reconstructive Pelvic Surgery.* 4th ed. Philadelphia: Elsevier; 2015:96–104.
10. Walters MD, Ridgeway BM. Surgical treatment of vaginal apex prolapse. *Obstet Gynecol.* 2013;121:354–374.
11. Walters MD, Unger CA. Description and classification of lower urinary tract and pelvic organ prolapse. In: Walters MD, Karram MM, eds. *Urogynecology and Reconstructive Pelvic Surgery.* 4th ed. Philadelphia: Saunders; 2015:109.

CHAPTER 19

BREAST DISEASE

Susan Park, MD

1. **How is the breast examination performed?**
   In general, be methodical and consistent. Palpation should be systematic and with variable pressure. Examine the patient while she is in the sitting and supine positions. Have the patient flex the pectoralis muscle to look for any skin retraction or dimpling. The areola should be compressed to identify any discharge as well as to evaluate for nipple retraction. To evaluate for lymph nodes, ask the patient to open the axilla by placing the ipsilateral hand behind her head.

2. **What physiologic changes occur in the breast during the luteal phase of the menstrual cycle?**
   Cyclic symptoms of increased sensitivity, pain, or even nipple discharge result from an increase in size, nodularity, and density. Breast volume increases an average of 25 to 30 mL. Breast examination is therefore best performed shortly after menses.

3. **How common is breast pain (mastalgia)?**
   Breast pain occurs in more than two thirds of menstruating women. Cyclic pain tends to be diffuse, bilateral, and associated with benign fibrocystic changes. Noncyclic breast pain is localized and may be associated with an identifiable cyst or mass. Pain alone is rarely a presenting symptom of malignant disease. Various treatments have been used for mastalgia and include analgesics, low-dose diuretics, danazol, and reduced caffeine intake.

4. **What is mastitis?**
   Mastitis refers to the inflammation of breast tissue. It can be categorized as infectious or noninfectious. Noninfectious mastitis may warrant workup for possible malignancy. **Lactational mastitis** occurs in 2% to 10% of breastfeeding women and manifests with fever and a tender, red, engorged breast. Treatment is directed against *Staphylococcus aureus* (including methicillin-resistant *S. aureus* [MRSA]), and women are encouraged to continue breastfeeding.

5. **What is galactorrhea, and what are common causes?**
   Galactorrhea refers to spontaneous milky, nonbloody discharge from the nipple. It results from increased prolactin levels. Dopamine exerts negative feedback on prolactin release, and thyrotropin-releasing hormone (TRH) promotes prolactin release. Therefore, medications that have dopamine antagonist activity (e.g., antipsychotics or other phenothiazine drugs) or conditions in which the patient would have high levels of TRH (hypothyroidism) can cause galactorrhea. Pregnancy, oral contraceptives, and prolactinomas can also cause galactorrhea.

6. **What is the most common cause of bloody nipple discharge?**
   Bloody discharge is most commonly the result of a breast neoplasm, and the most frequent neoplasm is a benign intraductal papilloma.

7. **What are fibrocystic changes of the breast?**
   Fibrocystic changes are the most common benign breast conditions. They are characterized by fibrosis of breast stroma and the formation of cysts, and they typically affect women of reproductive age. Some women can palpate changes in the breast, but most women with fibrocystic change experience *cyclic* breast pain. Fibrocystic changes are not associated with an increased risk of breast cancer.

8. **How should a mass be described?**
   Size, contour, consistency, and mobility should be noted, along with any attachment to skin or underlying fascia. Careful examination of the axillary and supraclavicular lymph nodes should also be performed, and any nipple discharge or rashes should be noted.

9. **What is the differential diagnosis of a breast mass?**
   Breast cancer, fibrocystic disease, fibroadenoma, and trauma (fat necrosis); the frequency varies with age. Fibrocystic change is the most common cause of a breast mass.

10. **What important information should be obtained from a patient being evaluated for a breast mass?**

Most newly discovered breast masses are found by the patient herself. It is important to ask when the mass was first found, how it has changed, whether it changes with the menstrual cycle, and whether it is painful.

11. **What characteristics of a breast mass suggest malignancy?**

Palpable breast cancers usually have irregular or indistinct borders and may be attached to the skin, dermal attachments, or underlying fascia. More advanced local disease produces skin changes that result in retraction, dimpling, induration, edema ("peau d'orange"), ulceration, or inflammation. However, no physical characteristics can reliably distinguish between benign and malignant lesions—any breast mass should be examined by biopsy.

12. **What are the risk factors for breast cancer?**

Carcinoma of the breast, the most common malignant disease in women, occurs in 12% (1 in 8) of women during their lifetime. Risk factors include age, family history of breast cancer, history of breast cancer in the opposite breast, combined estrogen and progesterone hormone therapy (HT), early menarche or late menopause, nulliparity, radiation exposure, and a history of colon or uterine cancer. The Gail model is a computer model that combines various risk factors to produce an individualized risk assessment. It does not, however, include whether a woman has been tested for *BRCA* genes or used HT.

13. **What are the *BRCA* genes, and why are they important?**

The breast and ovarian cancer genes *BRCA1* and *BRCA2* are found on two separate chromosomes.

The lifetime risk of breast cancer in women with these mutations may be as high as 85%, and the lifetime risk for ovarian cancer is 20% to 40%. Women with a strong family history of breast or ovarian cancer may choose to be screened. Women who test positive require increased surveillance for cancer and are offered prophylactic mastectomy or oophorectomy after childbearing has been completed.

14. **Does the use of HT increase a woman's risk of breast cancer?**

According to the Women's Health Initiative (WHI), which was a large cohort study of women receiving HT after menopause, the risk of breast cancer (relative risk [RR]: 1.24; confidence interval [CI]: 1.02 to 1.5) is slightly increased with the use of a combination estrogen-progesterone regimen but not with estrogen alone. (The estrogen-only arm of the study actually showed a statistically insignificant decrease in risk, with an RR of 0.8 [CI: 0.62 to 1.04]). Women should consider their baseline risk of breast cancer before they take HT. A family history of breast cancer does not in itself preclude the use of HT.

Oral contraceptives have not been shown to increase the risk of breast cancer.

15. **Is there anything a woman can do to reduce her risk of developing breast cancer?**

For women at average risk, no proven methods exist because most of the risk factors (e.g., family history, age at menarche) are not able to be modified. For women at very high risk, tamoxifen has been shown to reduce the incidence of new hormone receptor–positive breast cancers. It has not, however, been shown to reduce deaths or the risk of hormone receptor–negative cancers. Prophylactic oophorectomy has been shown to decrease breast cancer risk by 50%, and prophylactic mastectomy decreases breast cancer risk by 90%.

16. **What are the current breast cancer screening guidelines?**

Mammography screening is associated with a 19% overall reduction of breast cancer mortality (≈15% for women in their 40s and 32% for women in their 60s), but it has disadvantages of false-positive results and overdiagnosis. At this time, a discrepancy exists among major organizations regarding breast cancer screening. Recommendations from the American Cancer Society, the American College of Obstetricians and Gynecologists, and the U.S. Preventive Services Task Force are summarized in Table 19-1. Screening magnetic resonance imaging (MRI) scans should be reserved for high-risk (>20%) women such as *BRCA* carriers.

17. **What initial diagnostic step should be taken to evaluate a newly discovered mass?**

A diagnostic mammogram should be the first imaging study to be performed, even if a patient has had a recent negative mammogram. Ultrasound can be used to determine whether a mass is solid or cystic, and it is the first-line imaging method for a woman who is pregnant or lactating.

Table 19-1. Current Breast Cancer Screening Guidelines

ORGANIZATION	MAMMOGRAM	CLINICAL BREAST EXAMINATION	BREAST SELF-EXAMINATION
American Cancer Society	Age 40 years and older annually	Age 20-39 every 1-3 years, then annually ≥40 years	Optional for age 20 years and older
American College of Obstetricians and Gynecologists	Age 40 years and older annually	Age 20-39 years every 1-3 years, then annually ≥40 years	Consider for high-risk patients
U.S. Preventive Services Task Force	Age 50-74 years biennially	Insufficient evidence	Not recommended

18. **If a breast cyst is aspirated, should the fluid be sent for microscopic examination?**
Only if it is bloody. Clear or yellow fluid does not need to be sent for cytologic analysis.

19. **What characteristics of an aspirated cyst require further workup?**
Aspiration of bloody fluid or a residual mass remaining after aspiration. Further diagnostic studies should also be performed if a cyst recurs.

20. **What are the advantages and disadvantages of fine-needle aspiration (FNA) of a breast mass over a core or excisional biopsy?**
Confirmation of any breast mass is made by either FNA or core biopsy. FNA is easily and safely performed in an office or clinic setting. It distinguishes cystic from solid masses and provides cells for subsequent cytologic evaluation. However, it requires considerable skill to obtain a satisfactory sample and has significant false-negative and false-positive rates. A core or excisional biopsy enables the pathologist to determine whether a malignant mass is invasive or in situ, whereas this determination may not be possible on the basis of an FNA.

21. **Does a normal-appearing mammogram in a woman with a palpable mass exclude the possibility of cancer?**
No. In general, the false-negative rate for mammograms is reported to be as high as 16%. Mammograms can be interpreted as normal even in the presence of clinically evident cancer; for this reason, any suspicious palpable mass should be examined by biopsy.

22. **In what settings are mammograms particularly difficult to interpret?**
Dense or very large breasts are difficult for radiologists to evaluate. This problem is found in 25% of women and is particularly common at younger ages.

23. **What is the role of ultrasound in the evaluation of solid breast masses?**
Ultrasound is useful for differentiating solid from cystic masses. The study can be used in women with large breasts who have deep, inaccessible lesions or who cannot undergo needle aspiration. It is also preferred in pregnant and lactating women as the primary workup.

24. **What is the approach to a woman whose mammogram shows a nonpalpable lesion that is read as "probably benign" by the radiologists?**
Two choices are possible: biopsy or repeat mammography within 6 months. Studies indicate that the second approach is probably safe, but it depends on the comfort of the physician with the mammographic appearance and the patient's ability to return for follow-up. The risk of malignancy in these cases is less than 2%.

25. **If a lesion is regarded as suspicious on a mammogram but is not palpable, what is the next step?**
Mammographic, ultrasound, or MRI localization techniques (including wires and dyes) can be used to perform an image-guided biopsy.

26. **What pathologic findings on breast biopsy put patients at a higher risk for subsequent development of breast cancer?**
Lesions with a proliferative pattern are associated with an increased risk for subsequent cancer, and lesions that show atypical hyperplasia have the highest relative risk (fivefold increase).

27. What are the major types of breast cancer?
- **Ductal:** Most breast cancers involve ductal tissue. Ductal carcinoma is divided into infiltrating ductal carcinoma and ductal carcinoma in situ (DCIS). DCIS identifies a woman at increased risk of invasive breast cancer. Most women with DCIS develop infiltrating carcinoma, and a few women have an invasive tumor present in the same breast at the time DCIS is diagnosed.
- **Lobular:** Approximately 10% of breast cancers are lobular. This category is subdivided into infiltrating lobular carcinoma and lobular carcinoma in situ (LCIS). LCIS is associated with an increased risk of invasive breast cancer in either the ipsilateral or contralateral breast. Compared with DCIS, the time to progression of LCIS is longer.

KEY POINTS: BREAST DISEASE

1. Breast pain occurs in more than two thirds of menstruating women; it tends to be diffuse, bilateral, and cyclic.
2. Fibrocystic changes are the most common benign breast conditions. Such changes are characterized by fibrosis of breast stroma and the formation of cysts, and they typically affect women of reproductive age.
3. The Gail model combines risk factors such as age, family history, personal history of breast biopsies, age of menarche, and age of menopause to assess an individual's breast cancer risk.
4. A palpable breast mass is initially evaluated with mammography or ultrasound, or both. FNA can be done to assess whether the mass is cystic or solid; if bloody fluid or solid tissue is obtained, it should be sent for cytologic examination. A core or excisional biopsy can enable a pathologist to determine whether a malignant mass is invasive.

BIBLIOGRAPHY

1. American Cancer Society. *Breast cancer early detection*, 2014. Available at http://www.cancer.org/acs/groups/cid/documents/webcontent/003165-pdf.pdf. Accessed November 18, 2014.
2. Dizon DS, Tejada-Berges T, Steinhoff MM, et al. Breast cancer. In: Barakat R, Markman M, Randall M, eds. *Principles and Practice of Gynecologic Oncology.* 5th ed. Baltimore: Lippincott Williams & Wilkins; 2009:897–945.
3. Grube BJ, Giuliano AE. Benign breast disease. In: Berek J, ed. *Berek and Novak's Gynecology.* 14th ed. Philadelphia: Lippincott Williams & Wilkins; 2007.
4. National Comprehensive Cancer Network. *Breast cancer risk reduction*, 2014. Available at http://www.nccn.org/professionals/physician_gls/pdf/breast_risk.pdf. Accessed November 18, 2014.
5. National Comprehensive Cancer Network. *Breast cancer screening and diagnosis*, 2014. Available at http://www.nccn.org/professionals/physician_gls/pdf/breast-screening.pdf. Accessed November 18, 2014.
6. Pace L, Keating N. A systematic assessment of benefits and risks to guide breast cancer screening decisions. *JAMA.* 2014;311:1327–1335.

CHAPTER 20

INTIMATE PARTNER VIOLENCE

Mae Zakhour, MD

1. **What are the characteristics of intimate partner violence (IPV)?**

   IPV includes threatened or actual physical, sexual, or psychological abuse by a current or former intimate partner. Most physical violence is accompanied by mental abuse and intimidation. IPV occurs among individuals of all ages, ethnicities, and socioeconomic classes and within both heterosexual and same-sex couples.

2. **What is the incidence of IPV?**

   It is difficult to determine the true incidence because IPV is likely underreported, but 200 million cases of IPV are estimated to occur in the United States annually. A female partner is the victim in approximately 90% of cases. In a survey conducted by the Centers for Disease Control and Prevention, 43.9% of women and 23.4% of men experienced sexual violence, and 19.3% of women and 1.7% of men reported a personal history of rape during their lifetime.

3. **What are "red flags" that should heighten suspicion for IPV?**

   Multiple injuries with inconsistent explanations of how they occurred, frequent emergency department or urgent care visits, missed appointments, significant difficulty with pelvic or rectal examinations, and the presence of an overly attentive or verbally abusive partner at clinic visits. The victim's partner may be reluctant to leave the room during an examination or may even refuse.

4. **What somatic complaints and psychological conditions are associated with IPV?**

   Victims of IPV have a higher incidence of multiple physical complaints, including headaches, chronic pain, insomnia, and irritable bowel syndrome. They also have a higher incidence of depression, suicidality, anxiety, eating disorders, substance use and abuse, and posttraumatic stress disorder.

5. **Who should be screened for IPV?**
   - Any patient who presents with signs or symptoms suggestive of IPV
   - Female trauma victims
   - Female patients in the emergency department
   - Women with chronic abdominal pain or chronic headaches
   - Women diagnosed with sexually transmitted infections

   All patients should be screened during an initial visit to a primary care provider or on presentation to a hospital, and pregnant women should be screened at their initial prenatal visit. Although studies have demonstrated that routine screening of asymptomatic patients increases detection of IPV, no studies have yet shown that screening improves health outcomes for the victim or the perpetrator.

6. **How should screening for IPV be performed?**

   It is important that patients feel safe and comfortable when asked questions about IPV. Partners and family members should be asked to leave the room before questioning. Providers should ask open-ended and direct questions while assuring confidentiality. Examples include the following:
   - At any time, has a partner hit, kicked, or otherwise hurt or threatened you?
   - I see patients in my practice who have been hurt or threatened by someone they love. Is this happening to you?

7. **What is the incidence of IPV during pregnancy?**

   Between 1% and 20%. A high rate of underreporting is suspected. Physical abuse during pregnancy is frequently directed to the breasts and abdomen. Changes in violence patterns are variable during pregnancy and the postpartum period, with one fifth of women reporting increased abuse and one third reporting a decrease in abuse. Pregnant patients may feel additional pressure to stay in a relationship and conceal abuse.

8. Are any pregnancy complications associated with IPV?

IPV has been associated with poor weight gain, infection, anemia, tobacco use, stillbirth, pelvic fracture, placental abruption, fetal injury, preterm delivery, and low birth weight. The leading cause of maternal mortality is homicide, and most cases are associated with a history of IPV.

9. What is a safety plan?

A safety or "exit" plan should be developed with a patient after she has divulged a history of IPV. This plan can be implemented whenever a patient feels that violence is escalating and her life may be at risk or at any other time she feels ready to leave her partner. A safety plan should include preparing an emergency kit, identifying a safe place for her to go, and establishing a signal to alert children or neighbors to call 911. Emergency kits should include important documents such as birth certificates or passports, money, car keys, and necessary medications. If a patient does not have any nearby family or friends, information about the nearest shelters should be provided.

10. What are the three phases of the cycle of domestic abuse?

The three phases are tension building, acute battering, and perpetrator apology and remorse. During the tension building phase, tension between the couple escalates, and the victim may attempt to calm or please the batterer in hopes of preventing abuse. In the acute battering phase, the victim sustains verbal, sexual, or physical abuse. In the final phase, the batterer demonstrates remorse and may apologize, make false promises, or even give the victim gifts. This cycle tends to repeat itself, with the abuse often becoming more severe with time.

11. What resources should be provided to patients who are victims of IPV?

Providers should be aware of local resources such as community hotlines, shelters, support groups, and social welfare services. Patients should be provided with telephone hotline numbers in a confidential setting. Flyers in bathrooms or brochures in waiting or examination rooms are another way to help patients access these resources, which include the following:

- National Domestic Violence Hotline: 1-800-799-7233 (1-800-799-SAFE)
- National Sexual Assault Hotline (1-800-656-4673)

KEY POINTS: INTIMATE PARTNER VIOLENCE

1. IPV includes threatened or actual physical, sexual, or psychological abuse by a current or former intimate partner.
2. The cycle of abuse involves three phases: tension building, acute battering, and perpetrator apology and remorse.
3. It is important that patients feel safe and comfortable when asked questions about IPV and that confidentiality is assured.
3. Once a patient divulges a history of IPV, a safety plan should be developed, and she should be made aware of local resources.

BIBLIOGRAPHY

1. Alpert EJ. *Intimate Partner Violence: The Clinician's Guide to Identification, Assessment, Intervention, and Prevention.* 5th ed. Waltham, MA: Massachusetts Medical Society; 2010.
2. American College of Obstetricians and Gynecologists. Intimate partner violence. ACOG committee opinion no. 518. *Obstet Gynecol.* 2012;119:412–417.
3. Breiding MJ, Smith SG, Basile KC, Walters ML, Chen J, Merrick MT. *Prevalence and characteristics of sexual violence, stalking, and intimate partner violence victimization: national intimate partner and sexual violence survey, United States, 2011*;63. MMWR Surveill Sum; 2014:1–18.
4. Lentz GM. Rape, incest, and domestic violence. In: Katz VL, Lentz GM, Lobo RA, Gershenson DM, eds. *Comprehensive Gynecology.* 5th ed. Philadelphia: Mosby; 2007:208–211.
5. McCloskey LA, Williams CM, Lichter E, Gerber M, Ganz ML, Sege R. Abused women disclose partner interference with health care: an unrecognized form of battering. *J Gen Intern Med.* 2007;22:1067–1072.
6. Moyer VA. Screening for intimate partner violence and abuse of elderly and vulnerable adults: U.S. preventive services task force recommendation statement. *Ann Intern Med.* 2013;158:478–486.
7. Nelson HD, Bougatsos C, Blanzina I. Screening women for intimate partner violence and elderly and vulnerable adults for abuse: systematic review to update the 2004 U.S. Preventive Services Task Force Recommendation. *Ann Intern Med.* 2012;156:796–808.

CHAPTER 21

PUBERTY

Michelle S. Özcan, MD, and Travis W. McCoy, MD

1. **What is the definition of puberty?**
   Puberty is the process by which the body undergoes hormonal changes and physical development to reach full reproductive capacity. During this time, significant neuroendocrine and physiologic changes in the reproductive system not only lead to the ability to ovulate and menstruate in girls, but also cause accelerated linear skeletal growth and the development of secondary sexual characteristics, including breast development and the appearance of pubic and axillary hair.

2. **What are the physical signs of puberty, and when do they occur and in what order?**
   Puberty begins with an increase in linear growth velocity 1 to 2 years before the onset of breast budding **(thelarche)** or the appearance of pubic and axillary hair **(adrenarche)**. These changes are followed by a period of maximum growth velocity ($\approx$9 cm/year) and culminate in menarche.
   - Mnemonic of order of puberty: **GTAPM**
     - Growth spurt
     - Thelarche
     - Adrenarche
     - Peak growth
     - Menarche

   The order of pubertal development varies based on race, as well as on individual characteristics. Thelarche typically precedes adrenarche in white girls, but the opposite is true in African-American girls. Approximately 10% of normal girls may experience menarche before adrenarche.

   The age of puberty has decreased since the original descriptions published by Marshall and Tanner in 1969. The Pediatric Research in Office Settings (PROS) study in 1997 provided more contemporary data, showing that the mean ages for thelarche, adrenarche, and menarche were 8.9, 8.8, and 12.2 years for African-American girls and 10, 10.5, and 12.8 years for white girls.

3. **What is Tanner staging?**
   In 1969, Dr. J.M. Tanner developed a system to grade the normal development of puberty by comparing breast and pubic hair development in girls (Table 21-1 and Fig. 21-1) and genital and pubic hair development in boys.

4. **What are the hormonal changes that occur with puberty?**
   Puberty and the menstrual cycle depend on a normally functioning hypothalamic-pituitary-ovarian (HPO) axis.

   The first neuroendocrine change to occur in puberty is an increase in the amplitude of gonadotropin-releasing hormone (GnRH) pulses from the hypothalamus as it becomes less sensitive to negative feedback from low levels of estrogen. This change triggers an increase in luteinizing hormone (LH) release from the pituitary beginning at night, with a lesser increase in follicle-stimulating hormone (FSH) pulses.

   These pulses stimulate the growing ovarian follicles to release estradiol, which ultimately initiates an LH surge capable of triggering ovulation. Progesterone is released from the corpus luteum following ovulation (in the luteal phase of the cycle).

   During this time ($\approx$6 to 8 years of age), the adrenal gland is also starting to produce increased levels of androgens independent of the HPO axis, which leads to adrenarche.

5. **What factors determine when puberty starts?**
   Family history, race, geographic factors, and body composition all play roles in the timing of initiation of puberty. A family history of early puberty, African-American race, and living closer to the equator, at lower altitude, and in urban settings predispose to early puberty. Adipose tissue contains the enzyme

Table 21-1. Classification of Female Breast and Pubic Hair Development

CLASSIFICATION	DESCRIPTION
Breast Growth	
B1	Prepubertal: elevation of papilla only
B2	Breast budding
B3	Enlargement of breasts with glandular tissue, without separation of breast contours
B4	Secondary mound formed by areola
B5	Single contour of breast and areola
Pubic Hair Growth	
PH1	Prepubertal: no pubic hair
PH2	Labial hair present
PH3	Labial hair spreading over mons pubis
PH4	Slight lateral spread
PH5	Further lateral spread to form inverse triangle and reach medial thighs

Modified from Roy S. Puberty. In: Mishell DR Jr, Davajan V, eds. *Infertility, Contraception, and Reproductive Endocrinology.* 4th ed. Malden, MA: Blackwell Scientific; 1997:225-226.

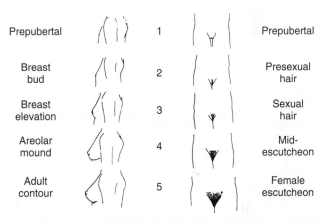

Prepubertal	1	Prepubertal
Breast bud	2	Presexual hair
Breast elevation	3	Sexual hair
Areolar mound	4	Mid-escutcheon
Adult contour	5	Female escutcheon

Figure 21-1. Pubertal staging according to Tanner stage. *(From Ross GT, Vande Wiele R. The ovary. In: Williams RH, ed. Textbook of Endocrinology. 5th ed. Philadelphia: Saunders; 1974. As redrawn in Rosenfeld RL, Cooke DW, Radovick S. Puberty and its disorders in the female. In: Sperling MA, ed. Pediatric Endocrinology. 4th ed. Philadelphia: Saunders; 2014.)*

aromatase, which catalyzes the conversion of testosterone to estradiol, thus increasing the likelihood of early puberty in obese women. Conversely, Frisch and Revelle proposed that a critical body fat content of 17% to 22% is necessary to initiate puberty; girls with anorexia nervosa, poor nutrition, excessive stress, or excessive exercise may suppress their HPO axis and experience delayed puberty or amenorrhea.

6. **What are the age limits for the normal onset of puberty?**
   The generally accepted range for the onset of puberty is between 8 and 14 years. The Pediatric Research in Office Settings (PROS) study in 1997 showed that approximately 50% of African-American girls had initiated puberty by age 8 years, and 40% of white girls had initiated puberty by age 9 years. Based on these results, revised guidelines recommend that puberty be considered precocious when thelarche or adrenarche begins before age 6 years in African-American girls or age 7 years in white girls. Girls who do not have any secondary sexual characteristics by age 13 years or no menses by 15 years of age with normal development of secondary sexual characteristics are considered to have delayed puberty.

7. Which patients should be evaluated for precocious puberty and for delayed puberty?
   - Precocious puberty
     - All girls younger than 6 years of age with breast or pubic hair development
     - Girls younger than 8 years of age with both breast and pubic hair development
     - Girls younger than 8 years of age with only breast or pubic hair development: careful history and examination with a bone age determination and close follow-up
   - Delayed puberty
     - No breast development by age 13 years
     - Absence of menarche by age 15 years
     - Absence of menarche within 3 years of thelarche
     - Absence of menarche by age 14 years if hirsutism is present or there is concern for an eating disorder, excessive exercise, or outflow tract obstruction

8. Is precocious puberty more common in girls or boys, and what about delayed puberty?
   Precocious puberty is up to 23 times more common in girls, but delayed puberty is more common in boys. Girls progress faster through puberty than boys by completing puberty in an average of 3 years as opposed to 5 years for boys. The incidence of precocious puberty in girls in the United States is approximately 1 in 10,000.

9. What are the classes of precocious puberty?
   - **GnRH-dependent (central):** caused by early activation of the HPO axis. Pulsatile GnRH release triggers LH and FSH release, which leads to gonadal sex steroid production. Puberty begins earlier, but it usually proceeds at the normal pace.
   - **GnRH-independent (peripheral):** resulting from excess sex steroid exposure independent of hypo-thalamic GnRH release. This exposure can originate from the gonads, adrenals, or from exogenous administration.

10. What is the difference between GnRH-dependent and GnRH-independent precocious puberty?
    GnRH-dependent ("central" or "true") precocious puberty is characterized by early activation of the HPO axis. This leads to breast and pubic hair development in girls and to pubic hair development and testicular enlargement in boys. The puberty is characterized as "isosexual," meaning that the changes are consistent with the child's sex.

    GnRH-independent ("peripheral" or "pseudo") precocious puberty refers to pubertal changes that are independent of the HPO axis; instead, they are the result of exposure to hormones that derive from the gonads, the adrenals, or the environment. Exposure to external hormones can sometimes cause activation of the HPO axis and lead to a mixed picture. This type of precocious puberty can be "iso-sexual" or "contrasexual," meaning that the changes are inconsistent with the child's sex—virilization in girls exposed to androgens (e.g., acne, hirsutism, clitoromegaly, voice deepening) or feminization in boys exposed to estrogens.

11. What is incomplete precocious puberty?
    Incomplete precocious puberty refers to isolated premature thelarche or adrenarche with a normal bone age and laboratory values. Usually, it simply represents a variant of normal pubertal develop-ment. These changes still require evaluation and close follow-up at a minimum, however, because they may sometimes progress to complete precocious puberty.

12. What are the causes of GnRH-dependent precocious puberty, and how are they treated?
    Up to 90% of cases of GnRH-dependent precocious puberty are idiopathic. Idiopathic GnRH-depen-dent precocious puberty is treated when bone age is advanced by 1 year or more, when growth velocity is greater than 6 cm/year, or when predicted adult height is lower than the target range. Treatment is with long-acting GnRH agonists such as leuprolide acetate, which causes pituitary desensitization and downregulation of receptors leading to a decrease in gonadotropin release and subsequent hypogonadism. Breast development should cease, and growth velocity and the pace of advancing bone age should decrease. The patient should be monitored every 3 to 6 months, and treatment should be stopped when epiphyses fuse or pubertal and chronologic ages are appropriately matched.

    Cerebral disorders account for 7% to 10% of cases of GnRH-dependent precocious puberty. These disorders can result from congenital malformations (hamartomas), tumors, hydrocephalus, infiltrative lesions, irradiation, infection, or neurofibromatosis. Treatment targets the specific pathologic process and may include surgical intervention, radiation therapy, or GnRH agonists.

13. **What are the causes of GnRH-independent precocious puberty, and how are they treated?**
    The causes of GnRH-independent precocious puberty can be separated by origin.
    - Gonadal causes
      - **Functional ovarian follicular cysts:** the most common cause of GnRH-independent precocious puberty. These cysts are usually self-limited, and bone age is usually not advanced.
      - **Ovarian tumors:** most commonly granulosa cell tumors (which secrete estradiol), but also Leydig cell tumors and gonadoblastomas. These tumors are treated surgically.
      - **McCune-Albright syndrome:** caused by a G-protein mutation that leads to continuous endocrine activation. The most common manifestations are precocious puberty, café-au-lait spots, and polyostotic fibrous dysplasia of the bone. Patients may also have gigantism, Cushing syndrome, thyrotoxicosis, or adrenal hyperplasia. Treatment is aimed at blocking estrogen production with aromatase inhibitors such as testolactone or letrozole or blocking the effects of estrogen with a selective estrogen receptor modulator (SERM) such as tamoxifen. Bisphosphonates may also be useful for polyostotic fibrous dysplasia.
    - Adrenal causes
      - **Adrenal androgen-secreting tumors** and **congenital adrenal hyperplasia (CAH):** Tumors are surgically excised, and CAH is treated with glucocorticoids.
    - Ectopic causes
      - **Human chorionic gonadotropin (hCG)–secreting tumors** are treated surgically.
    - Exogenous causes
      - Young children are extremely sensitive to the effects of low levels of estrogen, and exposure to **exogenous estrogens** in medications, personal care products, and environmental pollutants may cause precocious puberty. Treatment consists of removing the offending agent.

14. **What is the only form of precocious puberty in which bone age is delayed instead of advanced?**
    Severe primary hypothyroidism can cause precocious puberty through high serum levels of thyroid-stimulating hormone, which is structurally similar to FSH. Girls may present with breast development, galactorrhea (thyrotropin-releasing hormone stimulates prolactin secretion), and menstrual bleeding in the setting of delayed bone age.

15. **What are the essential parts of the history and physical examination in a patient with precocious puberty?**
    The history should focus on the timeline of pubertal changes, family history of pubertal milestones or any reproductive abnormalities, possible exposure to medications or environmental estrogens, history of trauma or central nervous system (CNS) insults, and any symptoms of thyroid disease, CNS lesions (headaches, seizures), or abdominal pain. The physical examination should include measurements of height and weight, as well as a review of growth charts with calculation of the patient's percentile for age and growth velocity (cm/year). Tanner staging should be performed along with a skin examination for acne or café-au-lait spots, and potential masses should be ruled out with thyroid, neurologic, abdominal, and pelvic examinations.

16. **What laboratory and imaging studies should be ordered?**
    - The most important primary test is a **bone age radiograph of the left hand and wrist** to assess for increased skeletal maturity.
    - **FSH** and **LH** should be evaluated; prepubertal levels of FSH are typically higher than LH levels, and this situation is reversed in puberty. A **GnRH stimulation test** can differentiate between GnRH-dependent and GnRH-independent causes—after stimulation, LH is elevated in GnRH-dependent precocious puberty.
    - In girls with GnRH-dependent precocious puberty, a **magnetic resonance imaging (MRI) scan of the head** is indicated, as well as possibly **thyroid function tests** if clinically indicated.
    - In girls with GnRH-independent precocious puberty (normal basal and stimulated LH levels), laboratory workup should include **serum estradiol, testosterone and hCG, dehydroepiandrosterone sulfate** (DHEA-S; adrenal production can result in premature adrenarche), **17-hydroxyprogesterone** (CAH), and late afternoon **cortisol** (Cushing syndrome).
    - A **pelvic ultrasound scan** should be obtained in all girls with precocious puberty to evaluate for functional ovarian cysts or tumors. Prolonged or repeated exposure to sex steroids can induce secondary premature maturation of the HPO-gonadal axis.

17. **What effect does estrogen have on bone?**
    Estrogen increases linear bone growth in the axial skeleton but promotes epiphyseal plate closure in long bones. Patients with precocious puberty therefore have an initial growth advantage, but they ultimately have short stature if the condition is left untreated.

18. **How can delayed puberty be classified, and what are the most common causes?**
    - Hypergonadotropic hypogonadism (increased FSH, decreased estradiol): 43% of cases
      - Ovarian failure: 65% will have an abnormal karyotype, Turner syndrome being the most common. Other causes of gonadal failure include idiopathic conditions, iatrogenic causes (e.g., gonadectomy or gonadotoxic chemotherapy), congenital abnormalities, and genetic abnormalities (Table 21-2).

Table 21-2. Causes of Delayed Puberty

HYPOGONADOTROPIC HYPOGONADISM (↓FSH, ↓ESTRADIOL)	HYPERGONADOTROPIC HYPOGONADISM (↑FSH, ↓ESTRADIOL)	EUGONADISM (NORMAL FSH, NORMAL ESTRADIOL)
Constitutional delay	Turner syndrome (or mosaicism)	Müllerian agenesis
GnRH deficiency (Kallmann syndrome)	Ovarian destruction	Transverse vaginal septum
Weight loss, excessive exercise, or anorexia nervosa	Pure gonadal dysgenesis	Androgen insensitivity syndrome
Pituitary insufficiency	Swyer syndrome (46XY)	Imperforate hymen
Prolactinoma	17-hydroxylase deficiency	
Hypothyroidism	X chromosome deletion	
Congenital adrenal hyperplasia	FSH receptor defect	
Craniopharyngioma	Myotonic dystrophy	
Cushing syndrome		
Congenital CNS defects		
Other hypothalamic or pituitary tumors		

CNS, Central nervous system; FSH, follicle-stimulating hormone; GnRH, gonadotropin-releasing hormone.

- Hypogonadotropic hypogonadism (decreased FSH, decreased estradiol): 31% of cases
  - The most common cause is functional GnRH deficiency, which can result from physiologic delay, malnutrition (e.g., anorexia nervosa), chronic illness, or excessive exercise. Other causes include hypothalamic or pituitary tumors, hypothyroidism, hyperprolactinemia, pituitary failure, or genetic defects such as Kallmann syndrome.
- Eugonadism (normal FSH and estradiol): 26% of cases
  - Congenital malformation (e.g., müllerian agenesis, imperforate hymen, transverse vaginal septum). These patients experience breast development but have primary amenorrhea.
  - Androgen insensitivity syndrome

19. **What are the components of the diagnostic workup of a patient with delayed puberty?**
    The history and physical examination should be used to evaluate breast development (a sign of estrogen exposure), height and weight, the presence or absence of a uterus, diet and exercise habits, systemic illnesses, medications, and timing of a growth spurt if one has occurred (a late growth spurt can indicate constitutional delay). A family history should focus on the pubertal history of siblings and parents, their reproductive history, and the presence of any chromosomal abnormalities. Neurologic symptoms (e.g., headache, visual disturbances, seizures) suggest a CNS disorder and prompt a visual field evaluation. Anosmia is suggestive of Kallmann syndrome (congenital GnRH deficiency caused by a variety of genetic mutations).
    Initial laboratory studies should include *prolactin, thyroid function tests, FSH, LH,* and *estradiol.* A low to low-normal FSH level in the setting of a low estradiol level is diagnostic of hypogonadotropic hypogonadism, and further diagnostic testing such as an MRI scan of the head and adrenal laboratory studies should be performed to determine the cause. A high FSH level in the setting of a low estradiol level is diagnostic of hypergonadotropic hypogonadism, and in these cases a karyotype should be obtained.

KEY POINTS: PUBERTY

1. In girls, the order of puberty is thelarche (breast budding), pubarche (pubic hair), maximum growth velocity, and then menarche (onset of menses).
2. Tanner stages are a uniform way to describe breast and pubic hair development.
3. Estrogen increases axial bone growth but fuses epiphyseal plates of long bones. This leads to short stature in patients with untreated precocious puberty.
4. Puberty is considered precocious when thelarche or adrenarche begins before the age of 6 years in African-American girls or the age of 7 years in white girls.
5. Puberty is considered delayed when girls have no secondary sexual characteristics by the age of 13 years or no menses by 15 years of age in the presence of normal secondary sexual characteristics.
6. Precocious puberty is idiopathic in 75% to 90% of girls.
7. The most common causes of delayed puberty are gonadal dysgenesis (Turner syndrome), constitutional delay, and müllerian agenesis.

BIBLIOGRAPHY

1. Frisch RE, Revelle R. Height and weight in menarche and a hypothesis of menarche. *Arch Dis Child.* 1971;46:695.
2. Fritz MA, Speroff L, eds. *Clinical Gynecologic Endocrinology and Infertility.* 8th ed. Philadelphia: Lippincott Williams & Wilkins; 2011.
3. Herman-Giddens ME, Slora EJ, Wasserman RC, et al. Secondary sexual characteristics and menses in young girls seen in office practice: a study from the Pediatric Research in Office Settings network. *Pediatrics.* 1997;99:505–512.
4. Kaplowitz PB, Oberfield SE. Reexamination of the age limit for defining when puberty is precocious in girls in the United States: implications for evaluation and treatment. *Pediatrics.* 1999;104:936–941.
5. Lentz GM, Lobo RA, Gershenson DM, Katz VL, eds. *Comprehensive Gynecology.* 6th ed. Philadelphia: Mosby; 2013.
6. Marshall WA, Tanner JM. Variations in the pattern of pubertal changes in girls. *Arch Dis Child.* 1969;44:291–303.

CHAPTER 22

AMENORRHEA

Michelle S. Özcan, MD, and Travis W. McCoy, MD

1. What is amenorrhea?
   Amenorrhea is the absence of menstruation in a woman of childbearing age. It is divided into two types: primary and secondary.

2. What is the difference between primary and secondary amenorrhea?
   - **Primary amenorrhea** is defined as the initial absence of menstruation by age 15 years in the presence of secondary sexual characteristics (breast development, pubic hair, growth acceleration), or within 5 years of initial breast development (see Chapter 21). The incidence of primary amenorrhea is 0.1%.
   - **Secondary amenorrhea** is defined as the absence of menses for longer than 6 months or the absence of menses for at least three previous cycle intervals in a woman who was previously menstruating. The incidence of secondary amenorrhea is 0.7%.

3. What are the most common causes of primary amenorrhea?
   The most common cause of primary amenorrhea is gonadal dysgenesis, such as in Turner syndrome. This accounts for more than 40% of cases. Müllerian agenesis (Mayer-Rokitansky-Küster-Hauser Syndrome) is the second most common cause, accounting for 15% of patients with primary amenorrhea.

4. What is the most common cause of secondary amenorrhea?
   Pregnancy.

5. How can the causes of amenorrhea be categorized?
   The causes of amenorrhea can be categorized as disorders of the following:
   - Uterus or outflow tract
   - Ovary
   - Pituitary
   - Hypothalamus or central nervous system
   - Endocrine system
   Table 22-1 is an overview of the causes of primary and secondary amenorrhea.

6. What are the first steps in determining the cause of amenorrhea?
   A careful history and physical examination are the first steps to narrow the differential diagnosis. Pregnancy should always be excluded. The following should be considered:
   - Does the patient have evidence of normal pubertal development? Breast development signals exposure to estrogen, and normal pubic or axillary hair signifies androgen production or exposure.
   - Is the reproductive tract normal on examination?
   - Is any evidence of hirsutism, excess androgens, or excess cortisol present?
   - Does the patient have a history of emotional, physical, or nutritional stress?
   - Are any signs of a hypothalamic or pituitary problem noted? Ask whether the patient has had any headaches, seizures, visual field defects, vomiting, changes in sleep or appetite, or galactorrhea.
   - Is the patient taking any medications, or has she received chemotherapy or radiation therapy?

7. What initial blood tests should be performed in a patient with amenorrhea?
   - A pregnancy test is performed.
   - Thyroid function tests are used to rule out hypothyroidism.
   - Prolactin level: Evaluate for hyperprolactinemia, which can occur even in the absence of galactorrhea. If hyperprolactinemia is identified, a magnetic resonance imaging (MRI) scan of the brain with intravenous (IV) contrast should be performed to rule out a prolactinoma.
   - Follicle-stimulating hormone (FSH) level: Determine whether failure of the hypothalamic-pituitary axis or ovary exists. High FSH levels indicate that the hypothalamus is functioning properly but with no feedback inhibition response from the ovaries. This condition indicates primary ovarian failure. Low or low-normal levels of FSH indicate hypothalamic dysfunction.

Table 22-1. Common causes of Primary and Secondary Amenorrhea

Common Causes of Primary Amenorrhea	
CATEGORY	**APPROXIMATE FREQUENCY (%)**
Absent Breasts and Increased FSH	**40**
45 X and variants	20
46 XX	15
46 XY	5
Absent Breasts and Low or Normal FSH	**30**
Constitutional delay	10
Prolactinoma	5
PCOS	3
Stress or anorexia	3
CAH	3
Kallmann syndrome	2
Breast Development Present	**30**
Müllerian agenesis	10
Androgen insensitivity	9
Constitutional delay	8
Transverse vaginal septum	2
Imperforate hymen	1

Common Causes of Secondary Amenorrhea	
CATEGORY	**APPROXIMATE FREQUENCY (%)**
Low or Normal FSH	**66**
Chronic anovulation (PCOS)	
Hypothyroidism	
Hyperprolactinemia	
Other pituitary tumor/disorder	
Cushing syndrome	
Weight loss/anorexia	
Nonspecific hypothalamic	
Ovarian Failure (High FSH)	**12**
46 XX	
Abnormal karyotype	
Anatomic	**7**
Asherman syndrome	
Hyperandrogenic States	**2**
Ovarian tumor	
Nonclassic CAH	
Undiagnosed Conditions	

Data from Current evaluation of amenorrhea. ASRM educational bulletin. *Fertil Steril.* 2008;90:S219-S225.
CAH, Congenital adrenal hyperplasia; *FSH,* follicle-stimulating hormone; *PCOS,* polycystic ovarian syndrome.

8. In what two syndromes does the patient have breast development but no uterus is present?
    1. In **müllerian agenesis**, the ovaries develop appropriately but the uterus does not; sometimes the vagina is absent as well. Because of the presence of estrogen, breast development is normal. Associated renal anomalies are common (horseshoe kidney, pelvic kidney, unilateral renal agenesis, ureteral duplication) and should be ruled out with a renal ultrasound scan or intravenous pyelography.
    2. In **androgen insensitivity syndrome (AIS)**, an X-linked recessive defect exists in androgen receptors. This disorder causes genotypic males (46 XY) to be phenotypically female because

target tissues cannot respond to circulating androgens (female external genital development is the default). These patients have gonads, and male levels of testosterone and dihydrotestosterone are present. Wolffian duct development, however, fails to occur because of the receptor defect. Müllerian structures (uterus and upper vagina) also do not develop because antimüllerian hormone (AMH) is still produced by the gonads. Patients have a 20% chance of gonadal malignancy (dysgerminoma or gonadoblastoma), and the gonads should be removed after the patient reaches sexual maturity. Breast development occurs normally because of estrogen produced by the peripheral conversion of androgens. The absence of androgen action results in absent or scant pubic and axillary hair.

9. What tests should be performed on an otherwise normal 15-year-old girl with primary amenorrhea with no evidence of breast growth or pubic hair? (The vagina and uterus are present.)

An absence of breast development indicates a lack of estrogen, so an **FSH level** is needed.

- Elevated FSH (hypergonadotropic hypogonadism) indicates gonadal failure. A **karyotype** should be performed and often shows an X chromosome abnormality, the most common being Turner syndrome. These patients should have an electrocardiogram, chest radiography, intravenous pyelography, and thyroid function tests to rule out other medical problems that coincide with gonadal dysgenesis 30% of the time. If any part of a Y chromosome is present in the karyotype, the gonads should be removed because of the risk of gonadal malignancy.
- Low or low-normal FSH (hypogonadotropic hypogonadism) can be seen in cases of constitutional delay, severe stress, or hypothalamic or pituitary dysfunction. **Thyroid function tests, IGF-1 (a reflection of growth hormone production),** and **prolactin** should be assessed. In cases of low FSH, MRI with IV contrast should be performed to evaluate for hypothalamic or pituitary masses (Fig. 22-1).

KEY POINTS: PRIMARY AMENORRHEA

1. Primary amenorrhea is classically defined as the absence of menses by age 13 years with no secondary sexual characteristics or by age 15 years with evidence of secondary sexual development.
2. Gonadal dysgenesis (e.g., Turner syndrome) and müllerian agenesis are the most common causes of primary amenorrhea.
3. Patients with müllerian agenesis and androgen insensitivity present with breast development but no uterus. These conditions can be differentiated with a karyotype or testosterone level.
4. Initial laboratory workup of amenorrhea should include FSH, TSH, and prolactin determinations.
5. Patients with primary amenorrhea and hypergonadotropic hypogonadism (elevated FSH) should have a karyotype performed.
6. Patients with primary amenorrhea and hypogonadotropic hypogonadism should have an MRI scan of the brain with IV contrast performed.

10. What are the hypothalamic causes of amenorrhea?
- **Dysfunctional gonadotropin-releasing hormone (GnRH) secretion:** can occur with polycystic ovarian syndrome, excessive exercise, eating disorders, and malnutrition
- **Isolated gonadotropin deficiency:** can be caused by Kallmann syndrome (lack of GnRH neurons, associated with anosmia) or be idiopathic
- **Infection:** tuberculosis, encephalitis or meningitis, syphilis, or sarcoidosis
- **Neoplasms:** craniopharyngioma, Langerhans cell histiocytosis, other tumors

11. What are pituitary causes of amenorrhea?
- **Cell damage leading to deficient luteinizing hormone and FSH secretion:** can occur with autoimmune disease, thrombosis, or hemorrhage (Sheehan syndrome, see Chapter 68)
- **Neoplasms:** most commonly prolactinoma, but also inactive adenomas or other hormone-secreting pituitary tumors including growth hormone leading to acromegaly and adrenocorticotropic hormone, with resulting Cushing syndrome

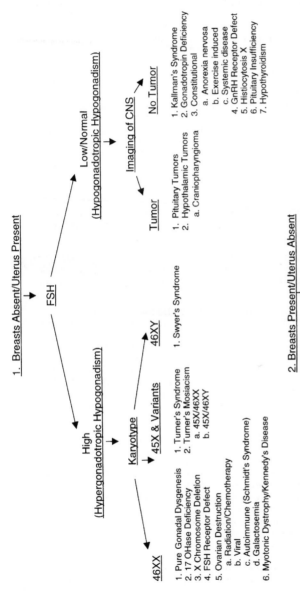

1. Breasts Absent/Uterus Present

FSH

High
(Hypergonadotropic Hypogonadism)

Karyotype

45X & Variants

1. Turner's Syndrome
2. Turner's Mosiacism
   a. 45X/46XX
   b. 45X/46XY

46XX

1. Pure Gonadal Dysgenesis
2. 17 OHase Deficiency
3. X Chromosome Deletion
4. FSH Receptor Defect
5. Ovarian Destruction
   a. Radiation/Chemotherapy
   b. Viral
   c. Autoimmune (Schmidt's Syndrome)
   d. Galactosemia
6. Myotonic Dystrophy/Kennedy's Disease

46XY

1. Swyer's Syndrome

Low/Normal
(Hypogonadotropic Hypogonadism)

Imaging of CNS

Tumor

1. Pituitary Tumors
2. Hypothalamic Tumors
   a. Craniopharyngioma

No Tumor

1. Kallman's Syndrome
2. Gonadotropin Deficiency
3. Constitutional
   a. Anorexia nervosa
   b. Exercise induced
   c. Systemic disease
4. GnRH Receptor Defect
5. Histiocytosis X
6. Pituitary Insufficiency
7. Hypothyroidism

2. Breasts Present/Uterus Absent

Karyotype/Testosterone Level

Male

Androgen Insensitivity Syndrome

Female

Uterovaginal Agenesis

Figure 22-1. Workup of primary amenorrhea. *CNS,* Central nervous system; *FSH,* follicle–stimulating hormone.

12. What are the causes of primary ovarian insufficiency (POI)?

POI is defined as ovarian failure before the age of 40 years. It is also referred to as premature ovarian failure. It has several causes:

- **Genetic defects,** including Turner syndrome and fragile X syndrome. If any XY cells are present on karyotype, the gonads should be removed immediately to decrease the risk of germ cell malignancy.
- **Toxins** can include chemotherapy, radiation, and certain viruses.
- **Autoimmune disease:** This can also cause thyroiditis, diabetes, and primary adrenal insufficiency (Addison disease).
- **Metabolic disorders:** These disorders include galactosemia.
- Up to 80% of the time, POI is **idiopathic.**

13. When should a karyotype be ordered in a patient with amenorrhea?

- Patients with primary amenorrhea who have breasts but no uterus (differentiates between androgen insensitivity and müllerian agenesis)
- Patients with primary amenorrhea and gonadal failure, to diagnose Turner syndrome or Swyer syndrome (XY gonadal dysgenesis)
- Patients with secondary amenorrhea who have POI or signs of Turner syndrome (e.g., short stature, webbed neck, high arched palate, shield chest)

14. What medications can cause amenorrhea?

- Medications that stimulate prolactin secretion: Prolactin has an inhibitory effect on GnRH secretion.
- Dopamine antagonists: Dopamine is a negative feedback inhibitor of prolactin release, so these medications lead to increased prolactin secretion. Antidepressants, (e.g., tricyclics), antipsychotics (e.g., risperidone and haloperidol), and some antiemetics (e.g., metoclopramide) are in this category.
- Selective serotonin reuptake inhibitors (SSRIs) and monoamine oxidase inhibitors (MAOIs) can induce amenorrhea through hyperprolactinemia. Other medications with this property include histamine receptor antagonists (H_2-blockers), reserpine, methyldopa, opiates, benzodiazepines, barbiturates, estrogens, and antiandrogens.

15. What causes athletic amenorrhea, and should it be treated?

In athletes, amenorrhea can result from high physiologic stress levels, energy deficit, or abnormal eating habits. Physiologic stress can increase catechol estrogens and β-endorphins and cause the hypothalamus to decrease the pulse frequency of GnRH release. Over time, the hypogonadotropic hypogonadism that ensues can lead to osteoporosis and stress fractures. The combination of disordered eating, amenorrhea, and osteoporosis is referred to as the *female athlete triad.* Athletic amenorrhea should be treated; patients should be encouraged to improve their diet, decrease stress levels, and decrease the amount of strenuous exercise if possible. Estrogen and progesterone should be replaced (oral contraceptives are a good option) if lifestyle changes are not effective.

16. What rare enzyme defects can cause amenorrhea?

Congenital adrenal hyperplasia (CAH) is an autosomal recessive disorder that can be caused by a variety of enzyme defects involved in steroidogenesis. Symptoms result from excessive or deficient production of mineralocorticoids, androgens, and estrogens. The most common enzyme deficiency in CAH is that of **21-hydroxylase.** Girls with classic CAH caused by 21-hydroxylase deficiency have ambiguous genitalia at birth as a result of exposure to androgens in utero, as well as salt wasting (hyponatremia and hypovolemia) from decreased mineralocorticoids. The nonclassic form of 21-hydroxylase deficiency, however, may manifest in adolescents or young adults with oligomenorrhea or amenorrhea and hirsutism. *17-Hydroxyprogesterone* is elevated in patients with 21-hydroxylase deficiency.

Another enzyme deficiency in CAH is that of **17α-hydroxylase,** which causes a lack of sex steroid and cortisol production and elevated mineralocorticoids. Girls with this defect have normally developed external genitalia but experience delayed puberty and primary amenorrhea because of a lack of estrogen production. Excess mineralocorticoids can also lead to hypertension, hypernatremia, and hypokalemia. These patients require exogenous estrogen and progesterone to attain sexual maturity and prevent osteoporosis.

Other enzyme defects include defects of **11β-hydroxylase** and **3β-hydroxysteroid dehydrogenase.**

KEY POINTS: SECONDARY AMENORRHEA

1. The most common cause of secondary amenorrhea is pregnancy.
2. Hypothalamic and pituitary causes of secondary amenorrhea include idiopathic conditions, eating disorders or excessive exercise, infection, and neoplasms (most commonly prolactinoma).
3. POI is usually idiopathic but can also result from Turner syndrome, fragile X syndrome, metabolic and autoimmune disorders, or chemotherapy or radiation therapy.
4. Medications that stimulate prolactin secretion include antipsychotics, antidepressants, gastrointestinal medications, antihypertensives, and hormones.
5. Nonclassic CAH caused by 21-hydroxylase deficiency can cause secondary amenorrhea and hirsutism. 17-Hydroxyprogesterone is elevated in these patients.

BIBLIOGRAPHY

1. Herman-Giddens ME, Slora EJ, Wasserman RC, et al. Secondary sexual characteristics and menses in young girls seen in office practice: a study from the Pediatric Research in Office Settings network. *Pediatrics.* 1997;99:505–512.
2. Current evaluation of amenorrhea. ASRM educational bulletin. *Fertil Steril.* 2008;90:S219–S225.
3. Lentz GM, Lobo RA, Gershenson DM, Katz VL, eds. *Comprehensive Gynecology.* 6th ed. Philadelphia: Mosby; 2012.
4. Fritz MA, Speroff L, eds. *Clinical Gynecologic Endocrinology and Infertility.* 8th ed. Philadelphia: Lippincott Williams & Wilkins; 2011.

CHAPTER 23

INFERTILITY

Lauren W. Sundheimer, MD, and Travis W. McCoy, MD

1. **What basic information should you provide a couple who has stopped using contraception and desires pregnancy?**
   Explain that the natural fecundity rate (chance per cycle of achieving pregnancy) is approximately 25% in young couples and decreases with age. Provide information about the proper timing of intercourse around ovulation. Discuss when a further workup is necessary (irregular cycles, history of pelvic infections, unable to conceive after 6 to 12 months of trying). Discuss the importance of avoiding smoking and limiting caffeine intake, both of which may decrease fertility. Recommend preconception use of folic acid (e.g., prenatal vitamins) to minimize neural tube defects.

2. **A couple has sought your opinion concerning infertility versus sterility. What do you tell them when asked about the chances of becoming pregnant?**
   With a fecundity rate of 25% in normally fertile couples, approximately 85% to 90% of couples will conceive within 1 year with regular, unprotected intercourse. Infertility is the inability to conceive after 1 year of regular intercourse without contraception in women younger than 35 years of age or after 6 months of regular intercourse without contraception in women 35 years old and older. This problem affects 10% to 15% of couples of reproductive age (i.e., 15 to 44 years old). *Primary infertility* applies to patients who have never conceived, whereas *secondary infertility* is the term reserved for patients who have previously conceived (including live born, ectopic, or abortion) and are currently infertile.

   Sterility implies an intrinsic inability to achieve pregnancy, whereas infertility implies a decrease in the ability to conceive. Sterility affects 1% to 2% of couples.

3. **Is fecundity related to age?**
   Yes. An inverse relationship exists between fecundity and the age of a woman. This is caused by a decrease in egg quality with age, likely as a result of deficient reproductive "machinery" within the egg, that leads to an increase in the proportion of aneuploid embryos created. In addition, the number of oocytes within the ovary declines because of progressive follicular atresia (by apoptosis). Fertility starts to decline in the mid-30s, with an increase in this decline in the upper-30s and a much more rapid decrease after age 40 years. In general, natural fertility is unlikely after age 43 to 44 years for most women.

   Sperm quality deteriorates somewhat as men grow older; the effect is slight, however, and generally does not become a problem before 60 years of age. Men can also have a decrease in testosterone production and subsequent reductions in sperm concentrations, motility (movement), and morphology (shape).

4. **What are three important goals that a generalist obstetrician-gynecologist should achieve in working with an infertile couple?**
   1. **Patient education:** A couple needs to know the basics of human reproduction, the chances of becoming pregnant, when it is best to have intercourse, common causes of infertility, investigative tests available, the cost and discomfort associated with tests, and the therapies available—along with their expected success rates.
   2. **Basic evaluation:** Essential elements include documentation of ovulation and tubal patency and testing for male factor problems. Peritoneal factors (adhesions and endometriosis) can also play a role, but weighing the costs of investigation and treatment against the potential benefit may be best left to a fertility specialist.
   3. **Emotional support and guidance:** The clinician should counsel the couple on how far to go with tests and when referral for further testing and treatment is appropriate.

5. **What are the general causes of infertility, and how common are they?**
   - Pelvic factors (tubal disease or endometriosis): 35%
   - Male factors: 35%
   - Ovulatory dysfunction: 15%

- Unexplained conditions: 10%
- Unusual problems: 5%

Overall, a cause for infertility can be found in 80% of cases. Infertility can result from one or both partners; an even distribution of male and female factors exists, including couples with multiple factors.

6. **What occurs during the initial assessment of an infertile couple?**
   An initial clinical assessment should begin with a thorough history and examination of both partners. Ovulation, tubal patency, uterine anatomy, and sperm should all be evaluated.
   - **Ovulation:** Irregular cycles or cycles more than 35 days in length are most likely nonovulatory. Regular cycles may still be nonovulatory. A menstrual history is reliable, but ovulation can also be proven with ultrasound examination or by measuring luteal phase progesterone.
   - **Tubal patency:** The initial evaluation is usually a **hysterosalpingogram (HSG)**, although false-negative and false-positive results are possible. HSG cannot show subtle tubal or ovarian adhesions that may affect anatomic positioning.
   - **Uterine anatomy:** This is evaluated with ultrasound. Myomas can sometimes affect fertility, and congenital anomalies can affect pregnancy outcomes.
   - **Sperm:** Assessment is recommended if a man has never fathered a pregnancy or if a pregnancy was in the distant past. Results can have a daily variation of up to 50%, however, and no result clearly indicates whether a man is fertile or infertile.

7. **What evidence from a patient's history is suggestive of ovulation?**
   Menses at regular monthly intervals, premenstrual **moliminal** symptoms (breast tenderness, bloating, mood changes), and **mittelschmerz** (localized lower quadrant discomfort during ovulation, not experienced by all women). A typical menstrual pattern involves sudden onset and several days of heavier bleeding that tapers off over the next several days.

8. **What methods can be used to establish that cycles are ovulatory, and what are their benefits and drawbacks?**
   - **Ultrasound:** Used to demonstrate mature follicles (18 to 22 mm) at approximately cycle day 12 to 14. This is the most reliable assessment and allows proper timing of intercourse, but it is more invasive and costly.
   - **Urine ovulation predictor kits (OPKs):** These kits detect the luteinizing hormone (LH) surge, which occurs about 24 hours before ovulation. They allow proper timing of intercourse, are easy to perform, and are cost effective, but they can also have false-negative results. False-positive results are less common.
   - **Luteal phase progesterone level:** When obtained approximately 1 week before expected menses, a level greater than 3 ng/mL confirms that ovulation has occurred. It does not allow for timed intercourse.
   - **Basal body temperature:** A sustained rise (>98° F) occurs after ovulation. This method has the lowest cost but is time consuming, can be difficult to interpret, and recognizes ovulation only after it occurs. It does not allow for timed intercourse.

9. **What clues in a patient's history should alert the physician to the possibility of a tubal factor?**
   A history of previous ectopic pregnancy, prior pelvic surgery, ruptured appendix, tuberculosis, septic abortion, or sexually transmitted infections (primarily *Chlamydia* infections) are risk factors for tubal factor infertility. However, 50% of women with tubal damage or pelvic adhesions have no history of these factors. Among women with no history of pelvic infection, 35% show serologic evidence of past exposure to *Chlamydia*.

10. **How can tubal patency be established?**
    Tubal patency can be assessed by an **HSG** or at the time of a laparoscopy. An HSG is a fluoroscopic examination of the uterus and tubes that is performed during the follicular phase of the cycle. It involves the transcervical injection of a radiopaque dye into the uterine cavity. At the time of laparoscopy, a water-based dye (indigo carmine or methylene blue) can be injected into the uterine cavity to visualize spillage out of the fallopian tubes directly. This technique is known as **chromopertubation**.

11. **What information can be obtained from an HSG?**
    HSGs are primarily used to document tubal patency, but they can also provide information about the shape of the endometrial cavity and tubal architecture. Endometrial cavity abnormalities manifest as filling defects and include submucosal leiomyomas (fibroids), endometrial polyps, or intrauterine adhesions (synechiae). Peritubal or pelvic adhesions may alter the filling characteristics and orientation of the fallopian tubes within the pelvis.

12. **What are the contraindications to an HSG, and any complications possible?**
Women with iodine allergies could have a reaction to the common iodinated contrast agent. In these cases, an option is to use a gadolinium-based dye (normally used in magnetic resonance imaging). Possible complications include pain (which can be minimized by premedication with a nonsteroidal agent) and development of acute salpingitis (1% to 3% of procedures). Acute pelvic infection is an absolute contraindication to HSG.

13. **What is a semen analysis, and what are normal results?**
A semen analysis is performed by evaluating sperm microscopically to assess concentration, percentage of sperm that are motile, and morphology. Sperm counts can vary by as much as 50% from day to day, so a single analysis provides only an estimate. Semen analysis results serve only as a proxy for the prediction of sperm function. Broad overlap exists between men who are fertile and those who are infertile, and caution must be used in counseling patients on the results of semen analysis. The lower limits of a normal semen analysis are listed in Box 23-1.

Box 23-1. Minimum Criteria for a Normal Sperm Analysis (5th Percentile)

- Volume: 1.5 mL
- pH: 7.2
- Sperm concentration: 15 million/mL
- Sperm motility: 40%
- Morphology: 4% normal (strict Kruger criteria)

---

14. **What is ovarian reserve, and how is it assessed?**
Assessment of ovarian reserve is an evaluation of the remaining egg follicle pool in the ovaries. A pelvic ultrasound scan is a simple way to measure the **antral follicle count,** and it also allows for early identification of pelvic disorders. The number of antral follicles (2 to 9 mm) is directly proportional to the number of remaining follicles. **Antimüllerian hormone (AMH)** is a direct marker of ovarian reserve. This hormone is made in small quantities by the follicle granulosa cells, and the level is directly proportional to the number of oocytes remaining. AMH has little cycle variability and can generally be measured at any point in the cycle. In the past, follicle-stimulating hormone (FSH) and estradiol levels in the early follicular phase (days 2 to 4) of the menstrual cycle were used. However, considerable daily and cycle-to-cycle variation limits interpretation.

15. **When is laparoscopy appropriate in an infertile woman?**
Laparoscopy allows for visualization of the internal female anatomy and assessment for peritubal or periovarian adhesions, endometriosis, and the external structure of the uterus. It is generally not part of an initial workup. If abnormalities are noted on an HSG, laparoscopy can be used for further assessment and treatment of problems such as distal tubal adhesions, occlusions, or hydrosalpinges. Hydrosalpinges can decrease pregnancy and embryo implantation rates and should be interrupted or removed. Endometriosis can also be diagnosed and treated at the time of laparoscopy, although fertility is only marginally improved.

16. **How does the treatment of proximal and distal tubal disease differ?**
In general, the most effective treatment of tubal factor infertility is **in vitro fertilization (IVF).** However, in some cases surgical repair is possible. Distal tubal disease can be treated with distal salpingostomy, in which the tube ends are opened and sutured open. However, with long-standing tubal closure and dilation, the tubal mucosa may be permanently damaged and not function. Proximal obstructions can sometimes be treated with hysteroscopic or radiologic tubal canalization, although the long-term effects of these procedures are limited. Tubal surgical procedures place a woman at risk for an ectopic pregnancy, adhesions, and reclosure of a salpingostomy. Midtubal disease is uncommon and not amenable to surgical repair. Patients with combination cases of distal and proximal disease should be treated with IVF.

17. **What is the impact of leiomyomas on fertility?**
Uterine leiomyomas are very common (see Chapter 5). In general, subserosal or pedunculated fibroids do not impair fertility. Submucosal fibroids that distort the uterine cavity have the greatest impact, leading to lowered pregnancy rates and increased risk of miscarriage. These tumors should be surgically removed. The most common procedure used is hysteroscopic myomectomy, if a significant portion extends into the endometrial cavity. Intramural or large submucosal fibroids can be addressed either laparoscopically or with laparotomy. In general, laparoscopic management is preferable because it has less recovery time and a lower incidence of severe pelvic adhesions

(which could affect tubal function and impair future fertility). However, pregnancy outcomes are equivalent with either procedure.

18. **Do congenital uterine anomalies cause infertility?**

Imperfect fusion of the müllerian duct system can cause a variety of congenital uterine anomalies. These anomalies range from a muscular septum that divides the uterine cavity to more extreme malformations such as bicornuate uterus (Fig. 23-1). Congenital uterine anomalies are associated with pregnancy loss but generally not infertility.

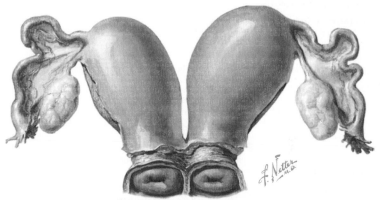

Uterus didelphys (uterus duplex separatus)

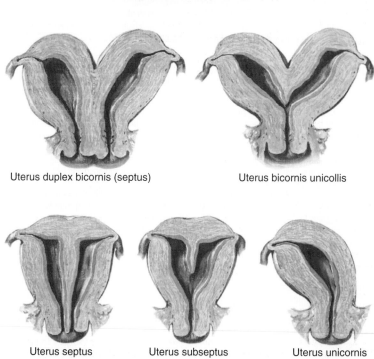

Uterus duplex bicornis (septus) Uterus bicornis unicollis

Uterus septus Uterus subseptus Uterus unicornis

Figure 23-1. Uterine anomalies: bicornuate, septate, and unicornuate uterus. *(From Smith RP. Netter's Obstetrics and Gynecology. 2nd ed. Philadelphia: Saunders; 2008.)*

19. **How are uterine malformations managed?**

    The data on management of uterine anomalies are limited by the fact that many women with uterine anomalies likely never come to medical attention. Even among women with known uterine anomalies, findings and clinical presentations vary widely. For women with a uterine septum, miscarriage rates are related to the extent of the septum, with complete septa leading to very high loss rates. The accepted therapy is hysteroscopic resection of the septum, which can reduce pregnancy loss rates. The management of a bicornuate uterus is controversial. Data showing the effectiveness of uterine reconstruction are limited, and this procedure is not generally performed anymore. Prophylactic cerclages can have some benefit in women with prior poor obstetrical outcomes. For further information on this topic, see Chapter 42.

20. **Can the cervix contribute to infertility?**

    Yes. Cervical factors such as structural abnormalities or abnormal mucus production can lead to impaired sperm penetration. Causes include scarring, stenosis, in utero diethylstilbestrol (DES) exposure, or earlier treatment for cervical dysplasia (i.e., loop electrode excision or conization). For suspected cervical issues, **intrauterine insemination (IUI)** can be used to bypass the cervix.

21. **Does endometriosis cause infertility?**

    Although endometriosis is a relatively common gynecologic condition (affecting 5% to 10% of women) and a documented cause of pelvic pain and dysmenorrhea, the exact relationship between endometriosis and infertility is unclear. Severe endometriosis can impair fertility through scarring and anatomic distortion. Milder endometriosis is thought to decrease fertility because of chronic inflammation, which creates a harsh pelvic environment for sperm and eggs. In women with long-standing infertility, endometriosis can be found in 50% to 70%. Although surgical therapy can slightly improve fertility, it is usually reserved for the treatment of pelvic pain.

22. **How is endometriosis treated surgically?**

    Nearly all cases of endometriosis can be treated laparoscopically. Because of improved visualization and patient outcomes, laparoscopy is the preferred route. Surgical techniques include excision of affected peritoneal tissue or the ablation of visible lesions with either cautery or laser. All have similar effects on fertility. Cautery and laser ablation can undertreat lesions that may invade the peritoneum, and more recent studies support better long-term results with excision.

23. **What are the most common endocrine disorders that can affect fertility?**

    Thyroid disorders, primarily severe hypothyroidism, can affect ovulation through inhibition of hypothalamic signaling. Hyperprolactinemia can also do the same. Uncontrolled diabetes raises the risk for miscarriage and birth defects.

24. **How is infertility related to polycystic ovarian syndrome (PCOS) managed?**

    Most fertility difficulties in women with PCOS result from anovulation, but it is important to rule out other causes because this may not be the only reason. Many women with PCOS can conceive easily with simple ovulation induction, but in other patients fecundity is still severely impaired. Lifestyle changes such as weight loss can help to restore ovulation and may improve pregnancy rates. Treatment of underlying insulin resistance with metformin may improve ovulation and has been used as an off-label adjunct (see Chapters 24 and 26 for further details).

    Ovarian drilling is a surgical method of treatment for women with PCOS who do not respond easily to medications. In this procedure, the surgeon uses a needle with electric current to puncture the ovary in multiple locations, thus leading to destruction of the ovarian cortex and stroma. The operation results in lower androgen levels which may improve ovulation. Risks include excessive destruction of tissue, possible decreased ovarian function, and the development of pelvic adhesions leading to tubal damage. This treatment is generally used as a last resort in women who cannot or will not progress to therapies such as IVF.

25. **How is unexplained infertility managed?**

    The diagnosis of unexplained infertility is assigned to couples with normal results of a standard infertility workup. In many cases, contributing factors are oocyte quality, deficient sperm function, or subtle pelvic issues. Treatment options include ovarian stimulation with insemination and IVF if this is not successful.

26. **What does the term assisted reproductive technology (ART) mean?**

    ART refers to any of a variety of procedures involving manipulation of gametes and embryos to treat infertility. Specific procedures most commonly include IVF and **intracytoplasmic sperm injection (ICSI)**.

Older procedures such as gamete intrafallopian transfer (GIFT) and zygote intrafallopian transfer (ZIFT) are rarely performed. ART is the fastest way to a pregnancy, although it is associated with increased cost. Patients must weigh the chance of success, costs, and infertility-related stress in making the decision to progress to ART.

KEY POINTS: INFERTILITY

1. Infertility is defined as inability to conceive after 1 year of regular intercourse without contraception in women less than 35 years of age and after 6 months in women 35 years old or older.
2. Causes of infertility most commonly result from defects in ovulation, oocyte quality, tubal function, peritoneal factors, or sperm function.
3. Initial evaluation of an infertile couple should include semen analysis, assessment of ovulation, and assessment of tubal patency.
4. Treatment options for infertility depend on the underlying cause and include ovulation induction, surgical intervention for tubal disease or endometriosis, intrauterine insemination, in vitro fertilization, and correction of male factors.

BIBLIOGRAPHY

1. Agarwal SK, Haney AF. Does recommending timed intercourse really help the infertile couple? *Obstet Gynecol.* 1994;84:307.
2. Al-Inany H. Laparoscopic ablation is not necessary for minimal or mild lesions in endometriosis associated subfertility. *Acta Obstet Gynecol Scand.* 2001;80:593–595.
3. Dechaud H, Anahory T, Aligier N, et al. Salpingectomy for repeated embryo nonimplantation after in vitro fertilization in patients with severe tubal factor infertility. *J Assist Reprod Genet.* 2000;17:200–206.
4. Fernandez H, Morin-Surruca M, Torre A, Faivre E, Deffieux X, Gervaise A. Ovarian drilling for surgical treatment of polycystic ovary syndrome: a comprehensive review. *Reprod Biomed Online.* 2011;22:556–568.
5. Ghahiry AA, Refaei Aliabadi E, Taherian AA, Najafian A, Ghasemi M. Effectiveness of hysteroscopic repair of uterine lesions in reproductive outcome. *Int J Fertil Steril.* 2014;8:129–134.
6. Golan A, Langer R, Neuman M, et al. Obstetric outcome in women with congenital uterine malformations. *J Reprod Med.* 1992;37:233–236.
7. Goodarzi MO, Dumesic DA, Chazenbalk G, Azziz R. Polycystic ovary syndrome: etiology, pathogenesis and diagnosis. *Nat Rev Endocrinol.* 2011;7:219–231.
8. Homer HA, Li TC, Cooke ID. The septate uterus: a review of management and reproductive outcome. *Fertil Steril.* 2000;73:1–14.
9. Jacobson TZ, Duffy JM, Barlow D, Farquhar C, Koninckx PR, Olive D. Laparoscopic surgery for subfertility associated with endometriosis. *Cochrane Database Syst Rev.* 2010;20:1398.
10. Johnson NP. Metformin use in women with polycystic ovary syndrome. *Ann Transl Med.* 2014;2:56–63.
11. Jones Jr HW, Toner JP. The infertile couple. *N Engl J Med.* 1993;329:1710.
12. Nawroth F, Schmidt T, Freise C, Foth D, Romer T. Is it possible to recommend an "optimal" postoperative management after hysteroscopic metroplasty? A retrospective study with 52 infertile patients showing a septate uterus. *Acta Obstet Gynecol Scand.* 2002;81:55–57.
13. Practice Committee of the American Society for Reproductive Medicine. Diagnostic evaluation of the infertile male: a committee opinion. *Fertil Steril.* 2012;98:294–301.
14. Practice Committee of the American Society for Reproductive Medicine. Diagnostic evaluation of the infertile female: a committee opinion. *Fertil Steril.* 2012;98:302–307.
15. Rossetti A, Sizzi O, Soranna L, et al. Fertility outcome: long-term results after laparoscopic myomectomy. *Gynecol Endocrinol.* 2001;15:129–134.
16. Sammour A, Tulandi T. Laparoscopic fertility-promoting procedures of the fallopian tube and the uterus. *Int J Fertil Womens Med.* 2001;46:145–150.
17. Tremellen K, Savulescu J. Ovarian reserve screening: a scientific and ethical analysis. *Hum Reprod.* 2014;29:2606–2614.
18. Vercellini P, Viganò P, Somigliana E, Fedele L. Endometriosis: pathogenesis and treatment. *Nat Rev Endocrinol.* 2014;10:261–275.

CHAPTER 24

OVULATION INDUCTION AND IN VITRO FERTILIZATION

Alexandra Walker, DO, and Travis W. McCoy, MD

1. **What is ovulation induction?**
   The practice of using medication to stimulate a woman's ovary to develop and release a mature egg.

2. **Before attempting ovulation induction, what type of preliminary evaluation should anovulatory women receive?**
   Testing for thyroid disease, hyperprolactinemia, and overt ovarian failure (thyroid-stimulating hormone, prolactin, follicle-stimulating hormone [FSH]) should be performed. In patients with long-standing anovulation without progestin treatment, endometrial sampling should be considered to rule out endometrial hyperplasia regardless of age.

   If a couple is unable to conceive after 1 to 3 months of successful ovulation, consideration should be given to performing a semen analysis and testing for tubal patency using a hysterosalpingogram (HSG). If patients have a history of pelvic infection or surgical intervention, it is reasonable to perform the HSG earlier.

3. **What is the basis for anovulation?**
   Anovulation is associated with either inadequate pituitary release of gonadotropins or ovarian failure. In most cases, hypothalamic signaling to the pituitary is inadequate, not allowing gonadotropins to be released in sufficient quantities to surpass the threshold needed for mature follicular development. The basis of ovulation induction therapy is to overcome this threshold by increasing pituitary release of gonadotropins (using oral medications) or directly replacing the gonadotropins (using injectable gonadotropins), or a combination of the two. For oral medications to be successful, the hypothalamic-pituitary axis must be intact (i.e., the patient does not have hypothalamic amenorrhea). For more information on anovulation, see Chapter 6.

4. **What are the roles of weight and insulin resistance in anovulation?**
   Most obese anovulatory women with polycystic ovarian syndrome (PCOS) have some component of insulin resistance, although the incidence in women of normal weight who have PCOS is much lower. This risk is related both to weight and to a family history of diabetes. Insulin acts as a direct stimulator of ovarian androgen production, thus worsening the effect of excess androgens in patients with PCOS. At a minimum, obese anovulatory women should be screened with a glycosylated hemoglobin (HbA1c) determination to rule out overt diabetes before conceiving, although a 2-hour glucose tolerance test is preferable.

   Weight loss, if possible, can be an effective therapy for anovulation. Even modest weight loss (5% to 10% of body weight) can often restore ovulatory cycles in obese anovulatory patients.

5. **What medications are used for ovulation induction?**
   Four general classes of medications are used: antiestrogens (clomiphene citrate), aromatase inhibitors (letrozole), gonadotropins (FSH or combinations of FSH and luteinizing hormone [LH]), and gonadotropin-releasing hormone (GnRH).

6. **Which patients are good candidates for oral ovulation therapy?**
   Women with oligo-ovulation (often associated with PCOS). Such women have an intact hypothalamic-pituitary axis, which is necessary for oral medications to work.

7. **How does clomiphene work?**
   Clomiphene is a selective estrogen receptor modulator, a weak estrogen that functions as an antiestrogen. At the hypothalamic level, clomiphene binds to estrogen receptors and causes an initial antagonistic effect, and it also interferes with receptor turnover, thus leading to receptor depletion. This effect causes the body to perceive circulating estrogen levels as lower than they actually are. This reduced negative estrogen feedback triggers GnRH stimulation, which stimulates pituitary gonadotropin release and subsequent follicular development.

8. **How do aromatase inhibitors work?**

   Aromatase inhibitors affect the peripheral production of estrogen from androgen precursors by blocking the enzyme aromatase. The decreased estrogen feedback leads to increased hypothalamic GnRH stimulation to the pituitary. These agents have no direct antiestrogenic effect.

9. **Does metformin have a role in ovulation induction?**

   By improving insulin sensitivity, metformin can improve the responsiveness to medication in some women with PCOS. Although some women may ovulate after long-term use of metformin alone, it is not recommended for use as a sole agent for ovulation induction.

10. **Is one oral ovulation medication better than the others?**

    Either clomiphene or letrozole can be used as first-line agents. Historically, clomiphene was considered a first-line agent, but later studies demonstrated that letrozole is associated with fewer side effects, lower risks of multiple gestations, the ability to achieve ovulation in a larger percentage of women than clomiphene, and slightly improved pregnancy rates.

11. **How are oral agents used?**

    Starting doses of clomiphene 50 mg or letrozole 5 mg/day are typically used for 5 days. If a patient is truly anovulatory, the starting day is not cycle specific, and inducing menses before starting therapy is not required (after first ruling out pregnancy). Ovulation generally occurs 9 to 12 days after the start of the medication.

12. **What steps can be taken if ovulation does not occur?**

    If ovulation does not occur, higher doses of clomiphene (100 to 150 mg) or letrozole (7.5 mg) can be successful, as can extending treatment courses from the normal 5 days up to 10 days. For women who do not respond to clomiphene, as many as two thirds will ovulate using letrozole. If a patient is ultimately not responsive to any oral therapy, exogenous gonadotropins are another option. They are usually administered under the supervision of a specialist.

13. **How effective are oral ovulation medications?**

    Overall, ovulation successfully occurs in 70% to 80% of women. Letrozole specifically can be expected to achieve ovulation in 85% to 90% of patients.

14. **Are pregnancy risks associated with oral ovulation agents?**

    Clomiphene use increases the risk of multiple gestation to 7% to 10%. Letrozole is associated with a 4% risk of multiple gestations. No evidence indicates that treatment with clomiphene or letrozole increases the risk of congenital anomalies, developmental delay, or learning disability. The miscarriage rate is not increased with either medication.

15. **How do you treat women with hypothalamic amenorrhea?**

    Ovulation induction with gonadotropins. Injections of FSH or FSH-LH combinations alone or in conjunction with oral ovulation agents are used. This technique requires an experienced reproductive endocrinologist and very close monitoring of follicular development, generally followed by serial transvaginal sonograms and estradiol levels. When dominant follicles are present, ovulation is induced by injecting human chorionic gonadotropin (hCG). Drawbacks to this method include increased cost of medications, a high risk of multiple gestation, and a risk of ovarian hyperstimulation.

16. **What is ovarian hyperstimulation syndrome?**

    Ovarian hyperstimulation can occur in patients undergoing ovulation induction, usually with gonadotropins. It is characterized by ovarian enlargement and increased capillary permeability, which leads to extracellular fluid shift and nausea or vomiting, dehydration, and ascites. In severe cases, hospitalization may be required to treat fluid and electrolyte imbalances. Rarely, patients may develop pleural effusions that necessitate drainage.

17. **What are the advantages and disadvantages of GnRH therapy compared with gonadotropins?**

    Exogenous GnRH is not currently available in the United States. Historically, it was sometimes used to induce ovulation by stimulating normal pituitary gonadotropin secretion. GnRH therapy requires a pump for continuous subcutaneous infusion, as opposed to more simple daily injections using gonadotropins. Compared with gonadotropin therapy, GnRH therapy led to more natural monofollicular ovulation, with decreased risks of hyperstimulation and multiple gestation.

18. **What is in vitro fertilization (IVF)?**

    IVF is an assisted reproductive technologies (ART) procedure in which eggs are fertilized with sperm outside the body and the resulting embryos are transferred into the uterus. It is the most commonly performed ART procedure.

19. **What general steps are involved in IVF?**

    IVF requires controlled ovarian stimulation with exogenous gonadotropins for 10 to 12 days, ultrasound-guided transvaginal egg retrieval, fertilization in the laboratory with sperm, embryo culture for 3 to 5 days, and then embryo transfer into the uterus.

20. **How successful is IVF?**

    Maternal age is one of the most important prognostic factors in IVF outcome. Success for a single IVF cycle is approximately 40% for women less than 35 years old. This number decreases substantially with age.

21. **What concerns exist regarding children born after ART?**

    Available studies indicate that ART is associated with a small increase in congenital anomalies. It carries an increased risk of multiple gestation, preterm delivery, and low birth weight, all of which, in turn, have additional complications.

22. **What are the indications for IVF?**

    Couples undergo IVF for various reasons. The most common are tubal factor infertility, male factor infertility, endometriosis, ovulatory dysfunction, and diminished ovarian reserve. Many couples undergo IVF for unexplained infertility.

23. **What screening tests should be performed before performing IVF?**

    - Semen analysis
    - Evaluation of ovarian reserve
    - Assessment of uterine cavity and tubal status by HSG, hysteroscopy, or sonohysteroscopy

24. **How is ovarian reserve assessed?**

    Ovarian reserve can be assessed using antimüllerian hormone (AMH) levels, antral follicle counts, and basal FSH levels. AMH is produced by each ovarian follicle and is directly correlated with ovarian reserve. Antral follicle count (AFC), which is the total number of antral follicles measuring 2 to 9 mm on both ovaries during the early follicular phase, is another way to assess ovarian reserve. An AFC of three to four or less predicts poor response to ovarian stimulation. FSH lower than 10 IU/L on cycle day 3 is considered normal; levels higher than 10 IU/L have a high specificity for predicting poor response to stimulation.

25. **What options are available to women with diminished ovarian reserve?**

    Ovarian reserve testing can provide important prognostic information and can guide fertility treatment choices. Many women with diminished ovarian reserve undergo successful IVF treatment, although they may not produce as many oocytes from stimulation. Women with grossly abnormal ovarian reserve testing are much less likely to achieve treatment success; these women may be better served by using donor eggs, which are associated with a much higher success rate. IVF with donor eggs involves stimulation of an egg donor, followed by egg retrieval, egg fertilization by the sperm of the infertile woman's partner, and embryo transfer to the prepared uterus of the recipient woman.

26. **What medications are used to produce mature eggs for use in an IVF cycle?**

    Ovarian stimulation is achieved using FSH alone or in combination with LH. A GnRH agonist or antagonist is used to inhibit premature ovulation of the developing follicle, and hCG is used to induce oocyte maturity before egg retrieval.

27. **What type of monitoring occurs during an IVF cycle?**

    During stimulation with gonadotropins, serial transvaginal ultrasound scans and serial measurements of serum estradiol are used to monitor progress. Medication doses and duration are adjusted based on these results. Once most follicles reach a certain diameter, hCG is administered to trigger the resumption of meiosis and completion of oocyte maturation. Oocyte retrieval is performed approximately 36 hours after hCG administration; if the oocytes are not retrieved, spontaneous ovulation will occur.

28. **What are reasons to cancel an IVF stimulation cycle?**

    Stimulation cycles are most frequently cancelled because of an inadequate response to stimulation. Some cycles are cancelled for excessive response.

29. **How is egg retrieval performed?**
Egg retrieval is generally performed using conscious sedation by ultrasound-guided transvaginal aspiration.

30. **At what stage of development are embryos transferred to the uterus?**
Embryos are transferred to the uterus on either day 3 or day 5. This transfer is performed transcervically and often under ultrasound guidance.

31. **How many embryos are returned to the uterine cavity at a time?**
This number varies; success rates must be balanced against the risk of multiple gestation. The number of embryos transferred is based on a patient's age and infertility treatment history, as well as the quality of the embryos and their stage of development. In general, patients less than 35 years old have one to two embryos transferred, and patients more than 35 years old have two to three embryos transferred.

32. **Can fallopian tube disease affect the success of IVF?**
Yes. Patients with a hydrosalpinx who undergo IVF have a 50% decreased pregnancy rate and live birth rate and a twofold increase in miscarriage. Salpingectomy or ligation of the hydrosalpinx restores the normal IVF pregnancy rate.

33. **What effect do uterine myomas have on IVF success?**
Submucosal myomas decrease IVF success significantly; subserosal myomas do not significantly affect it. For intramural myomas, the effect appears to be based on size and location. No compelling evidence indicates that removing submucosal myomas improves IVF outcomes, although such removal is routinely performed.

34. **What is intracytoplasmic sperm injection (ICSI), and when is it used?**
ICSI is a form of ART in which a microscopic needle is used to insert a single sperm directly into an egg's cytoplasm. It is used to address male factor infertility and is indicated when a man has abnormalities in sperm count, motility, or morphology. ICSI can also benefit couples with poor fertilization in previous IVF cycles.

35. **What options are available for men with no sperm (azoospermia)?**
Donor sperm can be used through intrauterine insemination (IUI) or along with IVF. In many cases, sufficient numbers of sperm are present in the epididymis or testicle and can be retrieved surgically. Because of the low numbers involved, retrieved sperm must be used in conjunction with IVF and ICSI.

36. **What is microsurgical epididymal sperm aspiration (MESA)?**
MESA is a procedure in which sperm are removed directly from the epididymis by microsurgical techniques for the purpose of ART. This procedure can be used in men who have had a vasectomy or who have congenital bilateral absence of the vas deferens (CBAVD). Most men with CBAVD are carriers for cystic fibrosis.

37. **What is testicular sperm extraction (TESE)?**
TESE is a procedure in which sperm is extracted directly from the testicles by using an open microsurgical technique. This procedure can be used in men with Klinefelter syndrome, congenital or acquired testicular failure, nonobstructive azoospermia, or those who have had a vasectomy. As with MESA, limited numbers of sperm are retrieved, and IVF and ICSI are required.

38. **What is preimplantation genetic diagnosis (PGD)?**
PGD is genetic testing before embryo implantation. It involves removal of cells from embryos to test for specific mutations and is useful in couples who are known carriers of a specific genetic abnormality. PGD can also be used to screen embryos for aneuploidy.

39. **Does cigarette smoking affect IVF success?**
Yes. Studies have shown that smoking significantly lowers the live birth rate per cycle and increases the odds of both spontaneous miscarriage and ectopic pregnancy. Smoking is also associated with diminished ovarian reserve.

40. **Does use of fertility treatment increase a woman's risk of cancer?**
No causal relationship has been established between fertility treatment and breast or ovarian cancer, although no long-term data are available. Prolonged treatment with ovulation induction is not recommended because continued treatment has little chance of increasing success.

KEY POINTS: OVULATION INDUCTION AND IN VITRO FERTILIZATION

1. Letrozole and clomiphene are first-line options for ovulation induction in women with an intact hypothalamic-pituitary axis.
2. Patients who fail to respond to oral ovulation medication should be referred to a fertility specialist for gonadotropin therapy.
3. Maternal age is the most important factor in determining the likelihood of IVF success.
4. IVF is the most effective treatment for couples with long-standing unexplained infertility.
5. Women who are older than 40 years of age or who have severely diminished ovarian reserve are most likely to have a successful pregnancy with donor egg IVF.
6. Although long-term data are not yet available, no known link exists between fertility treatment and cancer.

BIBLIOGRAPHY

1. Badawy A, Mosbah A, Tharwat A, Eid M. Extended letrozole therapy for ovulation induction in clomiphene-resistant women with polycystic ovary syndrome: a novel protocol. *Fertil Steril.* 2009;92:236.
2. Begum MR, Ferdous J, Begum A, Quadir E. Comparison of efficacy of aromatase inhibitor and clomiphene citrate in induction of ovulation in polycystic ovary syndrome. *Fertil Steril.* 2009;92:853.
3. Broekmans FJ, Kwee J, Hendriks DJ, Mol BW, Lambalk CB. A systematic review of tests predicting ovarian reserve and IVF outcome. *Hum Reprod Update.* 2006;12:685.
4. Centers for Disease Control and Prevention. 2007. *Assisted Reproductive Technology Success Rates. National Summary and Fertility Clinic Reports.* Atlanta, GA: Centers for Disease Control and Prevention; 2009.
5. Clark AM, Thornley B, Tomlinson L, Galletley C, Norman RJ. Weight loss in obese infertile women results in improvement in reproductive outcome for all forms of fertility treatment. *Hum Reprod.* 1998;13:1502.
6. Dickey RP, Holtkamp DE. Development, pharmacology and clinical experience with clomiphene citrate. *Hum Reprod Update.* 1996;2:483.
7. Gorlitsky GA, Kase NG, Speroff L. Ovulation and pregnancy rates with clomiphene citrate. *Obstet Gynecol.* 1978;51:265.
8. Hazout A, Bouchard P, Seifer DB, Aussage P, Junca AM, Cohen-Bacrie P. Serum antimüllerian hormone/müllerian-inhibiting substance appears to be a more discriminatory marker of assisted reproductive technology outcome than follicle-stimulating hormone, inhibin B, or estradiol. *Fertil Steril.* 2004;82:1323.
9. Hwu YM, Lin SY, Huang WY, Lin MH, Lee RK. Ultra-short metformin pretreatment for clomiphene citrate-resistant polycystic ovary syndrome. *Int J Gynaecol Obstet.* 2005;90:39.
10. Johnson N, van Voorst S, Sowter MC, Strandell A, Mol BW. Surgical treatment for tubal disease in women due to undergo in vitro fertilisation. *Cochrane Database Syst Rev.* 2010;1. CD002125.
11. Lobo RA, Gysler M, March CM, Goebelsmann U, Mishell Jr DR. Clinical and laboratory predictors of clomiphene response. *Fertil Steril.* 1982;37:168.
12. Mitwally MF, Casper RF. Use of an aromatase inhibitor for induction of ovulation in patients with an inadequate response to clomiphene citrate. *Fertil Steril.* 2001;75:305.
13. Mitwally MF, Biljan MM, Casper RF. Pregnancy outcome after the use of an aromatase inhibitor for ovarian stimulation. *Am J Obstet Gynecol.* 2005;192:381.
14. Practice Committee of Society for Assisted Reproductive Technology. Criteria for number of embryos to transfer: a committee opinion. *Fertil Steril.* 2013;99:44–46.
15. Purvin VA. Visual disturbance secondary to clomiphene citrate. *Arch Ophthalmol.* 1995;113:482.
16. Schenker JG, Yarkoni S, Granat M. Multiple pregnancies following induction of ovulation. *Fertil Steril.* 1981;35:105.
17. Somigliana E, Vercellini P, Daguati R, Pasin R, De Giorgi O, Crosignani PG. Fibroids and female reproduction: a critical analysis of the evidence. *Hum Reprod Update.* 2007;13:465.
18. Speroff L, Fritz MA. *Assisted reproductive techniques. Clinical Gynecologic Endocrinology and Infertility.* 8th ed. Philadelphia: Lippincott Williams & Wilkins; 2011:1331–1382.
19. Speroff L, Fritz MA. *Induction of ovulation. Clinical Gynecologic Endocrinology and Infertility.* 8th ed. Philadelphia: Lippincott Williams & Wilkins; 2011:1293–1330.
20. Strandell A, Lindhard A, Waldenstrom U, Thorburn J. Hydrosalpinx and IVF outcome: cumulative results after salpingectomy in a randomized controlled trial. *Hum Reprod.* 2001;16:2403.
21. Sunkara SK, Khairy M, El-Toukhy T, Khalaf Y, Coomarasamy A. The effect of intramural fibroids without uterine cavity involvement on the outcome of IVF treatment: a systematic review and meta-analysis. *Hum Reprod.* 2010;25:418.
22. Vandermolen DT, Ratts VS, Evans WS, Stovall DW, Kauma SW, Nestler JE. Metformin increases the ovulatory rate and pregnancy rate from clomiphene citrate in patients with polycystic ovary syndrome who are resistant to clomiphene alone. *Fertil Steril.* 2001;75:310.
23. Waylen AL, Metwally M, Jones GL, Wilkinson AJ, Ledger WL. Effects of cigarette smoking upon clinical outcomes of assisted reproduction: a meta-analysis. *Hum Reprod.* 2009;15:31–44.

CHAPTER 25

SPONTANEOUS ABORTION AND RECURRENT PREGNANCY LOSS

Paul Buzad, MD, and Travis W. McCoy, MD

1. **What is the definition of an abortion?**
   An abortion (miscarriage) is defined as a termination or loss of pregnancy before 20 weeks of gestation (as calculated from the date of the last menstrual period) or delivery of a fetus weighing less than 500 g.

2. **What are the different types of abortions?**
   - Spontaneous (complete or incomplete)
   - Induced
   - Threatened
   - Inevitable
   - Missed
   - Tubal (can occur with an ectopic pregnancy)

3. **What is the incidence of spontaneous abortions?**
   Spontaneous abortion is the most common complication of early pregnancy. Approximately 8% to 20% of all clinically recognized pregnancies and as many as 13% to 26% of unrecognized pregnancies end in miscarriage.

4. **When do most clinically recognized spontaneous abortions occur?**
   Eighty percent of recognized spontaneous abortions occur in the first trimester, and the incidence decreases with increasing gestational age.

5. **What is the most common presentation of spontaneous abortion?**
   Vaginal bleeding with or without pelvic cramping in the first trimester.

6. **What is the differential diagnosis of vaginal bleeding in the first trimester?**
   Vaginal bleeding is common in the first trimester, occurring in 20% to 40% of pregnant women; even heavy, prolonged bleeding can be associated with a normal outcome. The differential diagnosis includes the following:
   - Threatened abortion
   - Ectopic pregnancy
   - Vaginal lesions
   - Increased friability of the cervix
   - Infections (cervicitis, vaginitis, cystitis)

7. **What is the risk of spontaneous abortion in patients who experience first-trimester bleeding?**
   This outcome affects 25% of women with first trimester bleeding.

8. **What is the most common cause of spontaneous abortion?**
   Fetal genetic abnormalities are believed to account for as many as 75% of all spontaneous abortions. They are present in 70% of first trimester losses and in 30% of losses in the second trimester.

9. **What are the most common types of chromosomal anomalies found in spontaneously aborted fetuses?**
   - As a group, autosomal trisomies are the most common (49%). Within this category, **trisomy 16** is the most frequent.
   - Monosomy X (17%) is the most common single chromosomal abnormality. It is also known as Turner syndrome.
   - Polyploidies (19%)
   - Structural abnormalities (translocations, inversions) (10%)

10. What are other causes of spontaneous abortions?
    Box 25-1 provides a list of possible causes.

Box 25-1. Causes of Spontaneous Abortion

Genetic Causes (Chromosomal Abnormalities)
- Numeric (aneuploidy): trisomy, monosomy, polyploidy
- Structural: translocations, inversions

Uterine Conditions
- Congenital uterine anomalies
- Leiomyomas
- Intrauterine adhesions (synechiae)

Endocrine Disorders
- Hypothyroidism (uncontrolled)
- Diabetes mellitus (uncontrolled)
- Hyperprolactinemia

Autoimmune Disorders
- Antiphospholipid syndrome
- Lupus

Infections
- *Toxoplasma gondii*
- *Listeria monocytogenes*
- *Chlamydia trachomatis*
- *Ureaplasma urealyticum*
- *Mycoplasma hominis*
- Herpes simplex virus
- *Treponema pallidum*
- *Borrelia burgdorferi*
- *Neisseria gonorrhoeae*
- *Streptococcus agalactiae*

Medications and Substances
- Alcohol (>2 days/week)
- Heavy caffeine (>300 mg/day)
- Tobacco use
- Cocaine
- Anesthetic gases
- High doses of radiation
- Isotretinoin
- Methotrexate

---

11. What are the "most common" risk factors associated with spontaneous abortions?
    - Advanced maternal age
    - Previous spontaneous abortion
    - Maternal smoking of more than 10 cigarettes per day

12. What are the different types of abortions, and how is each type generally managed?
    Table 25-1 is an overview of treatment recommendations for each type of abortion.

13. How do I clinically differentiate among the different types of abortions when a woman presents with vaginal bleeding?
    A diagnostic flowchart is a helpful tool (Fig. 25-1).

Table 25-1. Management of Spontaneous Abortions

TYPE	DEFINITION	MANAGEMENT
Complete abortion	Spontaneous expulsion of all fetal and placental tissue from uterus; cervix closed on examination	Ultrasound scan to confirm an empty uterus; no further intervention necessary
Incomplete abortion	Passage of some but not all fetal or placental tissue from uterus; cervix dilated on examination	IV hydration, CBC, type and screen and crossmatch if necessary; if unstable, immediate suction curettage; if stable, medical management or suction curettage
Threatened abortion	Uterine bleeding <20 weeks of gestation without cervical dilation or effacement	Ultrasound scan to document fetal viability, close follow-up
Inevitable abortion	Uterine bleeding accompanied by cervical dilation, but no expulsion of fetal or placental tissue through cervical os	Expectant management; termination of the pregnancy can be considered, but normal ongoing pregnancy still possible
Missed abortion	Fetal death <20 weeks of gestation without expulsion of any fetal or placental tissue	Suction curettage or medical termination of pregnancy
Septic abortion	Any of the foregoing abortions, accompanied by fever and uterine infection	IV antibiotics followed by immediate suction curettage; considered an emergency

CBC, Complete blood count; IV, intravenous.

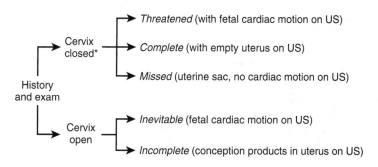

*Don't forget that ectopic pregnancy must be ruled out!

Figure 25-1. Diagnostic flowchart for spontaneous abortion. *US,* Ultrasound.

14. What is needed to evaluate a woman who presents with bleeding in early pregnancy?
    • History
      • Last menstrual period?
      • How much bleeding and for how long?
      • Cramping?
      • Passage of fetal tissue?
      • Fever, chills, abdominal tenderness?
    • Physical examination
      • Temperature and vital signs?
      • Abdominal tenderness?
      • Rebound or guarding?

- Speculum examination
  - Open cervix?
  - Active bleeding?
  - Passage of tissue?
  - Purulent discharge?
- Bimanual examination
  - Cervix: closed or dilated?
  - Positive or negative cervical motion tenderness?
  - Uterus: size, tenderness?
  - Adnexa: masses?
  - Tenderness?
- Laboratory tests
  - Complete blood count, platelets
  - Type and screen: Rh status; blood crossmatched if transfusion necessary
  - β-Human chorionic gonadotropin (β-hCG): serial levels needed to follow the trend of titers that can help make the diagnosis before detection of cardiac activity on ultrasound imaging
- **Imaging:** Transvaginal ultrasound (TVUS) is the most reliable and safe imaging modality to detect the earliest evidence of a gestation (see question 16).

15. What is the utility of quantitative hCG measurement in a patient with a threatened abortion?
In a normal early pregnancy, the hCG level should rise by approximately 66% every 48 hours and by approximately 53% at a minimum (99th centile). In patients with an abnormal pregnancy, the hCG level may still rise normally, rise slowly, plateau, or even fall.

16. What is the discriminatory zone?
Traditionally, a quantitative hCG level of 1500 mIU/mL has been called the **discriminatory zone** because this is the level at which one expects to visualize an intrauterine pregnancy if the pregnancy is normal. However, more recent data support a higher threshold, with 99% of gestational sacs visible with TVUS when the hCG level reaches 3500 mIU/mL. Absence of an intrauterine pregnancy on TVUS with an hCG level higher than the discriminatory zone is highly suggestive of an abnormal pregnancy (either an ectopic pregnancy or a nonviable intrauterine gestation).

17. Do Rh-negative women need Rho[D] immunoglobin for threatened, incomplete, and complete spontaneous abortions?
Yes. All Rh-negative women who experience pregnancy-related vaginal bleeding (including ectopic pregnancies) should receive Rho[D] immunoglobulin to prevent Rh isoimmunization. If the pregnancy is earlier than 12 weeks of gestation, minidose (50 μg) Rho[D] immunoglobin can be given if available. After 12 weeks of gestation, full dosing 300 μg is required.

18. How should women be followed after a complete abortion?
Their hCG levels should be followed on a weekly basis until hCG is no longer detectable. If the level plateaus, this should raise concern for a heterotopic pregnancy, retained placental tissue, or a gestational trophoblastic neoplasm. Heterotopic pregnancies occur when an intrauterine pregnancy and an ectopic pregnancy coexist. They are very rare, but women undergoing assisted reproductive technology (ART) are at higher risk compared with the general population.

19. What is the definition of recurrent pregnancy loss (RPL)?
RPL is defined as two or more failed pregnancies.

20. How often is an identifiable cause for RPL found?
An identifiable cause is found in approximately 50% of cases.

21. What does the initial workup for RPL include?
- Karyotype of both parents or products of conception (rule out genetic factors)
- Thyroid-stimulating hormone, glycosylated hemoglobin (HgbA1c), and prolactin (rule out endocrine factors)
- Ultrasound scan or saline-infusion sonogram (SIS) (rule out uterine abnormalities)
- Testing for antiphospholipid syndrome (APS; anticardiolipin antibodies, anti-β_2-glycoprotein antibodies, and lupus anticoagulant)

22. **What is the chance of a live birth after one, two, and three miscarriages?**
    - After one miscarriage, the chance of live birth is approximately 82%.
    - After two *consecutive* miscarriages, the chance of a live birth is approximately 73%.
    - After three *consecutive* losses, the chance of a live birth is 68%.

23. **What are the proposed mechanisms of antiphospholipid antibodies and lupus anticoagulant in RPL?**
    These antibodies block prostacyclin formation and result in thromboxane excess. (Prostacyclin is a vasodilator and inhibitor of platelet aggregation.) Thromboxane is a potent vasoconstrictor that promotes platelet aggregation, and its excess can increase the risk of thrombosis. Antiphospholipid antibodies and lupus anticoagulant may also bind to trophoblast cells and reduce proliferation, invasion, and the release of hCG.

24. **How are patients with APS treated?**
    Generally, patients with APS are placed on low-dose aspirin (50 to 100 mg) when conception is attempted. Subcutaneous unfractionated heparin or low-molecular-weight heparin (LMWH) is added on confirmation of intrauterine pregnancy.

25. **What is the role of empiric treatments for RPL?**
    In patients without a defined cause of RPL, the following empiric treatments have no significant benefit and are not recommended:
    - Aspirin
    - Anticoagulation (heparin)
    - Progesterone supplementation
    - Intravenous immunoglobulins

KEY POINTS: SPONTANEOUS ABORTIONS AND RECURRENT PREGNANCY LOSS

1. An abortion is defined as a termination or loss of pregnancy before 20 weeks of gestation (as calculated from the date of the last menstrual period) or delivery of a fetus weighing less than 500 g. Eighty percent of clinically recognized spontaneous abortions occur during the first trimester.
2. When differentiating the types of spontaneous abortions, it is important to consider whether the cervix is open or closed and whether any or all of the tissue has passed.
3. Fetal genetic abnormalities are the most common causes of spontaneous abortions, and they account for as many as 75% of spontaneous abortions in the first trimester. Autosomal trisomies are most common type of abnormality, but the *single* most common is monosomy X (Turner syndrome).
4. All Rh-negative pregnant women who experience uterine bleeding require Rho[D] immunoglobulin to prevent Rh isoimmunization.
5. RPL is defined as two or more failed pregnancies. Causes include genetic factors, uterine abnormalities, endocrine disorders, and APS.

BIBLIOGRAPHY

1. Barnhart KT, Sammel MD, Rinaudo PF, Zhou L, Hummel AC, Guo W. Symptomatic patients with an early viable intrauterine pregnancy: hCG curves redefined. *Obstet Gynecol.* 2004;104:50–55.
2. Doubilet PM, Benson CB, Bourne T, et al. Diagnostic criteria for nonviable pregnancy early in the first trimester. *N Engl J Med.* 2013;369:1443–1451.
3. Ku CW, Allen Jr JC, Malhotra R, et al. How can we better predict the risk of spontaneous miscarriage among women experiencing threatened miscarriage? *Gynecol Endocrinol.* 2015;31:647–651.
4. Practice Committee of the American Society for Reproductive Medicine. Definitions of infertility and recurrent pregnancy loss. *Fertil Steril.* 2008;89:1603.
5. Tulandi T, Al-Fozan H. *Definition and etiology of recurrent pregnancy loss.* UpToDate; 2014. Available by subscription at www.uptodate.com. Accessed October 27, 2015.
6. Tulandi T, Al-Fozan H. *Spontaneous abortion: risk factors, etiology, clinical manifestations, and diagnostic evaluation* UpToDate; 2014. Available by subscription at www.uptodate.com. Accessed October 27, 2015.
7. Vitzthum VJ, Spielvogel H, Thornburg J, West B. Prospective study of early pregnancy loss in humans. *Fertil Steril.* 2006;86:373–379.
8. Wang X, Chen C, Wang L, Chen D, Guang W, French J. Conception, early pregnancy loss, and time to clinical pregnancy: a population-based prospective study. *Fertil Steril.* 2003;79:577–584.
9. Yakut S, Toru HS, Cetin Z, et al. Chromosome abnormalities identified in 457 spontaneous abortions and their histopathological findings. *Turk Patoloji Derg.* 2015;31:111–118.

CHAPTER 26

HIRSUTISM AND POLYCYSTIC OVARIAN SYNDROME

Danny Younes, MD, and Travis W. McCoy, MD

1. **What is the definition of hirsutism, and what is virilization?**
   Hirsutism is excessive terminal hair growth in a male-pattern anatomic distribution generally attributed to hyperandrogenemia. It affects 5% to 10% of reproductive age women. Virilization describes the more severe signs and symptoms of excess androgens, characterized by clitoromegaly, temporal balding, voice deepening, and breast atrophy. This is different from hypertrichosis, which is an uncommon general increase in vellus body hair.

2. **What are the three types of body hair?**
   1. **Lanugo hair:** thin and faintly pigmented hair often found on neonates
   2. **Vellus hair:** fine, soft, nonpigmented hair found in most adult body regions
   3. **Terminal hair:** long, coarse, pigmented hair found at the scalp, axilla, pubic area of adults, and the male beard and chest

3. **What causes hirsutism?**
   - Increased exposure to androgens: secondary to exogenous androgen exposure, increased adrenal androgen production, increased ovarian androgen production, or alterations in binding globulins
   - Increased end-organ androgen sensitivity: secondary to increased 5α-reductase activity at the follicle (converts testosterone to more potent dihydrotestosterone [DHT])
   Androgens interact with the hair follicle, thus leading to a transformation from vellus to terminal hair.

4. **Which androgens are produced by the body?**
   - Ovary: testosterone (25%), androstenedione (50%), dehydroepiandrosterone (DHEA) (20%)
   - Adrenal gland: testosterone (25%), DHEA (50%), DHEA sulfate (DHEA-S) (100%)
   - Peripheral tissue conversion (adipose/skin): testosterone from androstenedione (50%), DHEA from DHEAS (30%), and DHT from testosterone

5. **What are the modulators of androgen action?**
   - Sex hormone–binding globulin (SHBG) (80%) and albumin (20%): bind to circulating androgens, thereby decreasing the amount of free androgens (only free androgens can act on target tissues)
   - 5α-reductase: converts testosterone to DHT (more potent and active) at the level of the skin

6. **What is the Ferriman-Gallwey scoring system?**
   A standardized grading system for scoring hirsutism. It is based on the distribution and degree of hair growth. A score less than 8 is normal; a score greater than 15 is severe. Providers can also consider patient-reported qualification of hirsutism ("patient-important hirsutism").

7. **What is the differential diagnosis for hirsutism?**
   - **Polycystic ovarian syndrome (PCOS)** (82% of cases): irregular menses, insulin resistance, obesity
   - **Idiopathic hyperandrogenemia:** normal menses, increased androgens
   - **Idiopathic hirsutism:** normal menses, normal androgen levels; likely caused by increased 5α-reductase activity in the skin
   - **Nonclassic congenital adrenal hyperplasia (NCCAH):** adult-onset increase in adrenal androgens, increased 17-hydroxyprogesterone (17-OH progesterone)
   - **Classic congenital adrenal hyperplasia (CAH):** increased adrenal androgens, ambiguous genitalia at birth, increased 17-OH progesterone
   - **Cushing syndrome:** central obesity, moon facies, violaceous striae, hypertension, high 24-hour urine free cortisol
   - **Hyperprolactinemia:** galactorrhea, amenorrhea, increased prolactin
   - **Androgen-secreting tumor (ovarian or adrenal):** sudden-onset hirsutism and virilization; very rare

8. **How should a patient with excessive hair growth initially be evaluated?**
   Workup is directed by the history and physical examination findings. Laboratory tests include total testosterone (>200 ng/dL suggests a tumor), DHEA-S (>700 µg/dL suggests an adrenal tumor), 17-OH progesterone (drawn during follicular phase of cycle, normally elevated after ovulation to rule out CAH), and prolactin.

9. **Which different medical treatments are available for hirsutism, and what are their mechanisms of action and adverse effects?**
   Table 26-1 is an overview of treatment options. Initial treatment is usually with a combined oral contraceptive pill (OCP). OCPs lower free ovarian and adrenal androgens by increasing SHBG. To block the effect of androgens, antiandrogens can be used in addition to OCPs. Spironolactone and finasteride are the most commonly recommended antiandrogens. Flutamide carries a risk of hepatotoxicity. Eflornithine is a topical cream. Because antiandrogens are teratogenic and can feminize male fetuses, they should not be used without OCPs.

Table 26-1. Medical Treatments for Hirsutism

TREATMENT	MECHANISM	SIDE EFFECTS
Combined oral contraceptive pill (OCP)	Increased SHBG Decreased ovarian androgen production	Headache GI upset
Spironolactone	Competitive inhibitor of androgen-receptors	Hyperkalemia **Teratogenicity**
Finasteride	5α-reductase inhibitor, targeted to type 2 isoenzyme	Hepatotoxicity **Teratogenicity**
Flutamide	Androgen receptor antagonist	Leukopenia Hepatotoxicity Photosensitivity **Teratogenicity**
Eflornithine	Topical; inhibitor of ornithine decarboxylase	Acne Erythema Burning sensation
Glucocorticoids*	Suppressors of adrenal androgen production	Weight gain Adrenal suppression

GI, Gastrointestinal; *SHBG*, sex hormone–binding globulin.
*Used only in cases of congenital adrenal hyperplasia.

10. **What adjuvant therapies are available?**
    - Short-term: shaving, epilation (plucking or waxing), chemical depilation (bleaching)
    - Long-term: electrolysis (galvanic or thermal), laser epilation, photoepilation, weight loss

11. **How soon is an effect on hirsutism seen once medical treatment has begun?**
    Treatment effect is usually not seen for 3 to 6 months, and it can often take longer. For this reason, medical treatment is more effective, to prevent progression of hirsutism.

12. **What is PCOS, and what causes it?**
    PCOS is a disorder characterized by chronic anovulation and increased androgen production, often associated with other metabolic derangements such as insulin resistance, hyperlipidemia, and obesity. It is considered a complex metabolic disorder, with numerous genetic and environmental factors interacting and contributing to the pathophysiologic features.

13. **What are the criteria for diagnosing PCOS?**
    PCOS is a diagnosis of exclusion; other underlying disorders must be ruled out first. Two sets of criteria are accepted:
    - **Rotterdam Consensus criteria (2003):** requires two or more of the following: anovulation or oligoovulation, clinical or biochemical evidence of hyperandrogenism, polycystic ovaries on ultrasound examination
    - **Androgen Excess and PCOS Society (2006):** requires evidence of hyperandrogenism with ovarian dysfunction

14. What findings are commonly associated with PCOS?
    - Irregular menses
    - Perimenarchal onset of symptoms
    - Insulin resistance (more pronounced in obese women)
    - Mildly elevated DHEAS and testosterone
    - Obesity (60% of patients)
    - Polycystic ovaries on ultrasound scan (not diagnostic, can be seen in women without PCOS as well)

15. What are the major disorders that should be ruled out before making a diagnosis of PCOS, and what tests can be used?
    - Thyroid dysfunction: check thyroid-stimulating hormone
    - Hyperprolactinemia: check prolactin
    - Ovarian failure: check follicle-stimulating hormone
    - Late-onset CAH (21-hydroxylase deficiency): check 17-OH progesterone during the follicular phase
    - Cushing syndrome, ovarian and adrenal neoplasms: total serum testosterone is markedly elevated

16. What are two mechanisms that lead to excessive androgen production by ovarian theca cells in PCOS?
    Hyperinsulinemia and excessive amplitude or increase pulse frequency of luteinizing hormone from the anterior pituitary.

17. How is PCOS related to obesity?
    PCOS involves many positive feedback mechanisms. Insulin resistance worsens hyperandrogenism, and both promote obesity. Obesity, in turn, worsens insulin resistance. Androgens and insulin resistance lower SHBG production in the liver, thus causing even greater amounts of free circulating androgens. Treatment should be directed at breaking these feedback loops by lowering androgens, increasing SHBG, and reducing insulin resistance.

18. What are the long-term consequences of PCOS?
    - Premature development of insulin-resistant diabetes
    - Hyperlipidemia
    - Hirsutism or acne
    - Anovulatory infertility
    - Increased risk of endometrial hyperplasia or endometrial cancer
    Long-term management should address these problems through the regulation of menses and treatment of any insulin-resistance, hyperlipidemia, and hirsutism.

KEY POINTS: HIRSUTISM AND POLYCYSTIC OVARIAN SYNDROME

1. Treatment of hirsutism should begin early to prevent progression. Medical treatments take months to produce a visible response and are more effective in preventing worsening of the condition.
2. Antiandrogen therapies are largely teratogenic and can feminize male fetuses; they should be used in conjunction with combined OCPs to increase efficacy and prevent pregnancy.
3. Treatment for PCOS should focus on reducing androgens and minimizing metabolic risks. Regulation of menses is critical to prevent endometrial hyperplasia and carcinoma.

BIBLIOGRAPHY

1. Azziz R, Sanchez LA, Knochenhauer ES, et al. Androgen excess in women: experience with over 1000 consecutive patients. *J Clin Endocrinol Metab*. 2004;89:453–462.
2. Bode D, Seehusen D, Baird D. Hirsutism in women. *Am Fam Physician*. 2012;85:373–380.
3. Carmina E, Rosato F, Jannì A, Rizzo M, Longo RA. Extensive clinical experience: relative prevalence of different androgen excess disorders in 950 women referred because of clinical hyperandrogenism. *J Clin Endocrinol Metab*. 2006;91:2–6.
4. Carr BR, Breslau NA, Givens C, Byrd W, et al. Oral contraceptive pills, gonadotropin-releasing hormone agonists, or use in combination for treatment of hirsutism: a clinical research center study. *J Clin Endocrinol Metab*. 1995;80:1169–1178.
5. Fauser BC, Diedrich K, Howles CM, et al. Contemporary genetic technologies and female reproduction. *Hum Reprod Update*. 2012;18:231.
6. Martin KA, Chang RJ, Ehrmann DA, et al. Evaluation and treatment of hirsutism in premenopausal women: an Endocrine Society clinical practice guideline. *J Clin Endocrinol Metab*. 2008;93:1105–1120.

7. Rotterdam ESHRE/ASRM-Sponsored PCOS consensus workshop group. Revised 2003 consensus on diagnostic criteria and long-term health risks related to polycystic ovary syndrome (PCOS). *Hum Reprod.* 2004;19:41–47.
8. Strauss JF. Some new thoughts on the pathophysiology and genetics of polycystic ovary syndrome. *Ann N Y Acad Sci.* 2003;997:42–48.
9. Teede H, Deeks A, Moran L. Polycystic ovary syndrome: a complex condition with psychological, reproductive and metabolic manifestations that impacts on health across the lifespan. *BMC Med.* 2010;8:41.

CHAPTER 27

PRECANCEROUS LESIONS OF THE LOWER GENITAL TRACT

Lisa Garcia, MD

1. **What is cervical dysplasia, and why is it clinically significant?**
   Cervical dysplasia is a precancerous lesion that, if left untreated, can progress to higher-grade lesions or cervical cancer. The progression to cervical cancer is a slow process, taking years to occur. Older terminology classified cervical dysplasia into cervical intraepithelial neoplasia (CIN) 1, 2, or 3; recommendations made in 2012, however, classify it into either low-grade or high-grade squamous intraepithelial lesions (LSIL and HSIL, respectively).

2. **What are risk factors for cervical dysplasia?**
   Infection with the human papillomavirus (HPV) is a necessary precursor for the development of both cervical dysplasia and most cases of cervical cancer (both squamous cell carcinoma and adenocarcinoma). Therefore, early coitarche and increasing numbers of sexual partners raise the risk of duration and frequency of HPV exposure, respectively, and increase the risk of cervical dysplasia. The most important non–HPV-related risk factor is smoking.

3. **How does infection with HPV result in cervical dysplasia?**
   HPV strains fall into two broad categories: low-risk strains and high-risk strains. Low-risk HPV strains (6, 11, 40, 42, 43, 44, 53, 54, 61, 72, 73, and 81) are associated with anogenital warts and low-grade cervical dysplasia (CIN 1/LSIL). High-risk HPV strains (16, 18, 31, 33, 35, 39, 45, 51, 52, 56, 58, 59, and 68) are responsible for high-grade cervical dysplasia and cancer. The virus integrates into the host cell's genome and causes loss of transcriptional regulation and overexpression of oncoproteins E6 and E7. HPV E6 protein binds to p53, and HPV E7 protein binds to retinoblastoma protein (Rb), thus disabling these tumor suppressor genes and ultimately leading to uncontrolled promotion of cell cycle progression. Most women infected with HPV, however, do not develop high-grade dysplasia or cervical cancer.

4. **How is HPV transmitted?**
   HPV is transmitted through sexual contact. *It is the most common sexually transmitted infection,* with 75% to 80% of persons infected by the age of 50 years. Barrier methods of contraception do not completely protect against transmission.

5. **What is the natural history of HPV infection?**
   HPV infection prevalence is highest in women 20 to 24 years old, and prevalence decreases with age. HPV infections are thought to be transient and cleared by immune-competent hosts within 6 to 24 months. Reactivation is possible, particularly in older persons. Infection with multiple strains of the virus is also possible. During transient infections, HPV can lead to cellular abnormalities of the cervix that resolve with clearance of the virus. Persistent infections increase the risk for high-grade dysplasia.

6. **Are any effective primary prevention strategies available to reduce HPV infection?**
   Three HPV vaccines are currently approved by the Food and Drug Administration (FDA): a bivalent vaccine against HPV types 16 and 18, a quadrivalent vaccine against types 16, 18, 6, and 11, and a vaccine against nine HPV strains (6, 11, 16, 18, 31, 33, 45, 52, and 58). In clinical trials, the efficacy of these vaccines in the prevention of high-grade dysplasia was 93% to 100% in HPV-naïve populations.

7. **Who should be vaccinated against HPV?**
   The Centers for Disease Control and Prevention (CDC) Advisory Committee on Immunization Practices (ACIP) recommends that all children—boys and girls—11 to 12 years old should be routinely offered HPV vaccination. Vaccination may begin as early as age 9 years and extend to age 26 years in women and age 21 years in men. Although 2015 ACIP guidelines state that men *may* be vaccinated through

age 26 years, it is explicitly recommended that men who have sex with men, or men who are immunocompromised, *should* be vaccinated through age 26 years.

8. **If someone is already HPV positive, does HPV vaccination still have a benefit?**
Because it is unlikely for patients to become infected with all the strains covered by the available vaccines, it is recommended that HPV-positive persons still be vaccinated. Vaccination does not, however, help clear an existing HPV infection.

9. **What screening tests are available for cervical dysplasia and cervical cancer?**
The three methods to screen for cervical dysplasia or cervical cancer are (1) cervical cytology (such as with a Papanicolaou [Pap] smear), (2) co-testing (cervical cytology combined with HPV testing), and (3) primary HPV testing. In resource-poor settings where cervical cytology or HPV testing is not available, visual inspection can be performed (aided by the use of various topical solutions that can be applied to the cervix to help identify areas of dysplasia).

10. **How frequently should screening for cervical dysplasia and cancer be performed?**
Frequency of cervical cancer screening depends on the method used. If cytology alone is used, testing should be performed every 3 years. If high-risk HPV co-testing is employed, testing can be extended to every 5 years. Primary HPV testing is performed every 3 years.

11. **At what age should cervical cancer screening begin?**
Cervical cytology alone should be used to screen women starting at age 21 years, irrespective of the age of coitarche or other risk factors. Specific guidelines dictate when co-testing or primary HPV testing can be initiated.

12. **What follow-up is recommended after an abnormal Pap smear or co-testing result?**
Abnormal Pap smears or co-testing results are managed according to guidelines set forth by the American Society for Colposcopy and Cervical Pathology (ASCCP). Depending on the severity of the abnormal result or the age of the patient, follow-up involves repeat cytologic examination or co-testing or, alternatively, colposcopy.

13. **What is colposcopy, and how is it used?**
Colposcopy is the visual inspection of the cervix with a colposcope, which is a specialized type of microscope. Colposcopy can also be used to evaluate the vulva, vagina, and perianal region. During colposcopy, topical solutions are applied to the cervix to aid in the detection of cervical dysplasia or cancer. Any areas that appear abnormal are examined by biopsy to obtain a histologic diagnosis.

14. **What region of the cervix is most vulnerable to the development of dysplasia?**
High-grade cervical dysplasia arises at the squamocolumnar junction (SCJ), which is the site of squamous metaplasia—the transition of columnar epithelium found in the endocervix to squamous epithelium found in the ectocervix. For a colposcopic evaluation to be considered complete or "satisfactory," the SCJ needs to be seen in its entirety.

15. **How do abnormal epithelial tissues appear on colposcopic examination?**
Abnormal epithelium reflects light after application of dilute acetic acid because of its high cellular count and increased nuclear content, thus giving it an opaque appearance. Patterns of abnormal ectocervical epithelium are described as acetowhite, and vascular abnormalities such as mosaicism and punctation can also be visualized. Early invasive cancer may have these abnormalities in a larger lesion with ulceration, increased vascularity, or areas of necrosis.

16. **If cervical dysplasia is found at the time of colposcopy, what treatment options are available?**
Low-grade cervical dysplasia can be safely observed without treatment; the risk of progression to cervical cancer in these cases is less than 1%. In the setting of high-grade dysplasia, treatment is recommended. Options can be categorized as either ablative or excisional. Both have similar efficacy, but not all patients are appropriate candidates for ablative therapies. Ablation should not be performed if discordance exists between the Pap smear result and the colposcopic findings (e.g., high-grade dysplasia found on a Pap smear but no evidence seen during colposcopy), the colposcopic examination is unsatisfactory, or the area of dysplasia is located within the endocervical canal.

17. **What are the risks associated with treatment for cervical dysplasia?**
Persistent disease or incomplete excision, cervical stenosis, and anatomic distortion are all risks of excision. The relationship between excisional procedures and preterm birth is controversial; historically,

these procedures were believed to increase the risk. More recent studies, however, suggest that the presence of dysplasia, rather than its treatment, increases the risk.

18. **When is a hysterectomy indicated for treatment of precancerous disease of the cervix?**
Hysterectomy is not a first-line treatment option for cervical dysplasia. It may be considered when dysplasia is present at the margins of a conization specimen and repeat excision would result in distorted cervical anatomy (which would make surveillance with colposcopy difficult).

19. **After treatment for dysplasia, how can recurrence be detected?**
Specific management algorithms for the follow-up of patients with high-grade dysplasia are available. HPV co-testing is typically recommended 1 and 2 years after treatment, with subsequent colposcopy if either cytologic findings or HPV test results are abnormal.

20. **What considerations should be made for a pregnant patient with abnormal cytologic findings?**
Pregnancy does not change the natural history of HPV infection or alter the risk of disease progression. The diagnostic management of abnormal cytologic findings in pregnancy is the same as for non-pregnant women, with the exception that endocervical sampling is not performed. For precancerous lesions, vaginal delivery and delay of treatment until after delivery are recommended. If a suggestion of invasive cancer exists, punch, wedge, or cone biopsy should be obtained. Increased vascularity of the cervix during pregnancy may increase procedure-associated blood loss in these cases.

21. **What is the importance of human immunodeficiency virus (HIV) status in precancerous disease?**
The prevalence of abnormal Pap smears, condyloma, and precancerous disease corresponds to the severity of immunodeficiency. HIV-infected women also have higher rates of persistence, recurrence, and progression of precancerous disease. Therefore, women are screened at 6-month intervals during the first year after their HIV diagnosis and yearly thereafter. More frequent screening is also recommended for women who have had a solid organ transplant, because of the required use of immunosuppressant medication.

22. **What are the risk factors for vaginal intraepithelial neoplasia (VAIN)?**
VAIN is found in women who have had cervical or vulvar intraepithelial neoplasia, have received previous radiation therapy for cervical cancer, or are immunosuppressed by medication or HIV infection. HPV has been implicated as the cause of vaginal neoplasia, and VAIN may be found in association with cervical or vulvar dysplasia.

23. **How can VAIN be diagnosed and treated?**
Most lesions are detected by colposcopy in the upper one third of the vagina and appear as acetowhite changes or areas of abnormal vasculature. Lugol solution may stain the lesions yellow. For lesions of VAIN II or greater, treatment consists of excisional or ablative therapy.

24. **What are the hallmarks of vulvar intraepithelial neoplasia (VIN)?**
VIN is classified as low grade or high grade with increasing degrees of atypia in the epithelium. Precancerous disease is associated with sexually transmitted infections, HIV infection, smoking, and other lower genital tract neoplasia. HPV is often found in VIN lesions.

25. **How does VIN manifest?**
Patients usually complain of chronic itching. Lesions may single or multiple and red, pigmented, or white. They can be flat or raised, and they can also involve the perianal region.

26. **How is VIN managed?**
After diagnosis is confirmed with punch biopsy, treatment options include wide local excision, laser ablation, or imiquimod. Recurrence is common, and reevaluation with colposcopy should be performed every 6 months.

KEY POINTS: PRECANCEROUS DISEASE OF THE LOWER GENITAL TRACT

1. HPV causes genital dysplasia and can lead to invasive cervical cancer.
2. The HPV vaccine prevents high-grade cervical dysplasia in 93% to 100% of HPV-naïve patients.
3. The SCJ must be viewed in its entirety for a colposcopic examination to be considered satisfactory.
4. High-grade cervical, vaginal, and vulvar dysplasia can be treated with either excision or ablation.

BIBLIOGRAPHY

1. American College of Obstetricians and Gynecologists. Screening for cervical cancer. ACOG practice bulletin no. 131. *Obstet Gynecol.* 2012;120:1222–1238.
2. American College of Obstetricians and Gynecologists. Management of abnormal cervical cancer screening test results and cervical cancer precursors. ACOG practice bulletin no. 140. *Obstet Gynecol.* 2013;122:1338–1367.
3. Centers for Disease Control and Prevention. Recommended Adult Immunization Schedule. Available at http://www.cdc.gov/vaccines/schedules/downloads/adult/adult-combined-schedule.pdf; 2015. Accessed October 28, 2015.
4. Diaz-Rosario LA, Kabawat SA. Performance of a fluid based, thin-layer Papanicolaou smear method in the clinical setting of an independent laboratory and an outpatient screening population in New England. *Arch Pathol Lab Med.* 1998;123:817–821.
5. Singer A, Monaghan J. *Lower Genital Tract Precancer: Colposcopy, Pathology, and Treatment.* 2nd ed. Oxford: Blackwell Science; 2000.
6. Solomon D, Schiffman M, Tarone R. ALTS Study Group. Comparison of three management strategies for patients with atypical squamous cells of undetermined significance: baseline results from a randomized trial. *J Natl Cancer Inst.* 2001;193:293–299.
7. Van Seters M, van Beurden M, ten Kate FJ, et al. Treatment of vulvar intraepithelial neoplasia with topical imiquimod. *N Engl J Med.* 2008;358:1465–1473.

CHAPTER 28

VULVAR AND VAGINAL CANCER

Ramy Eskander, MD

1. **How is vulvar dysplasia different from vulvar cancer?**
   Dysplasia refers to abnormally differentiated cells that are contained entirely within the epithelium and above the basement membrane. *Cancer* invades through the basement membrane.

2. **What is the incidence of vulvar cancer?**
   According to the American Cancer Society, an estimated 5150 new cases of vulvar cancer will be diagnosed in 2015; this number will account for 4% of gynecologic cancers. Approximately 1080 deaths will be caused by the disease, yielding a mortality rate of roughly 21%. The incidence appears to have increased during the last century; however, this may reflect the increasing average life span of women.

3. **What is the most common histologic type of vulvar cancer, and what are the other possible forms?**
   Squamous cell carcinoma is the most commonly diagnosed vulvar malignant disease and represents 85% of all vulvar neoplasms. It has a bimodal age distribution. A keratinizing subtype occurs in older patients (>60 years) and is related to chronic lichen sclerosus. In younger patients (30 to 40 years old), a warty or "bowenoid" subtype related to infection with human papillomavirus (HPV) types 16, 18, and 33 tends to occur.
   Other histologic tumor types include melanoma (5%), sarcoma (2%), basal cell carcinoma (2%), extramammary Paget disease of the vulva (<1%), and Bartholin gland carcinoma (<1%).

4. **What are risk factors for vulvar cancer?**
   Advanced age (the highest incidence occurs between ages 65 and 75 years), lichen sclerosus, obesity, hypertension, and diabetes are more commonly seen in patients with the keratinizing form of squamous cell vulvar cancer. Multiple risk factors related to persistent HPV infection (e.g., smoking) affect the risk of developing the warty subtype. For more information on the mechanism by which HPV causes dysplasia, see Chapter 27.

5. **What are the symptoms of vulvar cancer?**
   - Pruritus (most common)
   - Palpable mass
   - Pain
   - Bleeding
   - Ulceration
   - Dysuria

   In most patients, symptoms are mild and persist for months (or even years) before medical attention is sought.

6. **How is vulvar cancer diagnosed?**
   Diagnosis is made by vulvar biopsy; unfortunately, this is often delayed by weeks or months while topical medical treatments are attempted.

7. **What is the pattern of spread in vulvar cancer?**
   Most vulvar cancers behave similarly: relatively indolent growth followed by metastasis through lymphatic tissue. Lymphatic flow in the vulva runs anteriorly from the labia toward the mons, then laterally to the ipsilateral groin. The most common site of initial metastasis is to the superficial inguinal lymph nodes. From there, spread is usually through the fossa ovalis to the deep femoral lymph nodes, then proximally to the iliac chains. Lymph channels do cross the midline, and centrally occurring lesions have an increased incidence of contralateral groin involvement.
   Lymphatics in the anterior introitus and clitoris drain under the symphysis directly into the pelvic lymph channels, but pelvic metastasis without inguinal disease is exceedingly rare, and these lymphatics are of little clinical significance.

8. How is vulvar cancer staged?

Table 28-1 shows the International Federation of Gynecology and Obstetrics (FIGO) staging system. Vulvar cancer is surgically staged by a modified radical vulvectomy approach; the primary tumor is excised with lateral margins of at least 1 cm and down to the deep fascia of the urogenital diaphragm. When indicated, inguinofemoral lymphadenectomy (also known as "groin dissection") to assess the status of groin lymph nodes is also performed.

Table 28-1. International Federation of Gynecology and Obstetrics Staging of Vulvar Cancer*

Stage I: Tumor confined to the vulva

IA	Lesions ≤2 cm, confined to the vulva or perineum and with stromal invasion ≤1.0 mm
IB	Lesions >2 cm, or with stromal invasion >1.0 mm, confined to the vulva or perineum

Stage II: Tumor with extension to adjacent perineal structures (one third lower urethra, one third lower vagina, anus)

Stage III: Tumor with positive inguinofemoral lymph nodes

IIIA (i)	With one lymph node metastasis ≥5 mm
IIIA (ii)	With one or two lymph node metastases <5 mm
IIIB (i)	With two or more lymph node metastases ≥5 mm
IIIB (ii)	With three or more lymph node metastases <5 mm
IIIC	Any positive node or nodes with extracapsular spread

Stage IV: Tumor invading other regional (two third upper urethra, two thirds upper vagina), or distant structures

IVA (i)	Tumor invading upper urethral or vaginal mucosa, bladder mucosa, or rectal mucosa or fixed to pelvic bone
IVA (ii)	Fixed or ulcerated inguinofemoral lymph nodes involved by tumor
IVB	Any distant metastasis including pelvic lymph nodes

*The depth of invasion is defined as the measurement of the tumor from the epithelial stroma junction of the adjacent most superficial dermal papilla to the deepest point of invasion.

---

9. When is groin dissection necessary?

Ipsilateral groin dissection is required for lesions that are unilateral (>1 cm from midline) and invade more than 1 mm or are more than 2 cm in width. If these lymph nodes are negative for cancer, the risk for isolated contralateral metastasis is less than 1%. If any of the ipsilateral nodes are positive for cancer, the contralateral groin must also be surgically evaluated. Lesions that are less than 1 cm from the midline require bilateral dissection if groin evaluation is required.

In positive cases, prospective randomized trials have found that postoperative radiation to the groin and hemipelvis is superior to pelvic lymph node dissection.

10. How is vulvar cancer treated?

Surgical intervention remains the primary therapy for vulvar cancer. Traditionally, radical vulvar excision with bilateral inguinal and pelvic lymph node dissection was the standard of practice for all invasive lesions. This procedure provided excellent survival rates, but it carried considerable morbidity and was profoundly disfiguring. Wound breakdown rates could approach 50%. More recently, a more conservative approach through modified radical vulvectomy has demonstrated similar efficacy with substantially reduced morbidity. Sentinel lymph node biopsy instead of full inguinofemoral lymphadenectomy has also been increasingly used to help reduce morbidity.

11. Does a role exist for radiation therapy or chemotherapy?

Lesions demonstrating poor prognostic features can be treated with combination therapies using surgery, radiation, and chemotherapy. Radiation therapy is reserved predominantly for locally advanced disease. Chemotherapy is useful for disease that has metastasized out of the pelvis, when neither surgery nor radiation can address all the lesions. Response rates to chemotherapy alone are up to 30%, but the duration of response is generally short. A current area of investigation is use of chemotherapy as a radiation-sensitizing agent.

12. **What precautions should be taken when a lesion is near the urethra?**
Effort should be made to leave the urethra intact. If necessary, the distal 1 to 2 cm of the urethra can be excised without impairing continence. Care should be taken that the surgical repair is without tension; otherwise, stricture formation during and after healing may result.

13. **What are 5-year survival rates for vulvar cancer?**
    * Stage I: more than 90%
    * Stage II: 81%
    * Stage III: 48%
    * Stage IV: 15%

In most series, the presence of even one lymph node metastasis decreases survival rates in all stages by 50% or more. The presence of positive deep (pelvic) nodal metastases imparts an even more ominous prognosis, with fewer than 20% of patients surviving 5 years.

14. **What is vulvar Paget disease?**
Paget disease of the vulva is an intraepithelial lesion characterized by a superficial, velvety thickening with areas of intermixed redness and leukoplakia (the so-called "cake-icing effect"). Underlying adenocarcinomas were once reported in up to 20% of cases, thus prompting recommendations for radical excision. However, more recent studies suggest a much lower incidence; most lesions are now considered curable by simple local excision. Sampling of underlying tissue is generally performed to exclude occult cancer.

15. **What is the incidence of vaginal cancer?**
According to the American Cancer Society, an estimated 4070 new cases of vaginal cancer will be diagnosed in 2015, accounting for 1% to 3% of gynecologic cancers. Approximately 910 deaths will occur, yielding a mortality rate of roughly 22%. Secondary cancers of the vagina (from cervix, endometrium, vulva, bladder, urethra, and other locations) are more common than are primary vaginal malignant tumors.

16. **What are risk factors for vaginal cancer?**
Although vaginal epithelium is more stable than cervical epithelium and is less susceptible to HPV infection, vaginal cancer is associated with HPV infection. Exposure to diethylstilbestrol (DES) in utero is associated with an increased incidence of vaginal adenocarcinomas, specifically of the clear cell subtype.

17. **In what age group is vaginal cancer most common?**
Vaginal cancer has been reported in every decade of life, but it is predominantly a disease of older women; approximately 70% of patients are diagnosed after the age of 70 years. Two notable exceptions to this rule are sarcoma botryoides and vaginal endodermal sinus tumors, both of which demonstrate a predilection for infants and children.

18. **How does vaginal cancer manifest?**
The most common complaint is vaginal discharge, either with or without bleeding. Difficulty with voiding or intercourse is also reported because of the tendency of this cancer to restrict the normal caliber and plasticity of the vagina canal. The diagnosis is often delayed as a result of the subtle onset of symptoms, especially in women who are no longer sexually active.

19. **What is the pattern of spread in vaginal cancer?**
As with cancers of the cervix and vulva, the route of metastasis is primarily through lymph channels. Depending on the location of the lesion, vaginal cancer may spread through the pelvic or inguinal chain. In general, the distal third of the vagina drains to the femoral and external iliac nodes, the middle third drains to the internal iliac chain, and the proximal third drains to the common iliacs and presacral areas. However, any pelvic or inguinal lymph node chain may be primarily affected by extensive anastomoses among vaginal lymphatic channels.

20. **How is vaginal cancer staged?**
Table 28-2 provides an overview of vaginal cancer staging systems. As with cervical cancer, vaginal cancer is clinically staged. The FIGO clinical staging system permits use of physical examination, cystoscopy, proctoscopy, chest and skeletal radiography, and groin lymph node biopsy results.

Table 28-2. Vaginal Cancer Stages

TYPE	TNM	FIGO	DEFINITION
Primary tumor	TX		Primary tumor cannot be assessed
	T0		No evidence of primary tumor
	Tis	0	Carcinoma in situ
	T1	I	Tumor confined to the vagina
	T2	II	Tumor invading paravaginal tissues but not to the pelvic wall
	T3	III	Tumor extending to the pelvic wall
	T4	IVa	Tumor invading mucosa of the bladder or rectum or extending beyond the true pelvis
	—	IVb	Distant metastasis
Regional lymph nodes	NX	—	Regional lymph nodes cannot be assessed
	N0	—	No regional lymph node metastasis
Upper two-thirds of vagina	N1	—	Pelvic node metastasis
Lower one third of vagina	N1	—	Unilateral inguinal node metastasis
	N2	—	Bilateral inguinal node metastases
Distant metastasis	MX	—	Presence of distant metastasis cannot be assessed
	M0	—	No distant metastasis
	M1	—	Distant metastasis

FIGO, International Federation of Gynecology and Obstetrics; TNM, tumor, node, metastasis.

21. How is vaginal cancer treated?

Both stage I and in situ lesions can be managed with surgical excision. In some patients a radical hysterectomy can be performed to obtain adequate margins.

When deep invasion is present, external beam radiation to the whole pelvis is initially given to reduce the primary tumor volume and treat regional lymphatics. External beam therapy is then followed by intracavitary or interstitial treatment, which allows cytotoxic doses to be delivered directly to the tumor while minimizing collateral damage to surrounding tissues. Persistent or recurrent disease can be treated with exenterative procedures if no distant spread is noted and negative margins are thought to be achievable.

22. What are 5-year survival rates for vaginal cancer?
- Stage I: 75% to 95%
- Stage II: 50% to 80%
- Stage III: 30% to 60%
- Stage IV: 15% to 50%

KEY POINTS: VULVAR AND VAGINAL CANCER

1. Vulvar cancer is predominantly squamous cell and spreads through the lymphatics to the superficial inguinal nodes.
2. Vulvar cancer is diagnosed by biopsy and is surgically staged.
3. Paget disease may involve underlying adenocarcinoma; therefore, local excision is recommended.
4. Vaginal cancer is most commonly a secondary site of another cancer.

BIBLIOGRAPHY

1. American Cancer Society. *What are the key statistics about vaginal cancer?*, 2015. Available at http://www.cancer.org/cancer/vaginalcancer/detailedguide/vaginal-cancer-key-statistics.
2. American Cancer Society. *What are the key statistics about vulvar cancer?*, 2015. Available at http://www.cancer.org/cancer/vulvarcancer/detailedguide/vulvar-cancer-key-statistics.

3. Ferri F. *Ferri's Clinical Advisor 2016*. Philadelphia: Elsevier; 2016:1313–1314. e1.

4. Homesley HD, Bundy BN, Sedlis A, Adcock L. Radiation therapy versus pelvic node resection for carcinoma of the vulva with positive groin nodes. *Obstet Gynecol*. 1986;68:733–740.

5. Lanneau GS, Argenta PA, Lanneau MS, et al. Vulvar cancer in younger women: demographic features and outcome evaluation. *Am J Obstet Gynecol*. 2009;200:645.

6. Mutch DG. The new FIGO staging system for cancers of the vulva, cervix, endometrium and sarcomas. *Gynecol Oncol*. 2009;115:325–328.

7. Niederhuber J, Armitage J, Doroshow J, Kastan M, Tepper J, Abeloff M. Abeloff's Clinical Oncology. 5th ed. 87. Philadelphia: Saunders; 2014:1534–1574. e8.

CHAPTER 29

CERVICAL CANCER

Ramy Eskander, MD

1. **What is the difference between cervical dysplasia and cervical cancer?**
   Cervical dysplasia refers to a neoplastic process that has not violated the basement membrane. This is a premalignant condition, and for squamous cervical lesions it is referred to as *cervical intraepithelial neoplasia* (CIN). The term *adenocarcinoma in situ* is used for glandular lesions.
   CIN can be low (CIN 1) or high (CIN 2 or 3) grade. CIN 1 lesions usually regress, and the risk of progression to cervical cancer is minimal. CIN 2 and 3 lesions have a high risk of progression to cervical cancer if left untreated.
   The term *cancer* implies invasion through the basement membrane.

2. **What is the incidence of cervical cancer?**
   In the United States, cervical cancer is the eighth most common cancer in women and has a median age of diagnosis of 48 years. In 2014 an estimated 12,360 new cases and approximately 4020 deaths were reported.

3. **Is the incidence of cervical cancer changing?**
   The incidence of cervical cancer has dropped significantly since the 1960s as a result of the introduction of the Papanicolaou smear (usually referred to as the Pap smear or Pap test) and organized screening programs. However, it has recently reached a plateau. This finding is thought to reflect a persistent number of women who fail to be screened. For more information on screening, see Chapter 27.

4. **What is the cause of cervical cancer?**
   Human papillomavirus (HPV) is the major independent risk factor for cervical dysplasia, and several different "high-risk" subtypes having been identified (16, 18, 31, 45, 51 to 53, 58, and 59). The virus integrates into the host cell's genome, causes loss of transcriptional regulation and overexpression of oncoproteins E6 and E7, and ultimately leads to uncontrolled promotion of cell cycle progression. HPV E6 protein binds to p53, and HPV E7 binds to retinoblastoma protein (Rb), thereby disabling these tumor suppressor genes. However, most women infected with HPV do not develop high-grade dysplasia or cervical cancer.
   Environmental (e.g., cigarette smoking) and immunologic (e.g., chronic immunosuppression) factors have also been found to play important roles.

5. **What is the benefit of vaccination against the HPV virus?**
   The HPV vaccine significantly reduces the risk of high-grade cervical lesions, vulvar and vaginal lesions, genital warts, and Pap smear abnormalities. Clinical trials showed a 34% decrease in vulvar or vaginal dysplasia and a 20% decrease in cervical dysplasia, even in women with unknown HPV status. For young women without previous HPV exposure, vaccination had a 98% efficacy rate in preventing CIN 2. Women with a known history of dysplasia had a 44% prevention rate for CIN 2.

6. **How is cervical cancer diagnosed?**
   The diagnosis is made after a tissue biopsy demonstrates invasion through the basement membrane. A Pap smear cannot be used to diagnose cervical cancer; it is solely a screening tool.

7. **Do different histologic types of cervical cancer exist?**
   Yes. Squamous cell carcinoma (69% of all cervical cancers) and adenocarcinoma (25% of all cervical cancers) are the most common types and are associated with HPV infection. Other types include sarcomas, melanomas, neuroendocrine tumors, and lymphomas; they represent 6% of all cervical cancers and are not associated with HPV.

8. **How is cervical cancer staged?**
   Table 29-1 shows the International Federation of Gynecology and Obstetrics (FIGO) staging system. Staging for cervical cancer is clinical, meaning that it is primarily based on clinical examination and does not involve surgical exploration. A staging examination includes speculum, bimanual, and

Table 29-1. International Federation of Gynecology and Obstetrics Staging of Cervical Cancer

STAGE	CHARACTERISTICS
IA	Invasive cancer identified only microscopically; stromal invasion with maximal depth of 5.0 mm and maximal width of 7.0 mm
IA1	Stromal invasion no deeper than 3.0 mm and no wider than 7.0 mm
IA2	Stromal invasion depth >3.0 mm but no deeper than 5.0 mm, width ≤7.0 mm
IB	Grossly visible lesions confined to the cervix (even those with superficial invasion) or microscopic lesions larger than stage IA
IB1	Visible lesions ≤4.0 cm
IB2	Visible lesions >4.0 cm
IIA	No obvious parametrial involvement, but invasion past the cervix into the uterus or upper two thirds of the vagina
IIA1	Visible lesions ≤4.0 cm
IIA2	Visible lesions >4.0 cm
IIB	Obvious parametrial involvement
IIIA	Extension to the lower one third of the vagina but not to the pelvic sidewall
IIIB	Extension to the pelvic sidewall or hydronephrosis or renal damage
IVA	Extension into mucosa of the bladder or rectum or beyond the true pelvis
IVB	Spread to distant organs

rectovaginal examinations, palpation of groin and supraclavicular lymph nodes, examination of the right upper abdominal quadrant, and tissue diagnosis (i.e., cervical biopsy, cervical conization procedure, or endocervical curettings). According to the FIGO, the following procedures are permitted but not mandatory:

- Cystoscopy
- Proctoscopy
- Hysteroscopy
- Intravenous pyelogram to evaluate for urinary tract obstruction
- Plain chest radiograph and radiograph of the skeleton

In general, the cancer is strictly confined to the cervix in stage I. It invades beyond the uterus but not to the pelvic sidewall or to the lower one third of the vagina in stage II and to the pelvic sidewall or lower one third of the vagina in stage III. In stage IV, tumor has extended beyond the true pelvis or has clinically involved the mucosa of the bladder or rectum. Once assigned, the stage does not change based on progression or intraoperative findings.

9. **What are 5-year survival rates for cervical cancer?**
   The 5-year survival rates according to stage are as follows:
   - Stage I: 85% to 90%
   - Stage IIA: 75% to 85%
   - Stage IIB: 60% to 65%
   - Stage III: 25% to 35%
   - Stage IV: 8% to 15%

10. **What are the different treatment options for treating cervical cancer?**
    Surgical treatment is usually appropriate up to stage IIA; it does not confer any additional survival benefit over primary chemoradiation once parametrial involvement is obvious (stage IIB). The advantages of surgical treatment include ovarian preservation, avoidance of postradiation vaginal stenosis, decreased incidence of cystitis and enteritis, and the ability to assess pelvic and aortic lymph nodes. Avoidance of long-term radiation therapy spares the patient from side effects such as bowel obstruction, ureteral obstruction from fibrosis, and the risk of postradiation retroperitoneal or pelvic soft tissue sarcoma.

11. **What surgical procedure is typically performed in appropriate candidates?**
For early-stage disease (stage IA1) in patients who do not desire fertility preservation, simple hysterectomy is an acceptable option. For stage IA2 or IIA, radical hysterectomy with lymph node sampling is indicated; this procedure involves resection of the bilateral parametrial tissue, upper one third of the vagina, uterosacral ligaments, cardinal ligaments, and local blood supply. Lymph nodes from the pelvic (obturator, external iliac, hypogastric, and ureteral) and common iliac chains are removed. Unless obvious tumor involvement of the ovaries is present, oophorectomy is not necessary; the risk of future metastasis to this site is very low.

12. **What complications are associated with radical hysterectomy?**
The most common complication is transient bladder dysfunction, which results from interruption of the sensory and motor nerve supply to the detrusor muscles. The extent of dysfunction correlates with the extent of the dissection, but this complication is usually self-limited. Less frequent complications include lymphocyst formation, lymphedema, surgical site or urinary tract infection, venous thromboembolic events, and intraoperative hemorrhage. Ureteral fistula secondary to devascularization of the ureter is uncommon but possible.

13. **What if a patient with cervical cancer desires to preserve her fertility?**
For stage IA1 cancer without lymphovascular space invasion, cervical conization is an option. This modality can be used only if surgical margins of the cone specimen are free of disease. If patients are diagnosed with stage IA2 and IB1 disease without lymph node involvement *and the tumor is no larger than 2 cm*, radical trachelectomy is an option. This procedure includes removal of the cervix, upper vagina, and tissue adjacent to the cervix and upper vagina; the uterine corpus and ovaries are preserved.

14. **When is radiation therapy appropriate in the treatment of cervical cancer?**
Radiation therapy is appropriate for patients with locoregionally advanced disease (spread to the sidewall or lymph nodes) that is confined to the pelvis—generally stages IB through III. It may also be appropriate for early-stage disease in patients who are unable to tolerate surgical treatment or in older patients for whom neither ovarian preservation nor maintenance of sexual function is important. Radiation therapy can also be used for symptomatic control of metastasis or bleeding from a central tumor.

15. **How is radiation therapy given for cervical cancer?**
Radiation therapy is typically given in two phases. During the first phase, the entire pelvis receives external beam radiation to reduce tumor volume and sterilize the regional lymph nodes. Brachytherapy is the second phase and involves the insertion of a catheter through the cervix into the uterine cavity; radiation can be administered directly to the tumor by placing a radiation source (usually cesium or iridium) in the lumen of the catheter.

Multiple well-designed, prospective studies have demonstrated radiation therapy to be more effective with concomitant chemotherapy. Intravenous cisplatin (a platinum-based agent) is the most widely studied of the "radiation-sensitizing" chemotherapy agents, but optimal dosing remains under investigation.

16. **What complications are associated with radiation therapy?**
Radiation therapy has few acute side effects and is generally well tolerated. The most common complaints during treatment are fatigue, watery diarrhea, radiation cystitis, and a sunburn-like skin reaction. Long-term side effects are uncommon, but can include the following:
- Infertility
- Small bowel obstruction (especially if paraaortic lymph nodes are irradiated)
- Large bowel stricture
- Chronic intermittent enteritis or cystitis
- Vaginal atrophy and stenosis
- Postradiation soft tissue sarcoma

17. **When is chemotherapy appropriate in the treatment of cervical cancer?**
Aside from treatment with radiation-sensitizing agents, chemotherapy is employed when the disease has spread beyond the pelvis. Because not all organs can tolerate the high radiation doses required to treat cancer, radiation therapy is no longer an option once the disease has spread outside the pelvis. Unfortunately, cervical cancer is relatively chemoresistant and has a low response rate (10% to 25%) to most agents.

18. **What considerations should be made for adenocarcinoma (as opposed to squamous cell carcinoma)?**
    Although treatment regimens and survival rates for patients with adenocarcinoma are the same as with squamous lesions, adenocarcinomas tend to manifest at more advanced stages. Conservative treatment of stage IA adenocarcinoma, however, is not recommended. Microinvasive adenocarcinoma is difficult to characterize pathologically, may be multifocal, and is not as reliably assessed by follow-up Pap smears.

19. **What is total pelvic exenteration, and who are candidates for this procedure?**
    Total pelvic exenteration involves removing the bladder and distal ureters, any remaining müllerian structures, the vagina, rectum, and sigmoid colon, and the muscles of the pelvic floor. In general, the classic "total" pelvic exenteration has been replaced by more conservative, less morbid approaches such as an anterior (bladder and müllerian structures) or posterior (sigmoid colon or rectum and müllerian structures) exenteration. Supralevator exenteration, which spares the musculature of the pelvic floor, is also possible.
    Pelvic exenteration is reserved for patients with central recurrence of disease after primary therapy. It can also be used to palliate severe symptoms such as from postradiation fistulas or hemorrhage from residual tumor.

20. **What is the success rate for pelvic exenteration?**
    The 5-year survival rate for patients after pelvic exenteration ranges from 20% to 60%, with many investigators reporting rates of approximately 50%. Patients with recurrent disease after an exenteration are candidates for chemotherapy only and have a 1-year mortality rate in excess of 90%.

KEY POINTS: CERVICAL CANCER

1. Regular screening with Pap smears has led to a significant decrease in the incidence of cervical cancer.
2. Cervical cancer staging is performed clinically and is not changed based on intraoperative findings.
3. The difference between cancer and CIN is invasion of the basement membrane.
4. Treatment of cervical cancer depends on stage; surgical treatment is usually appropriate up to stage IIA.

BIBLIOGRAPHY

1. American College of Obstetricians and Gynecologists. Screening for cervical cancer. ACOG practice bulletin no. 131. *Obstet Gynecol.* 2012;120:1222–1238.
2. American College of Obstetricians and Gynecologists. Management of abnormal cervical cancer screening test results and cervical cancer precursors. ACOG practice bulletin no. 140. *Obstet Gynecol.* 2013;122:1338–1367.
3. Creasman W. Preinvasive disease of the cervix. In: Di Saia P, Creasman W, Mannel RS, McMeekin DS, Mutch DG, eds. *Clinical Gynecologic Oncology.* 8th ed. Philadelphia: Saunders; 2012:1–30.
4. The FUTURE II Study Group. Quadrivalent vaccine against human papillomavirus to prevent high-grade cervical lesions. *N Engl J Med.* 2007;356:1915–1927.
5. The FUTURE II Study Group. Four year efficacy of prophylactic human papillomavirus (types 6, 11, 16, and 18) L1 virus–like particle vaccine against low-grade cervical, vulvar, and vaginal intraepithelial neoplasia and condylomata acuminata. *BMJ.* 2010;340:1–9.
6. Pecorelli S. Revised FIGO staging for carcinoma of the vulva, cervix and endometrium: FIGO Committee on Gynecologic Oncology. *Int J Gynaecol Obstet.* 2009;105:103–104.

CHAPTER 30

ENDOMETRIAL HYPERPLASIA AND UTERINE CANCER

Ramy Eskander, MD

1. **What is the incidence of endometrial cancer?**
   In 2014, approximately 52,600 cases of endometrial cancer were diagnosed in the United States. The incidence has been rising over the past few decades, and this increase is thought to reflect an aging, more obese population.

2. **What are risk factors for endometrial cancer?**
   Most endometrial cancers are thought develop as a result of exposure to unopposed estrogen, which occurs with both obesity (relative risk [RR]: 2 to 5) and anovulation (RR: 1.5). Other predisposing factors include early menarche (RR: 1.5 to 2), menopause after age 52 years (RR: 2 to 3), nulliparity (RR: 3), diabetes (RR: 2.7), hypertension (RR: 2.1), tamoxifen use (RR: 2 to 3), and hereditary cancer syndromes such as Lynch syndrome (60% lifetime risk).

3. **Is age associated with endometrial cancer?**
   Yes. Endometrial cancer is predominantly a disease of postmenopausal women. The mean age at time of diagnosis is 63 years, and only 5% of women are diagnosed with this disease when they are less than 40 years old.

4. **Does a reliable screening test exist for endometrial cancer?**
   No. Unlike with cervical cancer, no screening tests are available.

5. **How does endometrial cancer typically manifest?**
   In most cases (75% to 90%), women present with abnormal or postmenopausal uterine bleeding. Approximately 10% of patients may complain of leukorrhea (white vaginal discharge). Occasionally, patients with cervical stenosis do not have bleeding; they can develop hematometria or pyometria secondary to cervical obstruction.

6. **What should be in the differential diagnosis when evaluating a patient with post-menopausal bleeding?**
   - Endometrial or vaginal atrophy
   - Exogenous hormone replacement
   - Endometrial or cervical polyps
   - Endometrial hyperplasia
   - Endometrial cancer
   - Cervical or vaginal cancer
   - Urethral caruncles
   - Trauma

7. **How should a patient with abnormal uterine bleeding be evaluated?**
   A detailed history should be taken to identify risk factors. A physical examination should include a pelvic examination and palpation for lymph nodes, and an endometrial biopsy (EMB) should be performed in the following groups:
   - Less than 45 years old with risk factors or persistent bleeding
   - At least 45 years old without risk factors
   - Postmenopausal status regardless of age
   For more information on evaluation of a patient with abnormal uterine bleeding, see Chapter 3.

8. **Is an alternative to EMB available?**
   Yes. In postmenopausal patients, transvaginal ultrasound can be used to visualize the endometrium. If the endometrial stripe appears homogenous and measures less than 4 mm, atrophy is the most likely cause of bleeding, and EMB may be deferred. However, sampling for biopsy should be performed if

bleeding persists. Ultrasound should not be used to evaluate for endometrial cancer in premenopausal patients or patients with uterine abnormalities (e.g., fibroids, polyps).

Hysteroscopy with dilation and curettage (D&C) can be performed in both premenopausal and postmenopausal patients as an alternative to EMB, although this requires use of an operating room and carries risks associated with anesthesia. This procedure is more frequently performed after nondiagnostic EMB results.

9. **What is endometrial hyperplasia, and what is its significance?**
   Endometrial hyperplasia refers to the abnormal proliferation of hormonally sensitive endometrial glands and stroma. In the setting of persistent estrogen excess (whether exogenous or endogenous), nuclear atypia may develop. Hyperplasia with atypia is both a precursor and a marker of endometrial cancer; it has been associated with endometrial cancer in up to 42% of cases.

10. **How is endometrial hyperplasia treated?**
    Depending on age, comorbidities, and fertility desires, patients with hyperplasia may be treated with either progestin therapy or hysterectomy. Hyperplasia that is not atypical can often be successfully treated with oral contraceptive pills, periodic progesterone withdrawal, or the levonorgestrel intrauterine device. Hysterectomy is recommended for patients with atypical hyperplasia who have completed childbearing. Alternatives are high-dose progestins (megestrol acetate or the levonorgestrel intrauterine device) with repeat EMBs every 3 months.

    Patients with atypical hyperplasia who choose to defer hysterectomy because of fertility desires should be counseled that data in support of conservative management are limited, that the disease may not regress, and that recurrence is likely once treatment is discontinued.

11. **What are the two different types of endometrial cancer?**
    - Type I (endometrioid adenocarcinoma): This type represents 80% of all diagnosed endometrial cancers and is associated with excess estrogen. It is usually well differentiated and associated with an overall good prognosis (5-year survival of 85%). Type I is divided into grade 1, in which 95% or more of the neoplastic tissue forms in glands, and grade 2, in which only 50% to 94% does this. Grades 1 and 2 are known as low-grade tumors.
    - Type II (grade 3 endometrioid, serous, clear cell, squamous, transitional cell, mesonephric, or undifferentiated): This type represents 10% to 20% of all diagnosed endometrial cancers and is *not* related to estrogen exposure; malignant cells arise in an atrophic endometrial background. Poorly differentiated forms carry the worst prognosis (5-year survival of 35%). In grade 3 endometrioid cancer (high-grade), less than 50% of the neoplastic tissue forms in glands.

    Approximately 3% of endometrial cancers are sarcomas such as leiomyosarcoma and endometrial stromal sarcoma. Even fewer endometrial cancers are classified as carcinosarcomas.

12. **Can the endometrium be a site of metastatic disease?**
    Yes. Common malignant diseases that can metastasize to the endometrium include breast, ovarian, stomach, colon, and pancreatic tumors. Not all metastases to the endometrium are carcinomas, however.

13. **How is endometrial cancer staged?**
    Table 30-1 shows the International Federation of Gynecology and Obstetrics. Endometrial cancer is surgically staged with hysterectomy, bilateral salpingo-oophorectomy, and removal of pelvic and paraaortic lymph nodes. Because up to 90% of patients present relatively early with abnormal vaginal bleeding, approximately 75% of patients with newly diagnosed endometrial cancer will have disease limited to the uterus. Twenty percent of patients will have advanced-stage disease involving regional (local) organs and lymph nodes, and 5% will have distant metastases.

14. **How does endometrial cancer spread?**
    Endometrial cancer spreads most commonly by direct extension through the myometrium and uterine serosa and into adjacent organs. Malignant cells may also be shed from the fallopian tubes and seed the peritoneal cavity. Lymphatic spread to the pelvic and paraaortic lymph nodes can occur, as well as hematogenous dissemination to the lungs, liver, and brain.

15. **How is endometrial cancer treated?**
    The need for treatment after the initial surgical procedure with adjuvant chemotherapy or radiation therapy is determined by stage. Chemotherapy regimens may include carboplatin and paclitaxel or combinations of paclitaxel, doxorubicin, and cisplatin.

Table 30-1. International Federation of Gynecology and Obstetrics Staging of Endometrial Carcinoma

STAGE	CHARACTERISTICS
IA	Tumor confined to the uterus, no or less than one half myometrial invasion
IB	Tumor confined to the uterus, more than one half myometrial invasion
II	Cervical stromal invasion, but not beyond uterus
IIIA	Tumor invasion of serosa or adnexa
IIIB	Vaginal or parametrial involvement
IIIC1	Pelvic node involvement
IIIC2	Paraaortic involvement
IVA	Tumor invasion of bladder or bowel mucosa
IVB	Distant metastases including abdominal metastases or inguinal lymph nodes

16. **Does hormonal therapy have a role in the treatment of endometrial cancer?**
    Yes. Studies show a response rate of up to 78% with progesterone therapy in patients with atypical hyperplasia or stage I, noninvasive grade 1 endometrial cancer. Progestins have also been evaluated as possible adjuvant therapy to prevent recurrence. Only approximately 15% to 30% of patients may respond to progestin therapy in the context of recurrent disease, but side effects are minimal.

17. **What are prognostic indicators in endometrial cancer?**
    - Stage of disease at diagnosis (most significant prognostic factor)
    - Age (younger women have a better prognosis)
    - Type
    - Grade
    - Depth of myometrial invasion
    - Presence of intraperitoneal metastasis
    - Presence of lymph node invasion
    - Lower uterine segment and cervical stromal involvement
    - Positive pelvic washings

    For 5-year survival rates based on the stage at time of diagnosis, see Table 30-2.

Table 30-2. Five-Year Survival Rates for Endometrial Cancer Based on Stage at Time of Diagnosis

STAGE	SURVIVAL RATE
IA	88%
IB	75%
II	69%
IIIA	58%
IIIB	50%
IIIC	47%
IVA	17%
IVB	15%

18. **Does endometrial cancer have a genetic association?**
    Yes. Approximately 2% to 5% of all endometrial cancers result from Lynch syndrome, which confers a lifetime risk up to 60% (as opposed to 2.6% in the general population). These patients also have elevated lifetime risk of developing ovarian cancer (up to 12%) as well as colon (up to 90%) and stomach cancer (12%).

The mean age for diagnosis of endometrial cancer in patients with Lynch syndrome is 46 to 50 years; patients are advised to undergo screening with EMB starting at age 30 to 35 years. They may also consider risk-reducing hysterectomy and bilateral salpingo-oophorectomy once they have completed childbearing or after age 40 years.

KEY POINTS: ENDOMETRIAL HYPERPLASIA AND UTERINE CANCER

1. Physiologic states of unopposed or excess estrogen are risk factors for developing endometrial hyperplasia and subsequent uterine cancer.
2. Most cases of endometrial hyperplasia and cancer manifest with abnormal uterine bleeding.
3. Postmenopausal bleeding can be evaluated with either a transvaginal ultrasound scan or an EMB.
4. Endometrial hyperplasia can be treated with progestins.
5. Endometrial cancer is staged surgically, and treatment is based on stage.

BIBLIOGRAPHY

1. American Cancer Society. 2015 Demographic Data for Endometrial Cancer. March 17, 2015.
2. American Cancer Society. cancer.org. Survival by Stage of Endometrial Cancer. Available at http://www.cancer.org/cancer/endometrialcancer/detailedguide/endometrial-uterine-cancer-survival-rates.
3. American College of Obstetricians and Gynecologists. Lynch syndrome. ACOG practice bulletin no. 147. *Obstet Gynecol.* 2014;124:1042–1054.
4. American College of Obstetricians and Gynecologists. Diagnosis of abnormal uterine bleeding in reproductive-aged women. ACOG practice bulletin no. 128. *Obstet Gynecol.* 2012;120:197.
5. American College of Obstetricians and Gynecologists. Endometrial cancer. ACOG practice bulletin no. 149. *Obstet Gynecol.* 2015;125:1006–1026.
6. American Joint Committee on Cancer. Corpus Uteri. In: *AJCC Staging Manual.* 7th. New York: Springer; 2010:p.403.
7. Eskander R, Bristow R, Ward K, et al. Uterine corpus cancers. In: Eskander R, Bristow R, eds. *Gynecologic Oncology: A Pocketbook.* New York: Springer-Verlag; 2015:133–174.
8. FIGO Committee on Gynecologic Oncology. FIGO staging for carcinoma of the vulva, cervix, and corpus uteri. *Int J Gynaecol Obstet.* 2014;125:97–98.
9. Kimura T, Kamiura S, Yamamoto T, et al. Abnormal uterine bleeding and prognosis of endometrial cancer. *Int J Gynaecol Obstet.* 2004;85:145.
10. Pecorelli S. Revised FIGO staging for carcinoma of the vulva, cervix, and endometrium. *Int J Gynaecol Obstet.* 2009;105:103.

CHAPTER 31

OVARIAN CANCER

Ramy Eskander, MD, and Mae Zakhour, MD

1. **What is the incidence of ovarian cancer?**
   Ovarian cancer ranks fifth in cancer deaths among women and is the most lethal gynecologic malignant disease. Approximately 21,290 women are expected to receive the diagnosis of ovarian cancer in 2015, with approximately 14,180 deaths. The lifetime incidence of a woman's being diagnosed with ovarian cancer is 1 in 71.

2. **What are the different histologic subtypes of ovarian cancer?**
   Ovarian cancer is a diverse term describing several different histologic entities. Each type has a different natural history.
   - Epithelial: 70%
     - Serous
     - Mucinous
     - Clear cell
     - Endometrioid
     - Undifferentiated
     - Brenner
   - Germ cell: 15%
     - Dysgerminoma
     - Endodermal sinus
     - Embryonal
     - Choriocarcinoma
     - Immature teratoma
     - Gonadoblastoma
   - Sex cord stromal: 10%
     - Granulosa
     - Sertoli-Leydig
   - Metastatic tumors to the ovary: less than 3%
     - Breast
     - Gastrointestinal
     - Others

3. **What are the stages of ovarian cancer?**
   Table 31-1 shows the International Federation of Gynecology and Obstetrics (FIGO) staging system.

4. **How is ovarian cancer staged?**
   Ovarian cancer is staged surgically to assess the extent of disease spread. Components of surgical staging may include careful inspection of all peritoneal surfaces, pelvic and abdominal washings, random peritoneal biopsies, biopsy of suspicious lesions, pelvic and paraaortic lymph node sampling, total abdominal hysterectomy, and bilateral salpingo-oophorectomy. Procedures are performed only as necessary; either to assign a stage to describe the patient's disease accurately or to cytoreduce advanced ovarian cancer optimally. For example, if diffuse disease is noted intraoperatively, pelvic washings or lymph node sampling can be omitted from the surgical procedure. If no gross disease is identified outside the ovary, however, peritoneal washing, peritoneal biopsies, omentectomy, and lymph node dissection are advised because approximately 25% to 30% of patients with no gross disease are found to have microscopic disease on resected specimens.

5. **How do patients with epithelial ovarian cancer (EOC) present clinically?**
   Presentation of EOC can be either acute or subacute. In a few patients, EOC is diagnosed at the time of surgical intervention performed for other indications.

Table 31-1. International Federation of Gynecology and Obstetrics Staging of Ovarian Cancer

Stage I: Tumor confined to ovaries

IA	Tumor limited to one ovary, capsule intact, no tumor on surface, negative washings
IB	Tumor involving both ovaries; otherwise, like stage IA
IC	Tumor limited to one or both ovaries
IC1	Surgical spill
IC2	Capsule rupture preoperatively or tumor on ovarian surface
IC3	Malignant cells in the ascites or peritoneal washings

Stage II: Tumor involves one or both ovaries with pelvic extension (below the pelvic brim) or primary peritoneal cancer

IIA	Extension or implant on the uterus or fallopian tubes
IIB	Extension to other pelvic intraperitoneal tissues

Stage III: Tumor involves one or both ovaries with cytologically or histologically confirmed spread to the peritoneum outside the pelvis or metastasis to the retroperitoneal lymph nodes

IIIA	Positive retroperitoneal lymph nodes or microscopic metastasis beyond the pelvis
IIIA1	Positive retroperitoneal lymph nodes only
IIIA1(i)	Metastasis ≤10 mm
IIIA1(ii)	Metastasis >10 mm
IIIA2	Microscopic, extrapelvic (above the brim) peritoneal involvement with or without positive retroperitoneal lymph nodes
IIIB	Macroscopic, extrapelvic, peritoneal metastasis ≤2 cm with or without positive retroperitoneal lymph nodes; includes extension to capsule of liver or spleen
IIIC	Macroscopic, extrapelvic, peritoneal metastasis >2 cm with or without positive retroperitoneal lymph nodes; includes extension to capsule of liver or spleen

Stage IV: Distant metastasis excluding peritoneal metastasis

IVA	Pleural effusion with positive cytologic findings
IVB	Hepatic or splenic parenchymal metastasis, metastasis to extraabdominal organs (including inguinal lymph nodes and lymph nodes outside the abdominal cavity)

- Acute presentation
  - Pleural effusion, shortness of breath
  - Bowel obstruction
  - Venous thromboembolism or pulmonary embolism
- Subacute presentation
  - Abdominal pain, distention, bloating
  - Palpable adnexal, pelvic, or abdominal masses
  - Early satiety
  - Abnormal vaginal or rectal bleeding (evaluate uterine disease first)
  - Abnormal glandular cytology on Papanicolaou (Pap) smear (evaluate uterine or cervical disease first)
  - Paraneoplastic syndromes

6. What are the different subtypes of EOC?
   - Serous carcinoma: 40%
   - Mucinous carcinoma: 10% to 15%
   - Endometrioid carcinoma: 15%
   - Clear cell carcinoma: 6%
   - Undifferentiated: 15%
   - Brenner tumor: 1%

7. What are the risk factors and protective factors for development of EOC?
   - Risk factors
     - Family history of ovarian cancer
       - First-degree relative raises risk 3-fold above baseline

- Two or more first-degree relatives raise risk 4- to 15-fold above baseline
- Age (highest incidence in the seventh decade of life)
- Nulliparity
- Early menarche
- Late menopause
- Hereditary breast and ovarian cancer (e.g., *BRCA* germline mutation)
- Protective factors
  - Oral contraceptive pills associated with a 50% risk reduction after 5 years of use
  - Multiparity
  - Breastfeeding

8. **How is EOC diagnosed?**
A thorough history and physical examination are performed when ovarian cancer is suspected. Regardless of whether or not a pelvic mass is identified on examination, a pelvic ultrasound scan is performed for a more complete evaluation of the pelvic structures, especially if suspicion remains high. If an adnexal mass is identified, laboratory evaluation of tumor markers can be performed for risk stratification. The most common EOC tumor markers are cancer antigen 125 (CA-125), human epididymis protein 4 (HE4), and OVA1, a proprietary test combining levels of five ovarian CA biomarkers. CA-125 is most often elevated in serous ovarian cancers, but it has poor sensitivity in early ovarian cancer.
　　Other imaging modalities such as magnetic resonance imaging can be used, although it is not typically performed.
　　Primary peritoneal carcinoma, a pathologic twin of EOC but affecting the peritoneal lining as opposed to the ovary, is more difficulty to identify because often no discrete masses can be seen on ultrasound scans. In these cases, a computed tomography scan can be used to evaluate the peritoneal lining, as well as evaluate for the presence of ascites.

9. **What is the typical stage at presentation?**
- Localized (confined to primary site): 15%
- Regional (spread to regional lymph nodes): 19%
- Distant (cancer has metastasized): 60%
- Unknown (unstaged): 6%
The Surveillance, Epidemiology, and End Results (SEER) database is a program of the National Cancer Institute, and it does not use the FIGO classification for epidemiologic data. Instead, it uses the classification shown in the foregoing list.

10. **How does ovarian cancer spread?**
Ovarian cancer is spread by direct dissemination in the peritoneal cavity, where tumor cells adhere to surrounding organs through direct extension. Lymphatic spread occurs when tumor invades pelvic or paraaortic lymph nodes. Hematogenous spread, as manifested by lung or parenchymal liver metastasis, is rare.

11. **How is EOC treated?**
Treatment typically involves a combination of surgery and chemotherapy. Because survival has been inversely linked to postoperative residual tumor, the goal of surgical treatment is to achieve optimal cytoreduction, or up to 1 cm of residual disease. Further benefit has been demonstrated from achieving an *R0 cytoreduction*, defined as only microscopic residual disease. Surgical treatment of ovarian cancer is usually performed by laparotomy. Optimal cytoreduction may require resection of portions of the bowel, liver, spleen, and diaphragm, among other structures.

12. **How is chemotherapy used in EOC?**
After adequate cytoreduction, adjuvant chemotherapy (a taxane, e.g., paclitaxel, and a platinum agent, e.g., cisplatin) is used for patients with high-risk stage I disease and for all patients with stage II, III, and IV disease. In certain patients with advanced metastatic disease, neoadjuvant chemotherapy can be given preoperatively to decrease the tumor burden and optimize resection. In these patients, additional chemotherapy follows surgical treatment.
　　Although the response rate to chemotherapy is high (≈70%) and many patients experience complete remission, most ultimately develop resistance and die of disease recurrence.

13. **What prognostic factors affect disease outcome?**
- Stage at diagnosis
- Adequacy of tumor debulking at the time of surgical treatment

- Preoperative functional status
- Pathologic factors (e.g., tumor grade and histologic features)
- Age

14. **What are 5-year survival rates for EOC?**
SEER survival data from 2005 to 2011 are as follows:
- Localized: 92.1%
- Regional: 73.2%
- Distant: 28.3%
- Unstaged: 22.9%
At present, survival data based on the most recent FIGO staging system are not available.

15. **Are any cost-effective screening methods available for ovarian cancer?**
No. Transvaginal pelvic ultrasound scans can be useful and sensitive for the identification of complex adnexal masses; however, their sensitivity is unacceptably low. CA-125 is expressed in as many as 80% of nonmucinous ovarian cancers, but it is also elevated in many benign conditions (e.g., pregnancy, pelvic inflammatory disease, endometriosis, infertility, benign ovarian cysts, hepatitis, cirrhosis, heart failure, and renal failure).

16. **How is CA-125 used postoperatively?**
Following surgical treatment, CA-125 levels can be monitored for response to chemotherapy, particularly if they were elevated preoperatively.

17. **What are the hereditary syndromes associated with ovarian cancer?**
Approximately 10% of all ovarian cancers are considered hereditary, and they occur as part of three different syndromes: site-specific familial ovarian cancer, breast/ovarian familial cancer syndrome, and Lynch II syndrome. The responsible genes are transmitted in an autosomal dominant fashion with variable penetrance.
Hereditary breast/ovarian cancer syndrome is the most common, accounting for 75% to 90% of all hereditary cases of ovarian cancer. Families usually have multiple cases of breast and ovarian cancer diagnosed before the age of 50 years. Almost all families with this syndrome display mutations in the *BRCA1* and *BRCA2* genes. Evidence indicates that these patients have better prognoses than patients with sporadic ovarian cancer.
Site-specific ovarian cancer accounts for approximately 5% of cases of familial ovarian cancer and is thought to be a variation of hereditary breast/ovarian cancer syndrome. In this syndrome, only ovarian cancer is demonstrated in the family; the lack of breast cancer may be secondary to chance, incomplete family histories, or differences in the cancer risk associated with each specific gene mutation. *BRCA1* and *BRCA2* mutations are responsible for most of these cases.
Lynch II syndrome, also known as hereditary nonpolyposis colon cancer syndrome, is associated with mutations in the DNA mismatch repair genes and accounts for approximately 2% of hereditary ovarian cancers. These families display nonpolyposis colorectal cancer, as well as adenocarcinomas of the endometrium, ovary, stomach, skin, small bowel, and urinary tract.

18. **What are low-malignant-potential (LMP) tumors of the ovary?**
Also known as **borderline tumors**, LMP lesions are characterized by epithelium that displays characteristics of malignant carcinoma but without identifiable invasion. Approximately 15% of all ovarian malignant lesions are LMP tumors. Most patients are young at diagnosis, with a mean age of 45 years. However, pregnancy, oral contraceptives, and breastfeeding appear to be protective. LMP tumors have an excellent prognosis, with 5-year survival rates ranging from 95% to 100%.

19. **What are malignant germ cell tumors (MGCTs)?**
MGCTs are tumors that derive from primitive germ cells of the embryonic gonad (Fig. 31-1). They usually manifest in women in their late teens and 20s, and symptoms usually include increasing abdominal girth and acute-onset lower abdominal pain. Some patients may also present with abnormal uterine bleeding.

20. **What are the different histologic types of MGCT?**
- Dysgerminomas
  - This most common type of MGCT comprises up to 50% of all MGCTs.
  - The contralateral ovary is involved in approximately 15% of patients.

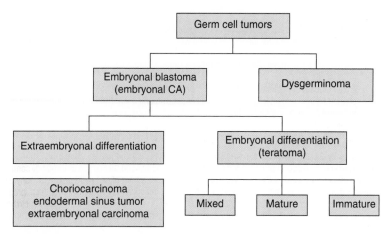

Figure 31-1. Classification schema of germ cell tumors of the ovary. *(From Bidus M, Elkas J, Rose GS. Germ cell, stromal, and other ovarian tumors. In: Di Saia P, Creasman W, eds.* Clinical Gynecologic Oncology. *8th ed. Philadelphia: Saunders; 2012.)*

- These tumors are sometimes associated with elevated serum lactate dehydrogenase (LDH) or human chorionic gonadotropin (hCG).
- They are among the more common ovarian tumors to be diagnosed during pregnancy.
- Patients often manifest with primary amenorrhea. In these cases, the diagnosis is often associated with gonadal dysgenesis and gonadoblastoma.
- Endodermal sinus tumors (also known as yolk sac tumors)
  - This is the second most common MGCT of the ovary, comprising approximately 25% of all tumors.
  - A common histologic finding is the **Schiller-Duval body**, an isolated papillary projection lined with tumor cells surrounding a single central blood vessel. Most secrete alpha-fetoprotein (AFP), thus making it a useful tumor marker.
  - Only 5% of cases are bilateral.
- Teratomas
  - They comprise approximately 20% of all MGCTs.
  - They arise from all three embryonic germ cell layers and are differentiated from their benign counterparts (mature cystic teratoma or dermoid cysts) by the presence of immature or embryonal structures.
  - Histologic grade is determined by the quantity of immature neural tissue present.
  - They are rarely bilateral (<5% of cases).
- Mixed germ cell tumors
  - They comprise approximately 8% of all GCMTs.
  - They include at least two different malignant germ cell components; the most common components are dysgerminoma and endodermal sinus tumors.
- Embryonal carcinoma
  - This is most commonly seen as a component of a mixed tumor; it is rare and aggressive in its pure form.
  - It may secrete estrogen and be associated with precocious puberty or irregular bleeding.
  - It often secretes hCG and AFP.
- Choriocarcinoma
  - Choriocarcinoma of the ovary is very rare.
  - Children with these tumors present with signs of precocious puberty.
  - Because cells secrete hCG, these tumors may be confused with ectopic pregnancy in adults.
- Polyembryoma
  - This rare tumor is characterized histologically by numerous structures resembling normal embryos.
  - Only a few have been reported in the literature, and most are associated with mixed tumors.
  - They have often metastasized to other structures in the pelvis and abdomen by the time of diagnosis.

- Gonadoblastoma
  - These rare tumors are associated with dysgerminomas.
  - Most of these tumors are diagnosed during workup for abnormal external genitalia, virilization, or primary amenorrhea.
  - The patient's karyotype often reveals either a single X chromosome (45,X) or mosaicism (45,X/46,XY).
  - Eighty percent of patients are phenotypic women; the rest are phenotypic men with hypospadias, cryptorchidism, and internal female sexual organs. Among phenotypic women, approximately half are normal in appearance and half are virilized, with primary amenorrhea or abnormal external genitalia.

21. How are MGCTs treated?
    The mainstay therapy for MGCTs is surgical resection. Because these tumors often affect younger women who may desire to preserve their fertility or ovarian function, the option of removing only the affected ovary is possible if the retained ovary appears grossly normal and without any evidence of disease. If surgical exploration reveals advanced disease, debulking with the goal of optimal cytoreduction if performed. Patients with stage IA dysgerminomas or stage IA grade 1 immature teratomas may be treated with surgical intervention alone; all other patients require adjuvant chemotherapy with bleomycin, etoposide, and cisplatin (BEP).

22. What are 5-year survival rates for MGCTs?
    Dysgerminomas have an excellent prognosis, and most are cured. Patients with stage IA disease have a 5-year survival rate greater than 95%, and patients with advanced disease have 5-year survival rates of 85% to 90%. For all other MGCTs, advanced-stage disease is associated with a 5-year survival rate of 60% to 80%.

23. How do patients with malignant sex cord stromal tumors (SCSTs) present?
    Malignant SCSTs of the ovary typically manifest in girls or women in their second or third decade of life, but these tumors demonstrate a bimodal distribution, with some cases arising in women in their fifth or sixth decade of life. Because of the production of ovarian sex steroids by these tumors, many of these patients present with symptoms of virilization, precocious puberty, or abnormal bleeding.

24. What are the different histologic types of malignant GCSTs?
    - Granulosa cell tumors
      - They secrete estrogen, but virilization occasionally occurs.
      - They have juvenile and adult variants.
      - The adult variant accounts for 95% of these tumors and occurs most often in postmenopausal women. Estrogen production results in hyperplasia or carcinoma of the endometrium, abnormal bleeding, and breast enlargement.
      - Juvenile variants usually manifest in women younger than 30 years of age. Children may show signs of precocious puberty. Older women may have amenorrhea or irregular bleeding.
      - Histologically, **Call-Exner bodies** are common.
    - Thecomas and fibromas
      - These are rarely malignant.
      - They are rare before puberty and usually manifest in perimenopausal or postmenopausal women.
      - Thecomas may produce estrogen.
      - Fibromas may cause **Meigs syndrome**, which mimics advanced-stage ovarian cancer with ascites and pleural effusions.
    - Sertoli-Leydig cell tumors (also known as androblastomas)
      - These are rare, with an average presenting age of 25 years.
      - Most are virilizing, some are estrogenic, and some produce no hormonal effects.
      - They may cause signs of pregnancy through progesterone production.

25. How are malignant SCSTs treated?
    Treatment is primarily surgical. Thecomas and fibromas are treated with unilateral salpingo-oophorectomy. Staging is important for patients with granulosa and Sertoli-Leydig cell tumors, and any disease identified outside the ovary should be debulked. Young patients may have a biopsy of the contralateral ovary in the absence of gross disease to attempt to preserve fertility. Adjuvant chemotherapy remains controversial, with several different regimens including BEP, VAC (vincristine, dactinomycin, and cyclophosphamide), and PVB (cisplatin, vinblastine, and bleomycin).

26. **What are survival rates for malignant SCSTs?**
    Overall, granulosa cell tumors have an excellent prognosis; 10-year and 20-year survival rates have been reported at 90% and 75%, respectively. Sertoli-Leydig cell tumors also have a good prognosis, with an overall 5-year survival of 70% to 90%. Granulosa cell tumors have a propensity for late recurrences and can even recur decades after the initial diagnosis. The median time to relapse, however, is approximately 5 years.

27. **Are stromal tumors associated with other cancers?**
    Because of the production of estrogen by stromal tumors, they are often associated with endometrial hyperplasia or carcinoma. As many as one in six patients with granulosa cell tumors will have concurrent endometrial cancer at the time of diagnosis.

28. **What tumors commonly metastasize to the ovary?**
    Approximately 5% of all tumors of the ovary are metastatic, the most common being breast cancer. Metastases from the gastrointestinal tract, colon, stomach, and uterus also occur.

29. **What is a Krukenberg tumor?**
    A Krukenberg tumor is metastatic adenocarcinoma to the ovary containing significant numbers of signet ring cells in a cellular ovarian stroma. Almost all these tumors metastasize from the stomach, but some arise in the breast, colon, or biliary tract. Rarely, these tumors spread from the bladder or cervix.

KEY POINTS: OVARIAN CANCER

1. No screening method exists for ovarian cancer; CA-125 is nonspecific, and transvaginal ultrasound is not cost effective.
2. Epithelial ovarian cancer usually manifests late in the disease course with nonspecific gastrointestinal symptoms.
3. Epithelial ovarian cancer is surgically staged and treated with a combination of cytoreductive surgery and chemotherapy.
4. MGCTs are tumors that derive from primitive germ cells of the embryonic gonads.
5. Sex cord and germ cell tumors are usually diagnosed in young women and tend to manifest at an early stage, thus allowing them to be highly curable.

BIBLIOGRAPHY

1. Bidus M, Elkas J, Rose GS. Germ cell, stromal, and other ovarian tumors. In: Di Saia P, Creasman W, eds. *Clinical Gynecologic Oncology*. 8th ed. Philadelphia: Saunders; 2012:329–356.
2. Cress RD, Chen YS, Morris C, Petersen M, Leiserowitz G. Characteristics of long-term survivors of epithelial ovarian cancer. *Obstet Gynecol*. 2015;126:491–497.
3. Eisenhauer E, Salani R, Copeland L. Epithelial ovarian cancer. In: Di Saia P, Creasman W, eds. *Clinical Gynecologic Oncology*. 8th ed. Philadelphia: Saunders; 2012:285–328.
4. Society of Gynecologic Oncology. FIGO Ovarian Cancer Staging. Available at https://www.sgo.org/wp-content/uploads/2012/09/FIGO-Ovarian-Cancer-Staging_1.10.14.pdf.
5. National Cancer Institute Surveillance, Epidemiology, and End Results Program. SEER Stat Fact Sheets. Ovary Cancer. Available at http://seer.cancer.gov/statfacts/html/ovary.html.
6. Zanetta G, Rota S, Chiari S, Bonazzi C, Bratina G, Mangioni C. Behavior of borderline tumors with particular interest to persistence, recurrence, and progression to invasive carcinoma: a prospective study. *J Clin Oncol*. 2015;19:2658–2664.

CHAPTER 32

GESTATIONAL TROPHOBLASTIC DISEASE

Ramy Eskander, MD

1. **What is the distinction between gestational trophoblastic disease (GTD) and gestational trophoblastic neoplasia (GTN)?**
   GTD is an abnormal proliferation of placental trophoblasts. It includes benign entities such as placental nodule and hydatidiform mole. GTN refers to malignant conditions such as invasive mole, choriocarcinoma, placental site trophoblastic tumor (PSTT), and epithelioid trophoblastic tumor (ETT).

2. **What is the incidence of GTD?**
   The incidence varies geographically. North American and European countries report low rates of 66 to 121 per 100,000 pregnancies, and Latin American, Asian, and Middle Eastern nations report rates of 23 to 1299 per 100,000 pregnancies.

3. **What are the different types of molar pregnancies?**
   Hydatidiform mole (HM) is the most common form of GTD, representing 80% of cases. It can be complete, partial, or invasive.
   - **Complete mole:** Has a diploid, 46,XX karyotype. It results from fertilization of an "empty" egg (maternal chromosomes are absent or inactivated) by a haploid sperm that then duplicates.
   - **Partial mole:** Has a triploid karyotype: 69,XXX, 69,XXY, or 69,XYY (rare). It results from fertilization of one egg by two haploid sperm.
   - **Invasive mole:** Can be either complete or partial. It is characterized by enlarged hydropic villi that invade into the myometrium, vascular spaces, or outside of the uterus. Invasive moles rarely resolve spontaneously and are considered a form of GTN.

4. **What is the clinical presentation of a molar pregnancy?**
   Women with HM typically present with symptoms or complications related to early pregnancy: abnormal vaginal bleeding, missed menses, positive pregnancy test, nausea, vomiting, or even hyperemesis gravidarum. If the diagnosis is delayed until the second trimester, symptoms can include uterine size greater than expected for the presumed gestational age, anemia, ovarian theca lutein cysts, hyperemesis, hyperthyroidism, preeclampsia, and even respiratory insufficiency. HM also may be suspected if the human chorionic gonadotropin (hCG) level is abnormally high for the presumed gestational age.

5. **How is a molar pregnancy diagnosed?**
   - **Complete moles** are usually diagnosed by ultrasound examination. Findings include the absence of an embryo or fetus and the presence of an intrauterine mass with many anechoic spaces. The characteristic appearance of a complete mole is frequently described as a "snowstorm" or "Swiss cheese" pattern (Fig. 32-1).
   - **Partial moles** often manifest similarly to a missed abortion. They may be difficult to diagnose before dilation and curettage (D&C) and subsequent histologic evaluation. On ultrasound scan, amniotic fluid volume may be reduced, and the placenta may have increased echogenicity or enlarged cystic spaces. Fetal tissue may be identified and may even be viable; growth restriction is common.

6. **How are molar pregnancies managed?**
   Dilation and curettage (D&C) should be performed in the operating room. If future fertility is not desired, a hysterectomy can be considered. A baseline chest radiograph, complete blood count (CBC), blood type, Rh status, aspartate aminotransferase (AST), alanine aminotransferase (ALT), creatinine, blood urea nitrogen (BUN), prothrombin time (PT), partial thromboplastin time (PTT), international normalized ratio (INR), and quantitative β-hCG should be collected.
   After the procedure, weekly β-hCG levels should be checked until they are undetectable for 3 consecutive weeks. Regular monthly β-hCG levels should then be obtained for 1 year. Because an

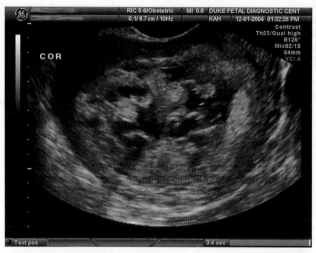

Figure 32-1. Transabdominal ultrasound scan of an unevacuated complete mole. *(Courtesy John Soper, MD. From Ko E, Soper J. Gestational trophoblastic disease. In: Di Saia PJ, Creasman WT, eds. Clinical Gynecologic Oncology. 8th ed. Philadelphia: Saunders; 2012.)*

early pregnancy may be confused with a recurrence, patients should be strongly urged to use birth control during this surveillance period.

If β-hCG levels plateau or rise, or if they persist for 6 months after the procedure, the patient should be evaluated for GTN. A plateau is defined as four β-hCG values within 10% of each other recorded weekly over a 3-week period. A rise is defined as three increasing β-hCG values by more than 10% recorded weekly over a 2-week period.

7. **Is GTN always preceded by a molar pregnancy?**
No. Only two thirds of GTN cases will follow this pattern. The remaining one third will develop after miscarriages, therapeutic abortions, or ectopic pregnancies.

8. **What is the risk of developing GTN after D&C for a molar pregnancy?**
For a complete mole, the risk is generally 15% to 20%. This rises to 40% among women with any of the following: age older than 40 years, uterine size larger than 20 weeks, or β-hCG higher than 100,000 at the time of diagnosis. After a D&C for a partial mole, the risk of GTN is 2%.

9. **How is GTN classified?**
GTN is classified as either nonmetastatic or metastatic. Metastatic GTN is further subdivided into high-risk and low-risk categories according to the World Health Organization (WHO) prognostic scoring system (Table 32-1). Patients should have a complete workup at the time of diagnosis to establish the severity of the disease and determine appropriate treatment. This evaluation includes a CBC, blood type, Rh status, quantitative β-hCG, AST, ALT, creatinine, BUN, PT, PTT, INR, chest radiograph, and computed tomography or magnetic resonance imaging (MRI) of the abdomen and pelvis. MRI of the brain may be considered.

10. **How is GTN treated?**
For nonmetastatic or low-risk GTN, single-agent chemotherapy with methotrexate or actinomycin-D is appropriate. Treatment is continued until β-hCG levels become undetectable. Eighty percent of these patients have a cured after a single administration, and nearly 100% have a cured within three.

High-risk GTN is treated with combination chemotherapy, most often EMA-CO (etoposide, methotrexate, actinomycin-D, cyclophosphamide, and vincristine). Once the β-hCG level becomes undetectable, treatment is continued for an additional two to three courses. The survival rate is approximately 70%.

As with molar pregnancies, β-hCG screening should occur monthly for 1 year, and patients should be strongly encouraged to use reliable birth control.

Table 32-1. World Health Organization Scoring System for Metastatic Gestational Trophoblastic Disease Based on Prognostic Factors

PROGNOSTIC FACTORS	Score*			
	0	1	2	3
Age (years)	≤39	>39	—	—
Antecedent pregnancy	Mole	Abortion	Term	—
Interval since antecedent pregnancy (months)	4	<4	7-12	>12
hCG (U/L)	$<10^3$	$10^3\text{-}10^4$	$10^4\text{-}10^5$	$>10^5$
Largest tumor	<3 cm	3-5 cm	>5 cm	—
Site of metastases	—	Spleen, kidney	Gastrointestinal tract, liver	Brain
Number of metastases	—	1-3	4-8	>8
Earlier chemotherapy	None	—	Single drug	≥2 drugs

hCG, Human chorionic gonadotropin.
*Scoring: 0 to 6 is low risk; 7 or higher is high risk.

11. **What is the pharmacologic basis for methotrexate, and what are its side effects?**
    Methotrexate is an antimetabolite that targets cells in the S-phase of the cell cycle. It binds to dihydrofolate reductase, thus preventing the reduction of dihydrofolate to tetrahydrofolic acid. This action, in turn, inhibits thymidylate synthetase and purine production and leads to decreased DNA, RNA, and protein production. The most common side effect of methotrexate is mucositis (patients typically complain of mouth sores). Less common side effects include nausea, vomiting, anorexia, thinning of hair, leukopenia, hepatotoxicity, and renal toxicity. In multidose protocols for high-risk GTN, leucovorin (calcium folinate) "rescue" is administered to replenish folate and minimize side effects.

12. **How should a woman with a history of GTN be counseled regarding future pregnancies?**
    Most pregnancies following treatment for a molar pregnancy or GTN—ideally after a year of surveillance—result in normal, healthy babies. The risk of a second molar pregnancy is 1% to 1.5% (10 to 15 times higher than the general population). A woman who has had two molar pregnancies has an 11% to 25% chance of having another, and the risk following three molar pregnancies is nearly 100%. Changing male partners does not affect risk.

KEY POINTS: GESTATIONAL TROPHOBLASTIC DISEASE

1. Most molar pregnancies manifest with symptoms similar to those of early pregnancy: abnormal vaginal bleeding, missed menses, positive pregnancy test, and nausea and vomiting.
2. Patients with molar pregnancies are treated with either a D&C or a hysterectomy.
3. Most cases of gestational trophoblastic neoplasia are preceded by a molar pregnancy. Common sites for metastatic disease are lung, pelvis (including vagina), brain, and liver.
3. Gestational trophoblastic neoplasia is treated with either single-agent (methotrexate) or combination chemotherapy.

BIBLIOGRAPHY

1. American College of Obstetricians and Gynecologists. Diagnosis and treatment of gestational trophoblastic disease. ACOG practice bulletin no. 53. *Obstet Gynecol.* 2004;103:1365–1377.
2. Creasman W. Preinvasive disease of the cervix. In: Di Saia PJ, Creasman WT, eds. *Clinical Gynecologic Oncology.* 8th ed. Philadelphia: Saunders; 2012:1–30.

NORMAL PHYSIOLOGY OF PREGNANCY

Stacy M. Yadava, MD

CHAPTER 33

1. **How soon after fertilization can β-human chorionic gonadotropin (hCG) be detected?**
   Levels of hCG can be detected by serum immunoassay (the most sensitive test) 7 days after fertilization, which is 4 to 5 days after implantation.

2. **What is the normal pattern of hCG rise in pregnancy?**
   Levels of hCG should rise by at least 66% every 48 hours during early pregnancy. This is the minimum rise known to result in a viable intrauterine pregnancy. In an ectopic pregnancy, levels usually rise more slowly or plateau (see Chapter 12 for more details). In cases of impending miscarriage (also known as spontaneous abortion), levels often decline.

3. **At what hCG level can fetal cardiac activity be seen on ultrasound imaging?**
   With modern imaging, a gestational sac can usually be seen when the hCG level reaches 3000 mIU/mL. If no evidence of intrauterine pregnancy is seen at this point, concern for an ectopic pregnancy should exist.

4. **What are the most common causes of false-positive and false-negative pregnancy test results?**
   With current immunoassay methods, false-positive results can be caused by hCG-producing tumors, pituitary hCG-like substances, and antibodies such as rheumatoid factor and antianimal antibodies (circulating human antibodies that react with animal proteins). False-negative test results generally occur in very early pregnancy when the hCG level is below the testing threshold. Blighted ova and ectopic pregnancies may also cause false-negative results.

5. **What changes occur to the reproductive tract during pregnancy?**
   - **Vagina:** Increased vascularity can result in a violet color, known as the **Chadwick sign.** Mucosal thickness also increases, and the presence of a thick white discharge **(leukorrhea)** is common.
   - **Cervix:** Increased vascularity occurs, as well as hypertrophy and hyperplasia of cervical glands. A mucus "plug" obstructs the cervical canal and remains present for the majority of the pregnancy.
   - **Uterus:** Following 12 weeks of gestation, the uterus is no longer contained within the pelvis. It enlarges in response to both stretching and hypertrophy. Estrogen and progesterone initiate these changes until 12 weeks of pregnancy, after which time the growing fetus exerts a direct stretching effect. The uterus also rotates to the maternal right (dextrorotation) as it enlarges because of the presence of the rectosigmoid colon in the left lower quadrant.
   - **Ovary:** The corpus luteum provides progesterone to maintain the pregnancy for 9 to 10 weeks of gestation. After that point, it involutes, and the placenta assumes this role.

6. **What changes occur in the cardiovascular system during pregnancy?**
   - Plasma volume increases by as much as 45%, and red blood cell mass increases by 250 to 450 mL (20% to 30%). This change results in dilutional anemia because the plasma volume expansion is greater than the red cell mass increase.
   - Cardiac output increases by 30% to 50% due to increases in heart rate and stroke volume.
   - Arterial blood pressure decreases, reaches a nadir at 24 to 32 weeks of gestation, and slowly rises back to nonpregnant values at term.
   - Systemic vascular resistance decreases.
   - Serum colloid osmotic pressure decreases, frequently contributing to edema later in pregnancy. There are no significant changes in pulmonary capillary wedge pressure or central venous pressure.

7. **Why does supine hypotension occur during pregnancy?**
In the supine position, compression of the inferior vena cava (IVC) by the gravid uterus can significantly decrease venous blood return to the heart and affect cardiac output. This produces symptoms in some women and can be avoided by having them lie in the left lateral position.

8. **What changes occur in the respiratory system during pregnancy?**
   - Changes in lung volumes
     - Functional residual capacity (FRC): decreases
     - Total lung capacity: decreases slightly at term
     - Vital capacity: unchanged
     - Inspiratory capacity: increases slightly
     - Expiratory reserve volume: decreases
     - Inspiratory reserve volume: unchanged
     - Residual lung volume: decreases
   - Changes in gas exchange
     - Oxygen consumption: increases
     - Tidal volume: increases
     - Minute ventilation: increases
     - Respiratory rate: unchanged

The increase in tidal volume results in hyperventilation and hypocapnia, which are compensated for by increased renal excretion of bicarbonate. Pregnancy is a state of compensated respiratory alkalosis; arterial pH is typically 7.44, and partial pressure of carbon dioxide is 28 to 32 mm Hg.

9. **What changes occur in the kidneys and urinary tract during pregnancy?**
   - Renal volume increases by approximately 30%.
   - Renal plasma flow and glomerular filtration rate (GFR) increase by more than 50%.
   - Ureteral tone decreases, and dilation of the urinary collecting system occurs in most (>80%) women. Dilation is more prominent on the right because of increased compression from the uterus and right ovarian vein (which crosses over the right ureter).
   - Although the filtered load of sodium increases, net retention occurs over the course of a pregnancy.
   - Glucose excretion increases dramatically and can result in glucosuria.
   - Urinary calcium excretion increases, although intestinal absorption also increases, and plasma levels of free (ionic) calcium remain stable.

10. **What are the effects of progesterone on the gastrointestinal and biliary systems?**
Increased progesterone causes delayed gastric emptying, reduced esophageal sphincter tone, decreased gut motility, and biliary stasis. Esophageal reflux and constipation are bothersome but normal complaints during pregnancy, and the risk of gallstones increases.

11. **What are common skin changes in pregnancy?**
Increased pigmentation from increased estrogen and progesterone is commonly seen in the areola, linea nigra, and perineum and may also result in melasma (darkening of facial skin). Striae gravidarum (stretch marks) frequently appear on the abdomen, breasts, and thighs. Pruritus gravidarum (itching with no skin changes) occurs in up to 15% of pregnant women and is thought to be secondary to changes in liver function. Symptomatic relief with a topical agent or oral antihistamine usually suffices, but ursodiol is generally prescribed in cases associated with abnormal liver function tests or serum bile acids.

12. **What changes occur in thyroid function in pregnancy?**
Transient suppression of thyroid-stimulating hormone (TSH) can occur in the first trimester secondary to high levels of hCG, which have structurally similar α subunits. Although free thyroxine (T_4) and triiodothyronine (T_3) levels remain unchanged, the total amounts of both hormones rise because of increased thyroid-binding globulin, which is secondary to increased estrogen levels. For more information on interpreting thyroid function tests in pregnancy, see Chapter 50.

13. **How is carbohydrate metabolism affected by pregnancy?**
Pregnancy is characterized by both hyperinsulinemia and increased insulin resistance. Lower fasting blood glucose levels and higher postmeal values are observed. In cases of pronounced insulin resistance, gestational diabetes may result. For more information on diabetes in pregnancy, see Chapter 48.

14. **What changes can be seen in coagulation parameters during pregnancy?**
    Pregnancy is a hypercoagulable state, with a fivefold increased risk of venous thromboembolism. This risk reflects increases in von Willebrand factor, fibrinogen (factor I), factors VII, VIII, IX, and X, decreases in protein S and fibrinolytic activity, and increases in platelet activation and venous stasis. For more information on venous thromboembolism in pregnancy, see Chapter 53..

KEY POINTS: NORMAL PHYSIOLOGY OF PREGNANCY

1. Plasma volume increases by as much as 45%, but red blood cell mass increases by only 20% to 30%, resulting in a dilutional anemia.
2. Pregnancy is a state of compensated respiratory alkalosis.
3. Renal plasma flow and glomerular filtration rate increase by more than 50%.
4. Increased progesterone causes delayed gastric emptying, reduced esophageal sphincter tone, decreased gut motility, and biliary stasis.
5. Pregnancy is a hypercoagulable state as a result of venous stasis, increased clotting factors and platelet activation, and decreased fibrinolysis.

BIBLIOGRAPHY

1. Barnhart KT, Sammel MD, Rinaudo PF, Zhou L, Hummel AC, Guo W. Symptomatic patients with an early viable intrauterine pregnancy: hCG curves redefined. *Obstet Gynecol.* 2004;104:50–55.
2. Braunstein G. False-positive serum human chorionic gonadotropin results: causes, characteristics, and recognition. *Am J Obstet Gynecol.* 2002;187:217–224.
3. Campion EW, Doubilet PM, Benson CB, Bourne T, Blaivas M. Diagnostic criteria for nonviable pregnancy early in the first trimester. *N Engl J Med.* 2013;369:1443–1451.
4. Centers for Disease Control and Prevention. Pregnancy Mortality Surveillance System. *Last updated.* September 16, 2015. Available at www.cdc.gov/reproductivehealth/maternalinfanthealth/pmss.html.
5. Constantine MM. Physiologic and pharmacokinetic changes in pregnancy. *Front Pharmacol.* 2014;5:65.
6. Cunningham FG, Leveno KJ, Bloom SL, Spong CY, Dashe JS, Hoffman BL, Casey BM, Sheffield JS, eds. Maternal Physiology. Williams Obstetrics. 24rd ed. New York: McGraw-Hill; 2013. Available at: http://accessmediicine. mhmedical. com.laneproxy.stanford.edu/content.aspx?bookid=1057&Sectionid=59789139.
7. Gordon M. Maternal physiology. In: Gabbe SG, Niebyl JR, Simpson JL, et al., eds. *Obstetrics: Normal and Problem Pregnancies.* 6th ed. Philadelphia: Churchill Livingstone; 2012:42–65.
8. Massey EW, Guidon AC. Peripheral neuropathies in pregnancy. *Continuum (Minneap Minn).* 2014;201:100–114.
9. Monga M, Mastrobattista JM. Maternal cardiovascular, respiratory, and renal adaptation to pregnancy. In: Creasy RK, Resnik R, Iams JD, Lockwood CJ, Moore TR, Greene MF, eds. *Creasy and Resnik's Maternal-Fetal Medicine: Principles and Practice.* 7th ed. Philadelphia: Saunders; 2014:93–99.

CHAPTER 34

PATHOPHYSIOLOGY OF THE PLACENTA

Carlos Rangel, MD

1. **What is a blastocyst, and how is it formed?**
   Mitotic division of the zygote results in the production of blastomeres. As the blastomeres continue to divide, they form a solid ball of cells called a morula. Fluid gradually accumulates between the blastomeres of the morula to form a blastocyst, which develops 96 hours after fertilization. At this time the conceptus is at the 58-cell stage, with a 5-cell inner mass and 53 trophoblasts.

2. **When does implantation occur, and when do the trophoblastic cells differentiate?**
   Six days after fertilization. By day 9, the trophoblastic cells differentiate into two layers: the inner cytotrophoblasts and the outer syncytiotrophoblasts. These two layers separate the maternal and embryonic circulatory systems.

3. **What is the origin of the fetal membrane?**
   The fetal membrane is composed of the chorion and amnion. The amniotic membrane originates from embryonic ectoderm and consists of a single layer of epithelial cells and a thin fibrous membrane. The chorion is composed of embryonic mesoderm and a double layer of trophoblasts.

4. **What is the yolk sac?**
   The yolk sac is a cavity outside the embryo and formed from embryonic endoderm; it is connected to the ventral surface of the embryo by a yolk sac stalk. The yolk sac is a site of early hematopoiesis and becomes incorporated into the primitive gut.

5. **What is the Nitabuch layer?**
   A layer of fibrinoid degeneration between the invading trophoblasts and the decidua basalis. This layer is where the placenta detaches from the uterus after delivery, and it is thought to play a role in preventing abnormally deep placental implantation.

6. **What are the main functions of the human placenta?**
   The human placenta functions as both a transport organ and an endocrine organ. Exchanges of nutrients, waste products, water, and oxygen all take place. The placenta also produces important hormones such as human chorionic gonadotropin (hCG), progesterone, estradiol, and human placental lactogen (hPL).

7. **What is hCG?**
   A glycoprotein produced by the syncytiotrophoblast, hCG is one of the earliest secretions by the conceptus. It has been detected as early as 3 to 4 days in some studies, and levels peak at 8 to 10 weeks of gestation. It functions to maintain the corpus luteum in early pregnancy (which produces progesterone) and may also play a role in promoting the differentiation of cytotrophoblasts into syncytiotrophoblasts.

8. **How is the hCG level used clinically?**
   Measurement of hCG during pregnancy has many uses. It can be used to follow suspected ectopic pregnancies (see Chapter 12), and higher than normal hCG levels may indicate a molar pregnancy (see Chapter 32) or multiple gestation. Low levels of hCG in early pregnancy indicate embryonic failure. In the second trimester, hCG levels are abnormally elevated in pregnancies complicated by trisomy 21 and monosomy X (Turner syndrome).

9. **What is hPL, and what is its function?**
   hPL is a glycoprotein made by syncytiotrophoblasts throughout pregnancy. It is also called human chorionic somatomammotropin. A polypeptide hormone, hPL has structural similarities to human growth hormone and prolactin. It plays a role in fetal growth and maternal metabolism and can lead to insulin resistance.

10. **What is relaxin, and where is it produced?**
    Relaxin is produced in several sites including the corpus luteum, the decidua, the atria of the heart, and the placenta. It appears to have a broad range of activities and to play a role in collagen remodeling, although it does not seem to be necessary for pregnancy maintenance or normal delivery.

11. **What are the physical measurements of a normal placenta?**
    A human placenta weighs between 450 and 550 g, with an average diameter of 20 cm and an average thickness of 2.5 cm.

12. **Can placental thickness be measured antenatally?**
    Yes. Placental thickness can be easily measured by ultrasound examination. Conditions such as intrauterine fetal infections, diabetes mellitus, and immune and nonimmune hydrops are associated with abnormally thick placentas (>4 cm).

13. **What is a battledore placenta?**
    Insertion of the umbilical cord at the margin of the placenta—also referred to as a **marginal cord insertion.** It is found in 7% of pregnant women, and its incidence is higher in multifetal gestations. It has no known clinical significance.

14. **What is a velamentous cord insertion?**
    When the umbilical cord does not insert directly into the placenta; instead, it separates into vessels that run through the fetal membranes immediately adjacent to the placenta. This occurs in 1% of singleton pregnancies. Vasa previa is a rare but serious condition in which fetal blood vessels are positioned over the internal os. Because the blood vessels are not protected by Wharton jelly, they can tear during labor and result in fetal exsanguination.

15. **What is placenta previa?**
    A condition in which the placenta covers the internal os. For more information on this topic, see Chapter 66.

16. **What are placenta accreta, increta, and percreta?**
    Placenta accreta is the term used when the placental villi are attached to the myometrium as a result of partial or complete absence of the decidua basalis and the Nitabuch layer. **Placental increta** occurs when placental villi invade the myometrium. When villi invade through the myometrium, the condition is known as **placenta percreta**. For more information on these topics, see Chapter 66.

17. **What is placental abruption?**
    Separation of a normally implanted placenta before the birth of the fetus. For more information on this topic, see Chapter 66.

18. **What is a succenturiate placenta?**
    A succenturiate placenta, or succenturiate placental lobe, is a condition in which an extra lobe of the placenta separated from it by space and connected to it by vessels. If unrecognized, this lobe may be retained at the time of delivery and cause postpartum bleeding and infection.

19. **What are the different types of placentation in twin pregnancy?**
    The three different types are dichorionic-diamniotic, monochorionic-diamniotic, and monochorionic-monoamniotic.

20. **Why is it important to know the chorionicity in twin gestations?**
    Perinatal mortality is highest for monochorionic-monoamniotic twins, and monochorionic-diamniotic twins are at increased risk for selective growth restriction and twin-to-twin transfusion syndrome (TTTS). For more information on this topic, see Chapter 60.

21. **What is the significance of a single umbilical artery?**
    Normally, three umbilical vessels are present: two arteries and one vein. The incidence of single umbilical artery (SUA) is approximately 1% of all singleton births. SUA has been associated with an increased rate of additional fetal malformations, most commonly in the renal, cardiovascular, gastrointestinal, and central nervous systems. If an additional abnormality is found, the risk of chromosomal abnormalities is increased.

KEY POINTS: PATHOPHYSIOLOGY OF THE PLACENTA

1. Implantation occurs 6 days after fertilization, after which trophoblastic cells differentiate into inner cytotrophoblasts and outer syncytiotrophoblasts.
2. The placenta functions as both a transport organ and an endocrine organ.
3. hCG is a glycoprotein made by the syncytiotrophoblast that serves to maintain progesterone production by the corpus luteum in early pregnancy. Peak concentration occurs at 8 to 10 weeks of gestation.
4. A velamentous cord insertion is when the umbilical cord inserts into the fetal membranes instead of the placental disk; vasa previa is when the exposed vessels lie over the internal os.
5. Normally the umbilical cord contains three vessels: two arteries and one vein. SUA is associated with an increased risk of additional malformations.

BIBLIOGRAPHY

1. Benirschke K. Twinning. In: Knobil E, Neill JD, eds. *Encyclopedia of Reproduction.* vol. 4. San Diego: Academic Press; 1998:887–891.
2. Benirschke K. Normal development. In: Creasy R, Resnik R, Iams JD, Lockwood CJ, Moore TR, eds. *Creasy and Resnik's Maternal-Fetal Medicine: Principles and Practice.* 7th ed. Philadelphia: Saunders; 2014.
3. Heifetz SA. The umbilical cord: obstetrically important lesions. *Clin Obstet Gynecol.* 1996;39:571–587.
4. Hull AD. Placenta previa, placenta accreta, abruptio placentae, and vasa previa. In: Creasy R, Resnik R, Iams JD, Lockwood CJ, Moore TR, eds. *Creasy and Resnik's Maternal-Fetal Medicine: Principles and Practice.* 7th ed. Philadelphia: Saunders; 2014.
5. Liu JH, Rebar RW. Endocrinology of pregnancy. In: Creasy R, Resnik R, Iams JD, Lockwood CJ, Moore TR, eds. *Creasy and Resnik's Maternal-Fetal Medicine: Principles and Practice.* 7th ed. Philadelphia: Saunders; 2014.

CHAPTER 35

PRECONCEPTION COUNSELING

Anna Karina Celaya, MD

1. **Why is preconception counseling important?**
   Preconception counseling offers the opportunity to:
   - Screen for and treat medical issues that place the mother and fetus at risk
   - Optimize chronic medical and psychological diseases before conception
   - Screen for substance or medication use that may be teratogenic
   - Screen for genetic disorders in high-risk populations
   - Educate patients on the importance of folic acid before and throughout pregnancy
   - Review the patient's obstetric history and discuss the risk of subsequent pregnancies
   - Assess immunization status and administer appropriate vaccines before conception
   - Evaluate for domestic violence, environmental exposures, and nutritional status
   - Refer the patient to subspecialists for further counseling when appropriate

2. **What relatively common medical conditions should be identified and addressed during preconception counseling?**
   - **Diabetes mellitus:** This is associated with an increased risk of birth defects that is further increased with poor glycemic control. Optimal blood glucose control, assessed by glycosylated hemoglobin (HbA1c), should be achieved before conception. The presence of end-organ damage should prompt referral to a subspecialist.
   - **Seizures:** Effort should be made to achieve good control with monotherapy. Many antiepileptics are teratogenic and should be avoided if at all possible (e.g., valproic acid, phenytoin). Adjustment of antiepileptic medication should be done in conjunction with a neurologist.
   - **Hypertension:** Angiotensin-converting enzyme (ACE) inhibitors and angiotensin receptor blockers (ARBs) are teratogenic and should be discontinued. Hypertension in pregnancy is associated with several pregnancy complications; for more information, see Chapter 49.

3. **What congenital defect can be potentially averted by preconception counseling?**
   Neural tube defects (NTDs). Supplementation with 0.4 mg folic acid on a daily basis reduces the risk of NTDs by 50%. Ideally, this regimen should be started a minimum of 1 month before conception. For women with a history of an earlier child with an NTD, 4 mg folic acid per day can reduce the recurrence rate by 72%. Women taking valproic acid or carbamazepine should also increase the daily dose of folic acid to 4 mg.

4. **What should women with phenylketonuria (PKU) be told before conception to minimize risk to their unborn children?**
   Women with PKU must follow a phenylalanine-restricted diet before conception. Otherwise, elevated phenylalanine levels can cause mental retardation, microcephaly, and cardiac defects (see Chapter 36).

5. **What laboratory tests may be indicated in preconception counseling?**
   - Complete blood count (CBC): can screen for hemoglobinopathies and anemia
   - Hepatitis B antigen, rubella, and varicella titers: nonimmune women should be vaccinated before pregnancy
   - Screening for human immunodeficiency virus (HIV) and other sexually transmitted diseases
   - Screening for specific genetic disorders, guided by family history and ethnic background
   - Papanicolaou smear
   - Diabetes screening in high-risk women

6. **What conditions should prompt cardiac testing (e.g., electrocardiogram, echocardiogram) before pregnancy?**
   - Pregestational diabetes
   - Chronic hypertension (>10 years, or >40 years of age)
   - Congenital heart disease

7. **How should the family history be assessed?**
Women should be asked whether they or their partners have any relatives with recognized genetic disorders, congenital defects (e.g., NTD, cardiac anomaly, cleft lip or palate), or chromosomal abnormalities. A first-degree family member with mental retardation of unknown cause should initiate screening for fragile X syndrome.

8. **What are the risks associated with advanced maternal age (≥35 years) in pregnancy?**
Approximately 10% of pregnancies occur among women of advanced maternal age. These pregnancies have higher rates of fetal growth restriction, aneuploidy, spontaneous abortion, preeclampsia, gestational diabetes, and medically indicated preterm delivery.

9. **Do any absolute contraindications to pregnancy exist?**
Yes. Because of extremely high mortality rates, women with Eisenmenger syndrome, pulmonary hypertension, or a history of peripartum cardiomyopathy without recovery of cardiac function are advised not to become pregnant. Women with Marfan syndrome who have aortic root dilation larger than 4 cm also fall into this category.

KEY POINTS: PRECONCEPTION COUNSELING

1. Preconception counseling provides an important opportunity to identify and address any health problems that may adversely affect a woman or her unborn child, or both.
2. Taken at least a month before conception, 0.4 mg folic acid on a daily basis reduces the risk of NTDs by as much as 50%. Women at high risk or who have already had a pregnancy with this complication are recommended to take 4 mg daily.
3. Pregnancy is not recommended for women with certain cardiac and pulmonary conditions.

BIBLIOGRAPHY

1. American College of Obstetricians and Gynecologists. The importance of preconception care in the continuum of women's health care. ACOG committee opinion no. 313. *Obstet Gynecol.* 2005;106:665–666.
2. American College of Obstetricians and Gynecologists. Moderate caffeine consumption during pregnancy. ACOG committee opinion no. 462. *Obstet Gynecol.* 2010;116:467–468.
3. American College of Obstetricians and Gynecologists. Smoking cessation during pregnancy. ACOG committee opinion no. 471. *Obstet Gynecol.* 2010;116:1241–1244.
4. American College of Obstetricians and Gynecologists. At-risk drinking and alcohol dependence: obstetric and gynecologic implications. ACOG committee opinion no. 496. *Obstet Gynecol.* 2011;118:383–388.
5. Cunningham FG, Leveno KJ, Bloom SL, Spong CY, Dashe JS, Hoffman BL, Casey BM, Sheffield JS. *Williams Obstetrics.* 24th ed. New York: McGraw-Hill Medical; 2014.
6. Institute of Medicine. *National Academy of Sciences. Fetal Alcohol Syndrome: Diagnosis, Epidemiology, Prevention and Treatment.* Washington, DC: National Academies Press; 1996.

CHAPTER 36

COMPREHENSIVE PRENATAL CARE

Hai-Lang Duong, MD

1. **What does prenatal care encompass?**

   Prenatal care is the careful, systematic assessment and follow-up of a pregnant patient to ensure the best possible health of the mother and her fetus. It is a preventive service and has been shown to be beneficial and cost effective; women receiving no or inadequate prenatal care have far more complications and poorer outcomes of pregnancy. Goals are threefold:
   1. To prevent, identify, or ameliorate maternal or fetal abnormalities that adversely affect pregnancy outcome, including socioeconomic and emotional factors, as well as medical and obstetric factors.
   2. To educate the patient about pregnancy, labor and delivery, and parenting in addition to ways she can improve her overall health.
   3. To promote adequate psychological support from her partner, family, and caregivers so she can successfully adapt to the pregnancy and the challenges of raising a family.

   Prenatal care commences with an extensive initial history and physical examination. Estimated gestational age and estimated date of delivery (EDD) are determined, and routine laboratory tests are drawn. In subsequent visits the physician explores any problems, documents fetal growth, and identifies potential complications. Assessment for risk factors is done at the initial visit and on each subsequent appointment. Weight gain and nutritional well-being are frequently evaluated, and patient education is provided on a timely basis.

2. **How often should patients be seen?**

   The American College of Obstetricians and Gynecologists (ACOG) recommends that pregnant women be seen for an extensive initial visit in early pregnancy and then every 4 weeks until 28 weeks, every 2 to 3 weeks to 36 weeks, and then weekly until delivery. For low-risk pregnancies, a national panel has suggested seven visits total for parous women (at 6 to 8, 14 to 16, 24 to 28, 32, 36, 39, and 41 weeks) and nine visits for nulliparous (two additional visits at 10 to 12 and 40 weeks). For high-risk patients, the schedule should be individualized and usually requires more visits.

3. **What historical information should be recorded at the initial prenatal visit?**
   - **Medical:** Many chronic medical conditions have an effect, often adverse, on pregnancy outcome; conversely, pregnancy usually has a distinct effect on the course of the condition itself.
   - **Surgical:** Be sure to note any earlier surgical or anesthetic complications and need for blood transfusion.
   - **Obstetric or gynecologic:** Some events in the patient's obstetric history often recur in subsequent pregnancies (e.g., fetal or neonatal death, low birth weight, preterm delivery, preeclampsia or hypertension, and postpartum hemorrhage). A history of recent infertility treatment, pelvic inflammatory disease, or ectopic pregnancy is also important for identifying early pregnancy complications such as tubal pregnancy or multiple gestations. A history of past sexually transmitted diseases should also be taken.
   - **Family history:** The history should focus on family members and relatives with cerebral palsy, mental retardation, neural tube defects, and other congenital malformations, as well as specific conditions such as cystic fibrosis, muscular dystrophy, and hemophilia. Inherited diseases are important to ask about because increasing numbers are amenable to prenatal diagnosis.
   - **Social:** Psychosocial background and lifestyle are also important because they frequently affect pregnancy and neonatal outcome. Be sure to ask about smoking, use of alcohol and illicit drugs, use of prescription and over-the-counter medications, employment and type of occupation, and the existence of problems at home such as domestic violence.

4. **What history elements should be obtained at subsequent prenatal visits?**

   A brief interval history should always be obtained, as well as a review of systems. Every patient should be asked about pain, contractions or cramping, pelvic pressure, bleeding, discharge, dysuria, gastrointestinal problems, presence and adequacy of fetal movements, and whether any other problems have arisen since the last visit. Smokers should be asked about their progress in smoking cessation. Patients with medical conditions or known complications should be asked specific questions regarding those problems.

5. **What physical examination components should be performed at an initial prenatal visit?**
   A general physical examination should always be performed at the first visit; this examination may be the only one for many women over a several-year period. Principal examination components include measurement of blood pressure and weight, heart and lung auscultation, palpation of the abdomen, and a breast examination.

   A routine pelvic examination can detect abnormalities of the vulva, vagina, cervix, uterus, and adnexa. It is important to estimate the size of the early gravid uterus in weeks and assess the cervix. A Papanicolaou (Pap) smear and cultures for sexually transmitted infections should be obtained, as well as evaluation of any abnormal vaginal discharge. Traditionally, clinical pelvimetry has been performed to determine pelvic adequacy in first pregnancies and for multiparous women who have experienced previous abnormal labor or difficult delivery. The only true test for pelvic adequacy, however, is a trial of labor.

6. **Which laboratory tests should be ordered at an initial prenatal visit?**
   The number of laboratory tested considered "routine" has increased with time, and these tests are listed in Table 36-1. Additional tests can be ordered as appropriate for women with health conditions.

Table 36-1. Prenatal Laboratory Tests

INITIAL VISIT	LATER IN PREGNANCY
Complete blood count	Aneuploidy screening
Urinalysis and culture	Dipstick urine analysis (every visit)
Blood type	Complete blood count (third trimester)
Antibody screen	Gestational diabetes screening (24-28 weeks)
Serologic test for syphilis	Group B streptococcus culture (36-37 weeks)
Rubella immunity	Antibody screening test (28 weeks; Rh-negative
Hepatitis B surface antigen	patients)
HIV testing	
Papanicolaou smear	
Gonorrhea and *Chlamydia* testing*	
Tuberculosis screening*	
Hemoglobin electrophoresis†	
Wet prep†	

HIV, Human immunodeficiency virus.
*In at-risk patients.
†As needed.

7. **How is gestational age determined?**
   An accurate last menstrual period (LMP) should be recorded at the first prenatal visit, along with the woman's normal menstrual cycle length and recent use of oral contraceptives. Careful determination of the EDD is needed so that therapeutic decisions at each stage of pregnancy are appropriately made. The EDD is initially calculated using the Naegele rule: take the first day of the LMP, add 7 days and 1 year, then subtract 3 months. This assumes that a term gestation is 280 days or 40 weeks from the start of the LMP, however, and that menstruation occurs every 28 days. Variations in cycle length and the timing of ovulation, use of oral contraception in the month preceding the LMP, and the appearance of menstrual-like bleeding during early pregnancy can render estimated dates of conception calculated with the method inaccurate.

   Ultrasound measurement of the embryo or fetus in the first trimester (<14 and 0/7 weeks of gestation) is the most accurate method of confirming the EDD based on LMP or giving a new EDD. A crown-rump length (CRL) is used to assess the gestational age in the first trimester; in the second and third trimesters, a collection of measurements known as **biometrics** (head circumference, biparietal diameter, abdominal circumference, and femur length) is used. If a significant discrepancy exists between an EDD based on ultrasound measurements and the EDD based on an LMP, the ultrasound results should be used. Ultrasound dating is also used when the LMP is unknown. For more information on ultrasound in pregnancy, see Chapter 38.

8. **What physical examination components are important on subsequent prenatal visits?**
Weight and blood pressure should always be recorded, and fetal heart rate should be assessed. The fundal height is measured in centimeters from the symphysis pubis to the top of the uterus. In a patient with a normal body habitus, serial measurements over the course of pregnancy provide an excellent assessment of fetal growth. Between 18 and 34 weeks, the height in centimeters roughly approximates the gestational week. Abnormal measurements should prompt a fetal ultrasound examination. Other examinations, including vaginal, are done as indicated by the patient's interval history.

   In the third trimester, Leopold maneuvers should be used to assess fetal position and estimate fetal size. These maneuvers involve palpation of the uterus to determine the following:
   - What fetal part lies in the fundus?
   - On which side is the fetal back?
   - What fetal part is oriented toward the pelvis, and is it engaged?
   - How far has the fetal presenting part descended into the pelvis?

9. **Why are a patient's prepregnancy weight and weight gain during pregnancy important?**
Women who are underweight or who have poor weight gain during pregnancy are at increased risk for fetal growth restriction, and a statistically significant relationship exists between poor maternal weight gain and preterm delivery. Excessive weight gain during pregnancy can lead to a large for gestational age (LGA) fetus, and prepregnancy obesity is associated with increased rates of spontaneous abortion, congenital anomalies, gestational diabetes mellitus, intrauterine fetal death, hypertensive disorders of pregnancy, cesarean delivery, thromboembolism, and postoperative wound infections.

   For more information on nutrition in pregnancy and recommended weight gain based on maternal body mass index, see Chapter 37.

10. **How is a complete blood count useful during pregnancy?**
Delivery is associated with a blood loss of 500 to 1000 mL; to avoid requiring a blood transfusion, patients who are anemic need to be identified well ahead of delivery. Most cases of anemia in pregnancy result from iron deficiency and improve with 60 to 100 mg/day of oral elemental iron supplementation. Microcytic anemia in the absence of iron deficiency should prompt testing for hereditary anemias (see later). A platelet count can identify women with thrombocytopenia and, in severe cases, prompt referrals to subspecialists.

11. **How are urinalysis and urine culture useful during pregnancy?**
All patients should have a urine sample collected on the first visit for urinalysis and urine culture. Detection of the approximately 5% of patients with asymptomatic bacteriuria can prevent progression to pyelonephritis, and women with group B streptococcus (GBS) bacteriuria can be identified (see later).

12. **What is the importance of the blood type and antibody screening tests?**
Rh-negative women must be identified so that they can be given Rh immune globulin (RhoGAM) at 28 to 30 weeks and within 72 hours of delivery to prevent Rh sensitization. The antibody screening test is done to detect any antibodies (e.g., Rh, Kell, Duffy, Lewis) that have the potential to cause hemolytic disease in the fetus and newborn infant. For more information on this topic, see Chapter 46.

13. **Are Pap smears interpreted any differently in pregnant women?**
No. Abnormal results should be managed according to guidelines published by the American Society for Colposcopy and Cervical Pathology (ASCCP). If colposcopy is indicated, endocervical curettage is not performed during pregnancy. For more information on this topic, see Chapter 27.

14. **How is hemoglobin electrophoresis useful during pregnancy?**
Sickle cell trait is estimated to be present in 8.5% of African Americans, and screening with hemoglobin electrophoresis should be performed. Women who carry the trait are more susceptible to urinary tract infections, and they should receive genetic counseling to understand their risk of having a child with sickle cell disease and obtain prenatal diagnosis if desired. Hemoglobin electrophoresis can also identify carriers of β-thalassemia, hemoglobin C, or rarer hemoglobinopathies. In patients with microcytic anemia, normal iron studies, and normal hemoglobin electrophoresis results, genetic testing for α-thalassemia should be performed.

15. **What is the purpose of the rubella antibody titer?**

    Congenital rubella syndrome is now rare because of widespread vaccination; however, many adults (10% to 15%) exhibit susceptibility on serologic testing. Because the rubella vaccine is live attenuated virus given as part of the MMR (measles, mumps, rubella) vaccine, women who are seronegative should be immunized post partum.

16. **Is serologic testing for syphilis still important?**

    Yes. Women who test positive should receive the fluorescent treponemal antibody (FTA) test; if the FTA test result is also positive, syphilis is diagnosed. For more information on this topic, see Chapter 55.

17. **Why test for hepatitis B?**

    Women who are chronic carriers of the hepatitis B virus have a high risk of vertical transmission to their infants during or after delivery. Many of these infants also become chronic carriers, and this in turn places them at risk for cirrhosis and hepatocellular carcinoma. The Centers for Disease Control and Prevention (CDC) recommend that all pregnant women be screened for the hepatitis B surface antigen and that all newborn infants receive vaccination against hepatitis B. Infants of antigen-positive mothers should be given hepatitis B immune globulin as well as the vaccine within the first 12 hours of life.

18. **Should pregnant women be screened for human immunodeficiency virus (HIV) infection?**

    Absolutely. The ACOG and the American Academy of Pediatrics now recommend screening all prenatal patients. Positive results from an initial enzyme-linked immunoassay (ELISA) test should be confirmed by Western blot analysis. Diagnosed women should then be assessed for viral load (by polymerase chain reaction [PCR]) and referred to appropriate subspecialists. At the time of delivery, women with a viral load of less than 1000 copies/mL are candidates for vaginal delivery. Women with higher viral loads should be delivered by cesarean section to reduce the risk of vertical transmission. All patients with a viral load greater than 400 copies/mL should be given intravenous zidovudine (formerly azidothymidine [AZT]) during labor or before a scheduled cesarean delivery. After birth, infants born to HIV-positive mothers should also be followed and treated by infectious disease specialists.

19. **Of what benefit are tests for other sexually transmitted diseases?**

    Testing for gonorrhea and *Chlamydia* should be done in at-risk patients (i.e., those <25 years old, unmarried, or with multiple sexual partners), and many authorities recommend routine testing for all pregnant women. Neonatal chlamydial infection occurs in 60% to 70% of infants passing through an infected birth canal. Conjunctivitis develops in 25% to 50% of exposed infants, and chronic pneumonia occurs in 10% to 20%. Before mandatory use of ophthalmic antibiotic prophylaxis after delivery, gonorrheal transmission at birth caused blindness in many newborn infants (**gonococcal ophthalmia neonatorum**). Gonococci can also cause chorioamnionitis after preterm premature rupture of membranes (PPROM), resulting in a high rate of prematurity and infant morbidity.

    Women who test positive for gonorrhea or *Chlamydia* infection should be treated and a test of cure obtained. Repeat testing should also be performed at 36 weeks of gestation. For more information on this topic, see Chapter 55.

20. **Which laboratory tests are repeated during the prenatal course?**

    - A complete blood count is generally repeated in the third trimester to identify women with anemia. It can be repeated more frequently in at-risk women.
    - Dipstick urine analysis for protein, glucose, leukocyte esterase, and nitrites is done at each prenatal visit. The presence of significant proteinuria (1+ or greater) should prompt further testing for preeclampsia, urinary tract infection, or renal disease. The presence of nitrites or leukocyte esterase should prompt further testing for urinary tract infection. Although glucose testing is performed, glucosuria has poor specificity and can be present in healthy pregnancy women.
    - Antibody screening test is repeated at 28 weeks of gestation in Rh-negative women.
    - Sexually transmitted disease testing is frequently repeated in the third trimester for at-risk women.

21. **Should pregnant women be screened for tuberculosis?**

    The incidence of tuberculosis nationwide has declined since 1992. However, this infection remains a problem for women born in foreign countries with high infection rates. Screening is therefore encouraged for women who have immigrated from Asia, Africa, or Latin America or for women who have other risk factors. Newborn infants are especially susceptible to tuberculosis, and active disease should be ruled out in women who screen positive. Treatment is acceptable in pregnancy if indicated; in the absence of active disease, it can be deferred until after delivery.

22. **Why is GBS screening done during pregnancy?**
GBS infection is a cause of neonatal sepsis and carries high rates of neonatal mortality and morbidity, especially in premature neonates. Eradicating the organism with an antibiotic (usually penicillin) at the time of delivery is the best means of preventing early-onset neonatal GBS sepsis. The CDC currently recommends routine screening of all mothers for GBS at 35 to 37 weeks; for women with unknown screening results or unknown GBS status, treatment is determined by risk factors (e.g., <37 weeks of gestation, membrane rupture >18 hours, maternal fever in labor). Intrapartum prophylaxis should be given to all patients with GBS bacteriuria or a history of a previous infant with GBS disease.

23. **Who should be screened for gestational diabetes (GDM), and how should this be done?**
The ACOG recommends that all pregnant women be screened for GDM, whether by clinical risk factors (Table 36-2), medical history, or laboratory screening tests. The most commonly used laboratory test is the 1-hour, 50-g glucose challenge test. It is performed at 24 to 28 weeks of gestation. Additional testing can be done at the initial prenatal visit for patients at high risk for gestational diabetes (e.g., history of GDM in a previous pregnancy, morbid obesity, strong family history). The literature does not clearly support using one cutoff value compared with another; screening thresholds of 130 to 140 mg/dL have been used, with varying sensitivity and specificity.

Patients with abnormal 1-hour test results should have a 3-hour, 100-g oral glucose challenge test; the test result is considered positive if the fasting level is higher than 125 mg/dL or if any two of the following are present:
- >95 mg/dL fasting
- >180 mg/dL at 1 hour
- >155 mg/dL at 2 hours
- >140 mg/dL at 3 hours

Table 36-2. Risk Factors for Gestational Diabetes*

HIGH RISK (ANY REQUIRED)	LOW RISK (ALL REQUIRED)
Previous macrosomic infant	<25 years of age
Previous stillbirth	Negative family history
Previous gestational diabetes	Normal body habitus
Family history of diabetes	Ethnic background with low prevalence
Obesity	No earlier poor obstetric outcomes associated with gestational diabetes
Ethnicity: Hispanic, African American, Native American, East or Southeast Asian, Pacific Islander	

*The presence of any high-risk factor should prompt further screening. For no additional screening to be considered necessary, all low-risk factors must be present.

24. **What is the purpose of nuchal translucency (NT) measurement and serum biochemical marker screening?**
The ACOG recommends that all pregnant women—regardless of age—should be offered aneuploidy screening before 20 weeks of gestation. The NT measurement is offered between 11 and 14 weeks of gestation; abnormally large (>3.5 mm) measurements indicate an increased risk for aneuploidy and congenital heart defects. Aneuploidy detection is improved when the NT is combined with biochemical serum markers in the first or second trimester. Various biochemical screening protocols are available, including the triple screen, the quad or quadruple screen, the first trimester combined screen, the sequential screen, and the integrated screen. Patients who screen

positive should be referred for genetic counseling and offered diagnostic testing with chorionic villus sampling or amniocentesis, depending on gestational age. For more information on this topic, see Chapter 39.

25. **Should a routine prenatal ultrasound scan be done?**
Yes. Ultrasound examination can show many major fetal anomalies. Ninety percent of infants with congenital abnormalities are born to women who do not have any risk factors, and pregnant women should have at least one ultrasound examination during pregnancy to assess fetal anatomy. This examination is generally done at 18 to 20 weeks of gestation. Ultrasound has not been shown to be harmful to a developing fetus.

26. **Should any routine medications be prescribed during pregnancy?**
Most authorities recommend supplemental iron because it is often difficult to meet the iron requirements of pregnancy by diet alone. Most prenatal vitamins contain 40 to 65 mg of elemental iron. Adequate intake of folic acid, a key component in neural tube development, should be started before pregnancy. For more information on this topic, see Chapter 37.

27. **Can pregnant women exercise during pregnancy?**
Yes. Most women can continue some form of exercise during pregnancy. For these women, aerobic exercise is recommended for at least 15 minutes three times per week. Women should continue activities they were familiar with before pregnancy, but avoid contact sports or activities with an increased risk of falling (e.g., skiing, horseback riding, gymnastics). For more information on this topic, see Chapter 37.

28. **Should pregnant women be screened for intimate partner violence (IPV) or domestic violence?**
Yes. The rate of IPV in pregnancy is estimated to be from 1% to 20%. As a group, victims of domestic violence are at high risk for poor pregnancy outcome and are likely to commence prenatal care late in pregnancy. The leading cause of maternal mortality is homicide, and most cases are associated with a history of IPV. For more information on this topic, see Chapter 20.

29. **What advice should be given to pregnant women regarding work outside the house?**
In general, women with low-risk pregnancies can continue working at their regular jobs as long as the job is not dangerous (physically or environmentally) or overly strenuous. Job requirements often can be modified to reduce the physical workload, or the patient can be transferred to a role that requires less strenuous work. Frequent breaks, elevation of legs, and changes in position are all helpful.

By federal law, employers offering medical disability compensation must treat pregnancy-related disabilities in the same manner as temporary disabilities (illness or injury) suffered by nonpregnant employees. Such temporary disability can result from pregnancy per se (e.g., musculoskeletal symptoms), complications of pregnancy, or hazardous occupational exposure during pregnancy. If employee disability coverage is not available, the patient may be eligible for state unemployment benefits, or she must use sick leave or vacation time or take an unpaid leave of absence. The Family and Medical Leave Act of 1993 provides that any pregnant woman working for a government or a company of more than 50 employees is allowed up to 12 weeks of nonpaid maternal leave, during which time the employer must continue her benefits and seniority and retain her job position or equivalent for when she returns.

30. **Which common complications of pregnancy can be prevented or minimized by good prenatal care?**
- Anemia from iron or folic acid deficiency
- Urinary tract infections and pyelonephritis
- Pregnancy-induced hypertension (preeclampsia)
- Preterm delivery
- Intrauterine growth retardation
- Sexually transmitted diseases and their effect on the newborn infant
- Rh isoimmunization
- Fetal macrosomia
- Breech presentation at term
- Hypoxia or fetal death from postterm birth

KEY POINTS: COMPREHENSIVE PRENATAL CARE

1. Prenatal care is intended to ensure the best possible health of the mother and her fetus. It is a preventive service and can prevent or minimize many common obstetric complications.
2. All pregnant women should be screened for HIV infection.
3. All pregnant women should be screened for gestational diabetes, whether by clinical risk factors, medical history, or laboratory screening tests. The most commonly used laboratory test is the 1-hour, 50 g oral glucose challenge test at 24 to 28 weeks of gestation.
4. Weight, blood pressure, dipstick urine analysis, fetal cardiac activity or heart rate, and fundal height should always be documented at each prenatal visit.
5. To decrease GBS neonatal sepsis, all pregnant women should be screened for this bacterium.

BIBLIOGRAPHY

1. American College of Obstetricians and Gynecologists. Exercise during pregnancy and the postpartum period. ACOG committee opinion no. 267. *Obstet Gynecol.* 2002;99:171–173.
2. American College of Obstetricians and Gynecologists. Ultrasonography in pregnancy. ACOG practice bulletin no. 101. *Obstet Gynecol.* 2009;113:451–461.
3. American College of Obstetricians and Gynecologists. Gestational diabetes mellitus. ACOG practice bulletin no. 137. *Obstet Gynecol.* 2013;122:406–416.
4. Centers for Disease Control and Prevention. Sexually transmitted diseases treatment guidelines, 2015. *MMWR Recomm Rep.* 2015;64:1–137.
5. Duff P. Maternal and fetal infections. In: Creasy RK, Resnick R, Iams JD, et al., eds. *Creasy and Resnick's Maternal-Fetal Medicine: Principles and Practice.* 7th ed. Philadelphia: Elsevier; 2014:802–851.
6. Eisenstat SA, Bancroft L. Domestic violence. *N Engl J Med.* 1999;341:886–892.
7. Kjos SL, Buchanan TA. Gestational diabetes mellitus. *N Engl J Med.* 1999;341:1749–1756.
8. McGregor JA, French J, Parker R, et al. Prevention of premature birth by screening and treatment for common genital tract infections: results of a prospective controlled evaluation. *Am J Obstet Gynecol.* 1995;173:157–167.
9. Schrag SJ, Zywcki S, Farley MM, et al. Group B streptococcal disease in the era of intrapartum antibiotic prophylaxis. *N Engl J Med.* 2000;342:15–20.
10. Stotland N, Bodnar L, Abrams B. Maternal nutrition. In: Creasy RK, Resnick R, Iams JD, et al., eds. *Creasy and Resnick's Maternal-Fetal Medicine: Principles and Practice.* 7th ed. Philadelphia: Saunders; 2014:131–138.
11. Wage and Hour Division, U.S. Department of Labor. The Family and Medical Leave Act. Available at www.dol.gov/whd/fmla. Accessed November 2, 2015.

CHAPTER 37

NUTRITION AND EXERCISE IN PREGNANCY

Maricela Rodriguez-Gutierrez, MD

1. **How do maternal body weight and weight gain during pregnancy affect outcomes?**

   Women who are underweight or who have poor weight gain during pregnancy are at increased risk for fetal growth restriction; this risk is even higher for women with both risk factors. A statistically significant relationship also exists between poor maternal weight gain and preterm delivery.

   Prepregnancy obesity is associated with increased rates of spontaneous abortion, congenital anomalies, gestational diabetes mellitus, intrauterine fetal death, hypertensive disorders of pregnancy, cesarean delivery, thromboembolism, and postoperative wound infections. Excessive weight gain during pregnancy can lead to a large for gestational age (LGA) fetus and even subsequent childhood obesity.

2. **What is the optimal amount of weight to gain during pregnancy?**

   The optimal amount is determined by a woman's prepregnancy body mass index (BMI). See Table 37-1 for more details. Assuming an average 1.1- to 4.4-pound weight gain in the first trimester, this translates to approximately 1 pound/week for underweight and normal weight women and approximately 0.5 pound/week for obese women in the second and third trimesters.

Table 37-1. Recommended Total Weight Gain Ranges for Pregnant Women by Prepregnancy Body Mass Index

WEIGHT STATUS	RECOMMENDED WEIGHT GAIN (POUNDS)
Singleton Pregnancy	
Underweight (BMI <18.5)	28-40
Normal weight (BMI 18.5-24.9)	25-35
Overweight (BMI 25-29.9)	15-25
Obese (BMI ≥30)	11-20
Twin Pregnancy	
Underweight	Insufficient data
Normal weight	37-54
Overweight	31-50
Obese	25-42

From Stotland N, Bodnar L, Abrams B. Maternal nutrition. In: Creasy RK, Resnick R, Iams JD, et al, eds. *Creasy and Resnick's Maternal-Fetal Medicine: Principles and Practice*. 7th ed. Philadelphia: Saunders; 2014:131-138. Adapted from Institute of Medicine. *Weight Gain During Pregnancy: Reexamining the Guidelines*. Washington, DC: National Academy Press; 2009. Copyright 2009 by the National Academy of Sciences. *BMI*, Body mass index.

3. **What is the average maternal weight gain during pregnancy?**

   It is 28 pounds. This weight gain is attributed to fetal weight, placental weight, amniotic fluid, breast enlargement, increased volume expansion, and maternal fat stores.

4. **What is the optimal diet during pregnancy?**

   Because energy requirements in pregnancy are increased by approximately 17% over the nonpregnant state, a woman of normal prepregnancy weight should consume an additional 300 kcal/day. In general, undernourished women require higher energy intake. Although total caloric intake varies based on BMI, the average recommendation is 2500 kcal/day.

Pregnant women need approximately 60 g of protein daily, 10 g greater than the requirement for nonpregnant women. Protein should comprise 20% of the diet, fat should comprise 30%, and carbohydrates the remaining 50%.

Ideal protein sources are lean meat, fish, skin-free poultry, eggs, dried beans, peas, and tofu. Carbohydrates should have a low glycemic index (e.g., brown rice, whole wheat baked products, boiled potatoes, green vegetables, and lentils).

The U.S. Department of Agriculture has created a website (www.choosemyplate.gov) that can help women make healthy choices and learn how to adjust their diet during pregnancy.

5. How do multiple gestations affect diet during pregnancy?

An additional 300 kcal and 10 g of protein per fetus beyond singleton are recommended. Daily caloric intake for women with twins should be 4000 kcal/day for underweight women, 3000 to 3500 kcal/day for women of normal weight, 3250 kcal/day for overweight women, and 2700 to 3000 kcal/day for obese women.

6. Is periconceptional nutrition important?

Yes. Organogenesis occurs early in the first trimester before many women are aware of the pregnancy, so nutritional status at the time of conception is very important.

Periconceptional supplementation with folic acid can reduce the incidence of neural tube defects by 50%. Women of childbearing age who have a chance of becoming pregnant should consume 0.4 mg of folate/day. Women with a history of pregnancy complicated by a neural tube defect or women taking anticonvulsants (e.g., valproate, carbamazepine) should consume 4 mg of folate/day from 1 month before conception occurs until the end of the first trimester. This reduces the risk of repeat neural tube defect by 72%. For twin pregnancies, the Society of Maternal-Fetal Medicine recommends 1 mg of daily folic acid supplementation throughout pregnancy. The neural tube closes between 18 and 26 days after conception; folic acid supplementation beginning after a diagnosis of pregnancy is usually too late to reduce risk.

Higher levels of glycosylated hemoglobin (hemoglobin A1c) are associated with progressively higher rates of congenital deformities. To reduce this risk, women with pregestational diabetes should be counseled to achieve optimal glycemic control before conception occurs.

Elevated phenylalanine can cause low birth weight (LBW), microcephaly, learning disabilities, and fetal cardiac defects. These risks can be significantly reduced if women with phenylketonuria (PKU) adhere to a phenylalanine-restricted diet for at least 3 months before conception occurs.

7. How much calcium is needed during pregnancy?

Large quantities of calcium are essential for the development of the fetal skeleton, fetal tissues, and hormonal adaptations during pregnancy. Studies suggest that inadequate calcium during pregnancy may be associated with gestational hypertension, preterm delivery, and preeclampsia. Fetal calcium needs are highest during the third trimester, when the fetus absorbs an average of 300 mg/day. The daily reference intake for calcium in women 19 to 50 years old is 1000 mg/day, and 1300 mg/day for girls and women 9 to 19 years old. Consuming at least three servings of dairy foods daily usually meets these requirements. Women with lactose intolerance may require a supplement or nondairy calcium-fortified foods. Calcium should be taken with adequate doses of vitamin D (600 IU daily), which stimulates increased intestinal absorption of calcium during the second and third trimesters. Vitamin D deficiency is common in pregnancy, especially in strict vegetarians or those who avoid dairy foods.

8. What problems are associated with megadose vitamin and mineral therapy?

High doses of certain supplements can cause harm. Excessive vitamin A in the first trimester is teratogenic and causes abnormalities of the cranial neural crest cells such as craniofacial and cardiac defects. The daily reference intake for vitamin A in pregnancy is 770 µg/day, and the tolerable upper intake has been established at 3000 µg/day. High doses of zinc suppress the immune system and compete with iron for absorption, and large amounts of fluoride during pregnancy have been associated with mottled teeth. Excessive vitamin C can interfere with copper metabolism.

9. Are herbal remedies safe in pregnancy?

Evidence is insufficient to support or refute the safety of all available herbal remedies and dietary supplements in pregnancy. The overall prevalence of herbal use anytime during pregnancy is 9.4%, and it is highest during the first trimester. It is important to review herb and supplement use with patients before conception occurs.

10. What are the guidelines for fluid requirements during pregnancy?

Pregnancy is associated with increased fluid requirements. An average of 9 L of fluid gained during gestation translates into a 30 mL/day requirement above the nonpregnant state. The current recommendation for water intake is drinking 8 to 10 glasses of water each day. Maternal fluid status may affect the regulation of amniotic fluid volume, and data demonstrate that acute changes in maternal osmolality alter fetal hydration. Hydration also helps alleviate constipation in pregnancy.

11. How much iron is needed in pregnancy?

Iron is an essential component of hemoglobin production, and its requirement almost doubles during pregnancy. Iron deficiency anemia increases the risk of maternal and infant death, preterm delivery, and low neonatal birth weight, and it has negative consequences for normal infant brain development and function. The prevalence of iron deficiency in pregnancy is higher in African-American women, low-income women, teenagers, women with less than a high school education, and women of high parity.

The Institute of Medicine recommends an iron intake of 27 mg/day during pregnancy. For women with multiple gestations or low preconception hemoglobin measurements, supplementation with 60 to 100 mg/day of elemental iron is recommended until hemoglobin levels are normal.

Iron supplementation can cause gastrointestinal side effects such as constipation and nausea. Constipation can be effectively treated with bulk laxatives, stool softeners, and increased fiber. If iron supplementation exacerbates nausea in early pregnancy, it can be deferred until the second trimester.

12. What foods are considered good sources of iron?

Foods with high iron content include oysters (cooked), lean red meats, tofu, legumes, and beans. Sources with moderate iron content include enriched grain products and cereals, and low-content sources include dairy products and light or white meats (e.g., chicken, salmon, and pork).

Iron supplements are best absorbed when taken with citrus juices because vitamin C enhances absorption. Antacids taken for heartburn can interfere with iron absorption, and tea and coffee can cut absorption of nonheme iron by more than half. Iron, whether dietary or supplemented, should not be consumed within 1 hour of calcium intake.

13. What special considerations apply to women with unusual diets?

Ovolactovegetarians consuming milk products, eggs, fish, and poultry generally meet suggested guidelines without the need for supplementation. More restrictive diets (lactovegetarian—no fish, eggs, or poultry; vegan—plants only) should prompt evaluation of vitamin B_{12} status and supplementation with calcium and iron. Vegan diets can also be low in omega-3 fatty acids; these can be obtained through foods such as algae, walnuts, avocado, and chia seeds.

Fasting for cultural reasons is common. Studies of pregnancy outcomes in healthy women who fasted during the month of Ramadan have not shown adverse fetal outcomes.

14. What are the nutritional concerns with adolescent pregnancy?

Recommendations for weight gain during pregnancy are the same for adolescents and adults. Adolescents need additional calcium during pregnancy because their own bones still require calcium deposition; adequate calcium intake in pregnant and nonpregnant adolescents is 1300 mg/day.

16. What are the nutritional concerns for pregnant women with a history of bariatric surgery?

Up to 80% of patients remain obese after bariatric surgery, and standard gestational weight gain guidelines still apply. The two major types of bariatric surgical procedures are (1) malabsorptive procedures such as the Roux-en-Y gastric bypass and (2) restrictive procedures such as laparoscopic adjustable gastric banding. Complications have been associated with both types during pregnancy, including small bowel ischemia and nutritional deficiencies. Generally, it is recommended to wait 12 to 24 months after bariatric surgery before conceiving, to avoid exposing the fetus to an environment of rapid maternal weight loss.

The most common nutritional deficiencies after Roux-en-Y gastric bypass surgery are protein, iron, vitamin B_{12}, folate, vitamin D, and calcium. Monitoring the blood count, ferritin, calcium and vitamin D levels every trimester may be considered. Nutrient deficiencies also can occur after restrictive surgical procedures, and early consultation with a bariatric surgeon is advisable because band adjustments may be necessary.

Dumping syndrome is characterized by fluid shifts from the intravascular compartment into the bowel lumen. It occurs in patients who have had gastric bypass procedures and is caused by ingestion of refined sugars or high-glycemic carbohydrates that the stomach rapidly empties into the small intestine. Distention of the small bowel causes abdominal cramping, bloating, nausea, vomiting, and diarrhea. Hyperinsulinemia and consequent hypoglycemia can also occur, resulting in tachycardia, palpitations, anxiety and diaphoresis. To avoid dumping syndrome, oral glucose challenge tests should not be used to screen for gestational diabetes. Monitoring blood glucose levels at home for a week is a commonly used alternative.

17. **Can fish be eaten during pregnancy?**

Yes, although with qualifications. Raw fish may contain parasites, are potential sources of food poisoning, and are not recommended during pregnancy. Fish with high levels of mercury should also be avoided; these include shark, swordfish, king mackerel, and tilefish. Safer alternatives include salmon, flounder, tilapia, trout, pollock, and catfish. White (albacore) tuna consumption should be limited to 6 ounces a week.

Fish are an excellent source of omega-3 fatty acids, which are important in fetal development. Some health authorities recommend at least 200 mg/day of docosahexaenoic acid (DHA) from either fish consumption or marine oil supplements. Seafood choices that are higher in omega-3 fatty acids include salmon, herring, mussels, trout, sardines, and pollock. To obtain the greatest benefits from omega-3 fatty acids, women should eat at least two servings of cooked fish or shellfish ($\approx$8 to 12 ounces) per week.

18. **What are the two major illnesses from food contaminants that can adversely affect pregnancy?**

1. **Listeriosis:** can cause spontaneous abortion, chorioamnionitis, stillbirth, and preterm delivery. To avoid listeriosis, pregnant women should be advised to wash vegetables and fruits and cook all meats. They should avoid processed, precooked meats such as deli meat and hot dogs, as well as soft cheeses (e.g., brie, blue cheese, and Camembert), unpasteurized or "raw" cheeses (e.g., queso fresco), and unpasteurized dairy products. Pregnant women are 13 times more likely to contract listeriosis compared with the general population.
2. **Toxoplasmosis:** can be passed to humans by water, dust, soil, and contaminated foods. Although cats are the main host of *Toxoplasma gondii,* toxoplasmosis most often results from eating raw or uncooked meat, eating unwashed fruits and vegetables, or handling contaminated soil. Most infected individuals do not have any recognizable symptoms and develop protective resistance to the parasite. However, infection during the first few months of gestation can result in stillbirth, intrauterine growth restriction, preterm delivery, or other serious fetal complications.

19. **Is caffeine intake acceptable during pregnancy?**

Yes. Most experts believe that consuming less than 200 mg of caffeine a day (a single 8-ounce cup of coffee) is safe.

20. **What is pica?**

Pica is the craving and eating of nonfood substances, such as cornstarch, dirt, clay, or ice cubes. Risk factors for this behavior include a family history of pica, rural residence, and African-American race. The cause is unknown, although iron deficiency anemia, cultural beliefs, and limited access to nutrition are thought to be possible causes. Dangers of this practice include ingestion of toxic substances and an increased risk of iron deficiency anemia through the binding of dietary iron by nonfood substances and reduced consumption of nutrient-rich foods. Appropriate management of pica is based on detection and counseling on its detrimental effects.

21. **What role does a perinatal nutritionist play?**

Perinatal nutritionists, a subgroup of the American Dietetic Association (ADA), specialize in the science of food and nutrition and are qualified to advise obstetric clients in various situations of nutritional risk. To obtain a list of perinatal nutritionists in a given area, call the ADA at 1-800-877-1600.

22. **What types of exercise are recommended during pregnancy?**

Aerobic exercise is recommended for at least 15 minutes three times per week, in addition to light strength training. Women should continue activities they were familiar with before pregnancy, but avoid contact sports or activities with an increased risk of falling (e.g., skiing, horseback riding, gymnastics). Scuba diving is not recommended because of the unknown effects of breathing compressed air and the risk of decompression sickness.

23. **What is the maximal pulse rate during exercise for pregnant women?**
The age-adjusted target heart rate should be reduced by 15 to 20 beats per minute. An easy rule is the "talk test," in which exercise intensity can be evaluated by the ability to maintain a conversation. If a patient is unable to converse, exercise intensity should be reduced.

24. **Does exercise cause miscarriage?**
No. In the first trimester, even vigorous exercise (e.g., daily running) has no effect on the rate of spontaneous abortion.

26. **Can exercise have a negative effect on the fetus?**
Yes. The risk of having a small for gestational age (SGA) infant is increased with high-intensity or frequent exercise (>5 days per week).

KEY POINTS: NUTRITION AND EXERCISE IN PREGNANCY

1. Recommended weight gain in pregnancy depends on prepregnancy BMI. On average, women gain 28 pounds.
2. Pregnant women need approximately an extra 300 kcal/day per fetus.
3. Nutritional status at the time of conception is important because organogenesis occurs early in the first trimester, before many women are aware of the pregnancy.
4. Light aerobic exercise is recommended for at least 15 minutes three times per week during pregnancy.

BIBLIOGRAPHY

1. American College of Obstetricians and Gynecologists. Bariatric surgery and pregnancy. ACOG practice bulletin no. 105. *Obstet Gynecol.* 2009;113:1405–1413.
2. Broussard CS, Louik C, Honein MA, et al. Herbal use before and during pregnancy. *Am J Obstet Gynecol.* 2010;202:443. e1-6.
3. Stotland N, Bodnar L, Abrams B. Maternal nutrition. In: Creasy RK, Resnick R, Iams JD, et al., eds. *Creasy and Resnick's Maternal-Fetal Medicine: Principles and Practice.* 7th ed. Philadelphia: Saunders; 2014:131–138.
4. Gabbe SG, Niebyl JR, Simpson JL, et al. *Obstetrics: Normal and Problem Pregnancies.* 6th ed. Philadelphia: Saunders; 2012:125–139.
5. Kilpatrick SJ, Safford KL. Maternal hydration and amniotic fluid index in women with normal amniotic fluid. *Obstet Gynecol.* 1993;81:49–52.
6. Kim SY, Sharma AJ, Sappenfield W, Wilson HG, Salihu HM. Association of maternal body mass index, excessive weight gain, and gestational diabetes mellitus with large-for-gestational-age births. *Obstet Gynecol.* 2014;123:737–744.
7. Luke B. Nutrition and multiple gestation. *Semin Perinat.* 2005;29:349–354.
8. Meizer K, Schultz Y, Boulvain M, Kayser B. Physical activity and pregnancy. *Sports Med.* 2010;40:493–507.
9. Waters TB, Huston-Presley L, Catalano PM. Neonatal body composition according to the revised Institute of Medicine recommendations for maternal weight gain. *J Clin Endocrinol Metab.* 2012;97:3648–3654.
10. Wolfe LA, Davies GAL. Canadian guidelines for exercise in pregnancy. *Clin Obstet Gynecol.* 2003;46:488–495.

CHAPTER 38

OBSTETRIC ULTRASOUND

Debra Linker, MD

1. **How does ultrasound technology work?**

   Ultrasound technology uses high-frequency sound waves to map tissues by measuring the reflection or "echo" of emitted sound waves and translating this into a pixelated image. Most obstetric ultrasound examination is performed at frequencies of 3 to 10 MHz. Abdominal probes have the highest penetration and operate at 2.5 to 5 MHz. Endocavitary probes (used for transvaginal ultrasonography) operate at 5 to 10 MHz.

   Higher-frequency sound waves (higher MHz) generate greater imaging resolution, at the expense of depth of penetration. For any given sound wave frequency, highly reflective tissues (e.g., bone or calcifications) have a higher signal intensity and appear more "echogenic" (white in color) on the translated image. Air also appears white because of high reflection of sound waves, whereas fluid reflects fewer sound waves and appears black or "hypoechoic".

2. **How is the ultrasound image oriented relative to the probe?**

   Ultrasound probes have a "marker" on one side that corresponds to a marker on the screen. By convention, the marker is oriented cephalad or to the patient's right side for abdominal or endovaginal ultrasound examination. The most superficial tissues are at the top of the image; the farther the tissue is from the transducer, the closer it will be to the bottom of the image.

3. **What is the role of ultrasound in establishing the estimated due date (EDD) of a pregnancy?**

   The Naegele rule is used to calculate the EDD based on the first day of the last menstrual period (LMP). Ultrasound measurement of the embryo or fetus in the first trimester (<14 and 0/7 weeks of gestation) is the most accurate method of confirming the EDD based on LMP. If a significant discrepancy exists between the EDD based on ultrasound measurements and the EDD based on LMP, the ultrasound results should be used. Ultrasound dating is also used when the LMP is unknown.

   In general, a significant discrepancy is considered to be more than 7 days in the first trimester, more than 10 days in the second trimester, and more than 21 days in the third trimester. A crown-rump length (CRL) is used to assess the gestational age in the first trimester; in the second and third trimesters, a collection of measurements known as **biometries** (head circumference, biparietal diameter, abdominal circumference, and femur length) is used.

4. **What is the Naegele rule?**

   A method used to calculate the EDD of a pregnancy by taking the first day of the LMP, adding 7 days and 1 year, and subtracting 3 months. Because this method is based on an average menstrual cycle length of 28 days and an average gestation of 40 weeks, it can be inaccurate because of varying cycle lengths and irregular ovulation.

5. **What is assessed in a first trimester ultrasound examination?**

   An ultrasound examination performed before 14 and 0/7 weeks of gestation should include the following:
   - Gestational sac location and number
   - Documentation of the size and shape of the yolk sac or sacs
   - Documentation of an embryo or fetus and number
   - Measurement of the CRL
   - Documentation of fetal cardiac activity for each embryo or fetus
   - If a multiple gestation is identified, documentation of chorionicity
   - Assessment of the uterus and adnexa

6. **What is assessed in a second trimester ultrasound examination?**

   An ultrasound examination performed at 18 to 20 weeks of gestation should include a detailed survey documenting the following:
   - Fetal number and presentation
   - For multiple gestations: chorionicity or amnionicity and comparison of fetal sizes

- Fetal cardiac activity, including any abnormalities of rate or rhythm
- Quantitative (amniotic fluid index or maximum vertical pocket) or qualitative assessment of amniotic fluid
- Placental appearance, location, and relationship with the internal cervical os
- Umbilical cord (number of vessels, assessment of placental cord insertion if possible)
- Fetal measurements (biparietal diameter, head circumference, abdominal circumference, femur length) and estimated fetal weight
- Anatomic assessment: head and neck (lateral cerebral ventricles, choroid plexus, midline falx, cavum septi pellucidi, cerebellum, cisterna magna, nose and upper lip, nuchal fold), heart (four-chamber view and ventricular outflow tracts), situs, abdomen (diaphragm, stomach, liver, kidneys, bladder, abdominal wall or cord insertion), spine, extremities, and sex
- Cervical length if abnormal
- Assessment of uterus and adnexa

7. **How does an early pregnancy typically appear on ultrasound examination?**
A gestational sac usually appears by 4 weeks of gestation. Visualization of a yolk sac or fetal pole inside the uterus, however, is needed to confirm an intrauterine pregnancy (Fig. 38-1). A yolk sac can be seen at 5 weeks of gestation and a fetal pole at 6 weeks, usually with cardiac activity. Absence of any of these findings may result from inaccurate gestational age calculation and should be correlated with a quantitative human chorionic gonadotropin (hCG) determination and clinical symptoms to rule out spontaneous or missed abortion or ectopic pregnancy.

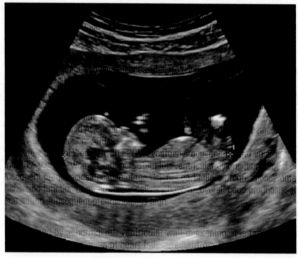

Figure 38-1. Fetal pole with crown-rump length measurement. *(From Bromley B, Shipp TD. First-trimester imaging. In: Creasy RK, Resnick R, Iams JD, et al, eds. Creasy and Resnick's Maternal-Fetal Medicine: Principles and Practice. 7th ed. Philadelphia: Saunders; 2014.)*

8. **What is nuchal translucency, and when is it measured?**
Nuchal translucency is the sonographic appearance of a collection of fluid under the skin behind the fetal neck in the first trimester. When measured in fetuses with a CRL between 45 and 84 mm (11 and 0/7 weeks and 13 and 6/7 weeks) by a certified provider, this measurement can be used alone or in combination with maternal serum biochemical markers to screen for fetal aneuploidy.

9. **What is a blighted ovum?**
A blighted ovum or anembryonic gestation is a fertilized ovum that has failed to develop a fetal pole. It is diagnosed if the mean gestational sac diameter reaches 13 mm or more without a visible yolk sac or more than 20 mm without a fetal pole. In the presence of borderline findings and a highly desired pregnancy, the ultrasound scan can be repeated in 1 week for confirmation.

10. **What ultrasound measurements are used to estimate fetal weight?**
    Most regression models use the following parameters to estimate fetal weight in the second and third trimesters:
    - Biparietal diameter (BPD): measured from the outer edge of the bony proximal calvaria to the inner edge of the distal calvaria, at the level of the thalami and cavum septum pellucidum, perpendicular to the falx cerebri and excluding the cerebellum (Fig. 38-2, *A*)
    - Head circumference (HC): measured at the same level of the BPD, around the outer edge of the bony calvaria (see Fig. 38-2, *A*)
    - Abdominal circumference (AC): including skin and soft tissues, on an axial view at the level of the fetal stomach and junction between the umbilical vein and portal sinus (Fig. 38-2, *B*)
    - Femur length (FL): measured on the long axis of the femoral shaft, excluding the distal femoral epiphysis (Fig. 38-2, *C*)

11. **How accurate is an estimated fetal weight obtained with ultrasound examination?**
    Accuracy is highly dependent on the operator's skill, but it generally varies 15% to 20% from the actual weight.

12. **What is the amniotic fluid index (AFI)?**
    The AFI is an ultrasonographic method of quantifying the amount of amniotic fluid. It is obtained by dividing the maternal abdomen into four quadrants and measuring the deepest vertical pocket in each quadrant (in centimeters). The AFI is the sum of these measurements. An alternative method to assess amniotic fluid is measuring the single maximum or deepest vertical pocket. It is most frequently used when the fundal height is not above the umbilicus or in multiple gestations.

13. **What are the definitions of oligohydramnios and polyhydramnios?**
    Polyhydramnios is an AFI greater than 25 or a maximum vertical pocket larger than 8 cm. Oligohydramnios is an AFI less than 5 cm or a maximum vertical pocket smaller than 2 cm.

14. **What is M-mode ultrasound?**
    M-mode is a setting that measures movement along a single ultrasound beam. It can be used to document fetal cardiac activity and assess the motion of the cardiac chambers and valves.

15. **What is the role of Doppler technology in obstetric ultrasound?**
    Doppler ultrasound can be used to assess the presence and direction of flow in maternal and fetal vessels as well as in the fetal heart. It can also quantitatively assess flow in fetal vessels (e.g., umbilical artery, middle cerebral artery, ductus venosus) to evaluate pregnancy complications such as intrauterine growth restriction, fetal anemia, fetal hypoxemia, and fetal cardiac anomalies.

16. **How can ultrasound examination help determine chorionicity in multiple gestations?**
    Chorionicity is best determined in the first trimester. In the first trimester, the presence of two gestational sacs indicates dichorionic twins. The presence of two yolk sacs in a single gestational sac suggests monochorionic, diamniotic twins. One yolk sac and one gestational sac in the presence of two fetal poles indicates monochorionic, monoamniotic twins. As pregnancy progresses, the insertion site of the dividing amniotic membrane into the placenta or placentas can help distinguish between a dichorionic gestation, which is associated with a "Y" or twin peak sign, and a monochorionic gestation, associated with a "T" sign (Fig. 38-3).

KEY POINTS: OBSTETRIC ULTRASOUND

1. Visualization of a yolk sac or fetal pole inside the uterus is needed to confirm an intrauterine pregnancy.
2. Ultrasound measurement of the embryo or fetus in the first trimester is the most accurate method of confirming the EDD based on the first day of the LMP.
3. Nuchal translucency is the sonographic appearance of a collection of fluid under the skin behind the fetal neck in the first trimester. It can be used alone or in combination with maternal serum biochemical markers to screen for fetal aneuploidy.
4. Most regression models to estimate fetal weight use the BPD, HC, AC, and FL.
5. The AFI is an ultrasonographic method of quantifying the amount of amniotic fluid.

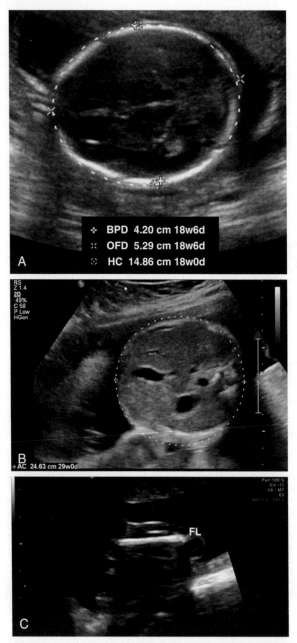

Figure 38-2. Fetal biometries. A, Head circumference (HC), biparietal diameter (BPD), and occiput frontal diameter (OFD). **B,** Abdominal circumference (AC). **C,** Femur length (FL). *(**A** and **C,** From Moore T. Performing and documenting the fetal anatomy ultrasound examination. In: Creasy RK, Resnick R, Iams JD, et al, eds.* Creasy and Resnick's Maternal-Fetal Medicine: Principles and Practice. *7th ed. Philadelphia: Saunders; 2014. **B,** From Bahtiyar M. Atlas of selected normal images. In: Copel JA, D'Alton ME, Gratacos E, et al, eds.* Obstetric Imaging. *Philadelphia: Saunders; 2012.)*

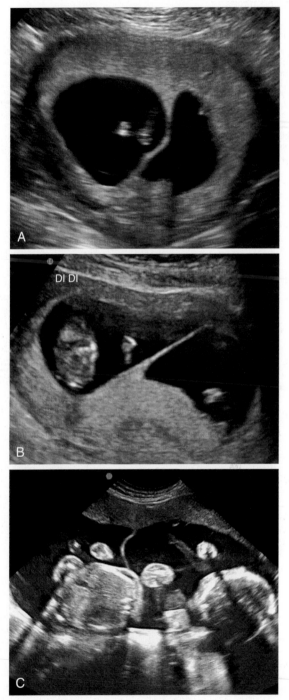

Figure 38-3. "Y" (**A** and **B**) and "T" (**C**) signs in determining chorionicity. *DI DI,* Dichorionic diamniotic. (*A and B,* From *Fuchs KM, D'Alton ME. Dichorionic diamniotic twin gestations. In: Copel JA, ed.* Obstetric Imaging. *Philadelphia: Saunders; 2012. C, From Fuchs KM, D'Alton ME. Monochorionic diamniotic twin gestations. In: Copel JA, D'Alton ME, Gratacos E, et al, eds.* Obstetric Imaging. *Philadelphia: Saunders; 2012.*)

BIBLIOGRAPHY

1. American College of Obstetrics and Gynecology. Ultrasonography in pregnancy. ACOG practice bulletin no. 101. *Obstet Gynecol*. 2009;113:451–461.
2. American College of Obstetrics and Gynecology. Method for estimating due date. ACOG committee opinion no. 611. *Obstet Gynecol*. 2014;124:863–866.
3. Gabbe SG, Niebyl JR, Simpson JL, et al., eds. *Obstetrics: Normal and Problem Pregnancies*. 6th ed. Philadelphia: Saunders; 2012.
4. Reddy UM, Abuhamad AZ, Levine D, Saade GR. Fetal Imaging Workshop invited participants. Fetal imaging. Executive Summary of a Joint Eunice Kennedy Shriver National Institute of Child Health and Human Development, Society for Maternal-Fetal Medicine, American Institute of Ultrasound in Medicine, American College of Obstetricians and Gynecologists, American College of Radiology, Society for Pediatric Radiology, and Society of Radiologists in Ultrasound Fetal Imaging Workshop. *Obstet Gynecol*. 2014;123:1070–1082.

CHAPTER 39

PRENATAL DIAGNOSIS

Isha Wadhawan, MD

1. **What is prenatal diagnosis?**
   Prenatal diagnosis is a set of screening and diagnostic tests used to determine a couple's risk of passing on genetic disease to the fetus and the fetus's risk of having a chromosomal or congenital abnormality.

2. **Who should be offered prenatal diagnosis?**
   Couples at risk for having a fetus with any of the following:
   - Chromosome abnormality
   - Congenital malformations
   - Genetic disease (e.g., hemoglobinopathy, cystic fibrosis, fragile X, Tay-Sachs)
   - Neural tube defect (NTD)

   Mothers with:
   - Teratogen exposure
   - Abnormal maternal serum screening tests
   - Abnormal ultrasound examination
   - Family history of chromosomal or congenital abnormalities
   - History of previous affected pregnancy (congenital malformation or chromosome abnormality)
   - Exposure to certain pathogens or infections during pregnancy (e.g., cytomegalovirus [CMV], *Toxoplasma*, rubella)

3. **What techniques are used most often for prenatal screening and diagnosis?**
   - Maternal serum screening
   - Cell free fetal DNA
   - Ultrasound examination
   - Chorionic villus sampling (CVS)
   - Amniocentesis

4. **What is the function of maternal serum screening?**
   These tests use biochemical markers in the maternal serum to calculate the risk for NTD and specific chromosome abnormalities (i.e., trisomy 21, trisomy 18, and trisomy 13).

5. **What biochemical markers are used in maternal serum screening?**
   - **First trimester screening:** maternal serum pregnancy-associated plasma protein-A (PAPP-A) and free human chorionic gonadotropin (hCG). Performed between 11 and 14 weeks of gestation, it assesses the risk of trisomy 21 and trisomy 18. When this screening is used in combination with ultrasound measurement of nuchal translucency (NT), the detection rate for trisomy 21 is 82% to 87%. NT alone has an 80% detection rate for trisomy 21 with a 5% false-positive rate.
   - **Second trimester screening:** maternal serum α-fetoprotein (AFP), hCG, unconjugated estriol (uE$_3$), and inhibin A; also known as the "quad" or "quadruple screen." Performed between 15 and 22 weeks, it assesses the risk of trisomy 21, 18, NTDs, and the rare disorder called Smith-Lemli-Opitz syndrome. In fetuses with trisomy 21, hCG and inhibin A are elevated, whereas estradiol and AFP are decreased. The detection rate for trisomy 21 is 81% to 83%.

   First and second trimester screening can be combined in different ways to improve detection rates:
   - Sequential screening: First trimester screening results are revealed to the patient, and she may opt for diagnostic testing if the risk is elevated.
   - Integrated screening: First trimester results are withheld from the patient and are combined with results from second trimester screening.

6. **What other information is used in maternal serum screening calculations?**
   - Maternal age
   - Gestational age
   - Ethnicity

- Diabetes mellitus
- Maternal weight
- Presence of a multiple gestation

7. **How are the biochemical markers in maternal serum screening reported and interpreted?**
   Analytes are reported as multiples of the median (MoM) for the gestation age at the time of sampling after adjusting for variables such as maternal weight, age, ethnicity, diabetes, and multiple gestation. Using the MoM for each analyte, risks for open NTD and common aneuploidies (21 and 18) are calculated.

8. **How can ultrasound findings be used to assist in prenatal diagnosis?**
   - **NT** measurement is frequently used in conjunction with first trimester maternal serum screening. Another marker that can be assessed in the first trimester is the presence or absence of the nasal bone. An abnormally large NT (>3.5 mm) and an absent nasal bone are each considered to increase the risk of aneuploidy. Even in the absence of aneuploidy, an elevated NT is associated with an increased incidence of cardiac defects.
   - A **detailed anatomy survey** is generally performed at 18 to 22 weeks as part of standard antenatal care. It can be used to detect numerous congenital malformations in multiple organ systems. Additionally, certain markers that have been associated with aneuploidy may be identified (see later) and prompt further testing.

9. **What are some of the ultrasound findings associated with trisomy 21?**
   - Small for dates fetus
   - Short long bones
   - Echogenic bowel
   - Echogenic intracardiac focus
   - Structural cardiac malformations
   - Thickened nuchal fold
   - Pyelectasis

10. **How is cell free fetal DNA testing in maternal serum useful in prenatal diagnosis?**
    Multiple groups have demonstrated that by using well-known molecular techniques such as massive parallel genomic sequencing and chromosome-specific sequencing, serum of pregnant women can be used to screen for aneuploidy in the fetus with a sensitivity greater than 98% and a false-positive rate of less than 0.5% for trisomy 21, which is the most common aneuploidy in liveborn infants. The American College of Obstetricians and Gynecologists (ACOG) now recommends offering cell free fetal DNA screening to high-risk women (e.g., age ≥35 years, abnormal ultrasound findings, history of previous affected pregnancy, positive serum screening results) after appropriate pretest counseling. Cell free fetal DNA is a screening test, and invasive testing is still needed to confirm positive results.

11. **What is genetic amniocentesis?**
    Amniocentesis is the sampling of amniotic fluid, which contains desquamated fetal cells that can be used for cytogenetic and molecular testing. It is offered after 15 weeks of gestation and is most often performed between 16 and 18 weeks. The risk of procedure-related pregnancy loss is very low (1 in 400 procedures). Amniotic fluid AFP and acetylcholinesterase can also be measured if concern exists for an NTD.

12. **What is CVS?**
    CVS is a procedure in which a small amount of placental tissue is sampled between 10 and 12 weeks of gestation. The tissue can be obtained by either a transabdominal or a transcervical approach and used for genetic diagnosis. The main advantage of this procedure is that it is performed earlier than amniocentesis and can allow for earlier pregnancy termination. In experienced hands, the fetal loss rate is similar to that from second trimester amniocentesis. Even if results are normal, second trimester AFP screening and ultrasound examination for fetal anatomic assessment are strongly recommended to rule out congenital malformations.

13. **What is preimplantation diagnosis?**
    Early in human gestation, a single cell at the eight-cell stage or a dozen cells at the blastocyst stage can be removed without subsequent damage to the fetus. These cells can provide sufficient DNA for polymerase chain reaction (PCR)–directed molecular analysis for heritable diseases or fluorescence in situ hybridization for aneuploidy. Preimplantation diagnosis is performed in conjunction with in vitro fertilization.

14. How should a couple with a previous child with spina bifida be screened?

If the couple has had a child with an isolated NTD, the risk for recurrence is approximately 3% for each pregnancy. Because serum screening may produce a false-negative result, a detailed ultrasound assessment of fetal anatomy should be performed, and amniocentesis for amniotic fluid AFP and possibly acetylcholinesterase should be offered for definitive diagnosis.

15. If a family history identifies a couple at risk for a specific genetic disorder, how should they be counseled?

First try to obtain medical records of the affected family members to confirm the diagnosis, and then determine the inheritance pattern and whether prenatal diagnosis is available for that condition. Counseling should include a calculated risk of the fetus inheriting the disorder, CVS- or amniocentesis-associated risks, and any limitations of the testing method. Referral to a geneticist or genetic counselor is often helpful. For more information on this topic, see Chapter 41.

KEY POINTS: PRENATAL DIAGNOSIS

1. Biochemical screening using maternal serum and antenatal sonography are well established screening tools for fetal abnormalities.
2. CVS is performed between 10 and 12 weeks; it involves sampling of placental tissue for genetic diagnosis.
3. Amniocentesis is performed after 15 weeks; it involves sampling of amniotic fluid for genetic diagnosis or biochemical assessment if concern exists for an open neural tube defect.
4. Assessment of cell free fetal DNA in maternal serum is a very sensitive screening tool for common aneuploidies in high-risk women.

BIBLIOGRAPHY

1. American College of Obstetricians and Gynecologists. Screening for fetal chromosomal abnormalities. ACOG practice bulletin no. 77. *Obstet Gynecol.* 2007;109:217–227.
2. American College of Obstetricians and Gynecologists. Invasive prenatal testing for aneuploidy. ACOG practice bulletin no. 88. *Obstet Gynecol.* 2007;110:1459–1467.
3. American College of Obstetricians and Gynecologists. Preimplantation genetic screening for aneuploidy. ACOG committee opinion no.430. *Obstet Gynecol.* 2009;113:766–767.
4. American College of Obstetricians and Gynecologists. Cell-free DNA screening for fetal aneuploidy. ACOG committee opinion no. 640. *Obstet Gynecol.* 2015;126:e31–e37.
5. Simson JL, Holzgreve W, Driscoll DA. Genetic counselling and genetic screening. In: Gabbe SG, Niebyl JR, Simpson JL, et al., eds. *Obstetrics: Normal and Problem Pregnancies.* 6th ed. Philadelphia: Saunders; 2012.
6. Simson JL, Holzgreve W, Driscoll DA. Prenatal genetic diagnosis. In: Gabbe SG, Niebyl JR, Simpson JL, et al., eds. *Obstetrics: Normal and Problem Pregnancies.* 6th ed. Philadelphia: Saunders; 2012.

CHAPTER 40

ANTEPARTUM FETAL SURVEILLANCE

Laurin Cristiano, MD

1. **What is antepartum fetal surveillance, and why is it performed?**
   Antepartum fetal surveillance refers to the assessment of fetal well-being before the onset of labor. Its purpose is to detect changes in fetal status so intervention can take place before irreversible morbidity or mortality. Testing methods are based on the physiologic relationships among fetal behavior, blood flow, and the level of hypoxemia or acidemia. With increasing physiologic stress, normal fetal behaviors such as fetal breathing and fetal movement are altered or disappear entirely. In the setting of chronic hypoxia, fetal blood flow changes in predictable patterns that can be detected with ultrasound examination using Doppler velocimetry. The most significant limitation of antepartum fetal surveillance is that it cannot predict fetal compromise in response to sudden events (e.g., placental abruption, sudden change in maternal health or status).

2. **What are the most commonly used tests in antepartum fetal surveillance?**
   - Nonstress test (NST)
   - Biophysical profile (BPP)
   - Modified biophysical profile (MBPP)
   - Amniotic fluid index (AFI) or deepest vertical pocket (DVP)
   - Umbilical artery Doppler velocimetry

3. **What is an NST?**
   The NST is an assessment of fetal well-being based on the association between fetal movement and fetal heart rate. A healthy, well-oxygenated fetus demonstrates movements, which cause accelerations in heart rate that can be detected with an external Doppler ultrasound transducer. A fetus experiencing physiologic stress decreases movement, thus resulting in fewer or absent heart rate accelerations.

4. **How is an NST performed?**
   An external Doppler ultrasound transducer is applied to a patient's abdomen for 20 minutes while the patient is at rest. A continuous graphic recording of fetal heart rate is produced and assessed for the presence of accelerations. The test result is considered "reactive" when two accelerations occur within a 20-minute period; because of fetal sleep cycles, the duration of the test can be extended up to 60 minutes to achieve two accelerations within a 20-minute period. If this does not occur, the test is considered nonreactive.

5. **How is a fetal heart rate acceleration defined?**
   Between 28 and 32 weeks of gestation, an acceleration is defined as an increase of 10 beats per minute higher than the baseline heart rate for at least 10 seconds' duration. After 32 weeks of gestation, an increase of 15 beats per minute higher than baseline for at least 15 seconds' duration is required.

6. **What if an NST is not reactive?**
   Although a high false-positive rate is associated with NSTs, a nonreactive test result should prompt additional evaluation. This is most often done with a BPP (see next question).

7. **What is a BPP, and how is it performed?**
   A BPP evaluates fetal well-being by using five different components. The first component is the NST; the remaining four are obtained with ultrasound examination:
   - Amniotic fluid
   - Fetal breathing

- Body or limb movements
- Fetal tone

Each component is given a score of 2 if normal and 0 if abnormal or absent. Scores are reported as a multiple of 2 out of 10 (e.g., 10/10, 8/10). When a BPP is performed without an NST, all 4 ultrasound components must be normal—otherwise, an NST should be added. Normal criteria for each component of a BPP are described in Table 40-1.

Table 40-1. Components of the Biophysical Profile

COMPONENT	NORMAL CRITERIA*
Amniotic fluid	Amniotic fluid index 5-25 cm, or a single deepest vertical pocket >2 cm
Fetal breathing	≥1 episodes of rhythmic fetal breathing movements of lasting 30 seconds or more within 30 minutes
Fetal body or limb movement	≥3 discrete body or limb movements within 30 minutes
Fetal tone	≥1 episodes of extension of a fetal extremity with return to flexion, or opening or closing of a hand
Nonstress test	2 accelerations within a 20-minute period

*For each component, two points are given if normal criteria are met.

8. **How is amniotic fluid volume assessed?**
   The AFI and DVP are two methods used to describe the amount of amniotic fluid.
   - **AFI:** With the patient supine, an ultrasound transducer is applied to the maternal abdomen and is positioned perpendicular to the floor. The abdomen is divided into 4 quadrants, and the deepest pocket not containing umbilical cord is measured in centimeters in each. The sum of all 4 quadrants is the AFI; values between 5 and 25 are considered normal.
   - **DVP:** This is performed similarly to the AFI, with the patient supine and the ultrasound transducer perpendicular to the floor. The largest vertical depth of amniotic fluid seen in any quadrant free of umbilical cord is measured and reported, and values between 2 and 8 cm are considered normal.

9. **What does amniotic fluid tell us about fetal well-being?**
   The primary determinant of amniotic fluid is fetal urine production; amniotic fluid volume is therefore a reflection of fetal perfusion over time, as well as the gastrointestinal and genitourinary systems. (For more information on this topic, see Chapter 45.) Abnormal values may reflect one of the following diagnoses:
   - AFI less than 5 or DVP less than 2 (oligohydramnios)
     - Obstructive anomalies along the genitourinary tract
     - Chronic fetal hypoxia; preferential shunting of blood to the heart and brain resulting in decreased renal perfusion
     - Premature rupture of membranes; may not be perceived by the patient if the size of the leak is small
   - AFI greater than 25 or DVP greater than 8 (polyhydramnios)
     - Obstructive anomalies of the gastrointestinal system; inability of swallowed amniotic fluid to pass though the esophagus, stomach, and duodenum possibly resulting in increased volume
     - Neurologic problems; inhibit or decrease fetal swallowing
     - Fetal polyuria secondary to maternal diabetes
   In general, the DVP has a lower false-positive rate and is associated with fewer unnecessary interventions compared with the AFI.

10. **What is a modified BPP?**
    A modified BPP has only two components: an NST and a DVP. (Fetal movement is inferred by a reactive NST result). A normal modified BPP requires a DVP greater than 2 cm and a reactive NST result, and it has been shown have the same predictive value as a contraction stress test (CST; see later).

11. How does a BPP score influence management?

Two key factors should be considered: (1) gestational age; and (2) which, if any, components are abnormal.

- **8/10 or 10/10:** considered normal as long as oligohydramnios is not present. No change in management is required. If oligohydramnios is present and membranes are not ruptured, term fetuses are delivered. Preterm fetuses with oligohydramnios require additional testing and potentially need to undergo delivery; expert consultation should be obtained.
- **6/10:** considered abnormal. The BPP should be repeated after a short period of time, usually within 6 hours. If the score normalizes, no change in management is necessary. Otherwise, term fetuses should undergo delivery, and additional testing and expert consultation should be obtained for preterm fetuses.
- **4/10:** acute fetal hypoxia likely. Move toward delivery.
- **2/10:** acute fetal hypoxia very likely. Delivery is usually by cesarean section.
- **0/10:** severe, acute hypoxia a certainty. Delivery of viable fetuses should occur immediately by cesarean section.

12. What is Doppler velocimetry, and how is it used?

Doppler velocimetry is the use of real-time ultrasound to evaluate flow patterns in blood vessels. The main vessel evaluated in fetuses is the umbilical artery, in which flow reflects downstream resistance in the placenta. Placental insufficiency can lead to fetal hypoxemia and acidemia.

13. How is umbilical artery velocimetry interpreted?

In a normal fetus with a healthy placenta, Doppler velocimetry demonstrates constant forward flow through the umbilical artery during both parts of the heart cycle (Fig. 40-1, *A*). As resistance in the placenta increases, less forward flow occurs during the filling phase of the heart cycle, and the ratio between the velocity of flow during systole and the velocity of flow during diastole (S/D ratio) increases (Fig. 40-1, *B*).

In cases of severe placental insufficiency, forward flow through the umbilical arteries ceases during diastole. This is referred to as *absent end-diastolic velocity* (Fig. 40-1, *C*). In the most severe cases, backward flow is observed during diastole. This is known as *reversed end-diastolic velocity* and is a sign of impending fetal demise (Fig. 40-1, *D*).

14. How does umbilical artery velocimetry influence management?

Absent end-diastolic velocity requires frequent surveillance and expert consultation. In the term or near-term fetus, delivery should be considered. In the preterm fetus, administration of steroids for fetal lung maturity in preparation for likely delivery is usually indicated.

Reversed end-diastolic velocity is a critical finding; most fetuses decompensate within days. Term or near-term fetus should undergo delivery immediately. Along with expert consultation, a thorough assessment of the preterm fetus should be performed to help decide whether to delay delivery for steroids or proceed immediately.

15. What is a CST?

A CST is used to evaluate the fetal response to uterine contractions, either spontaneous or induced. A fetal heart rate monitor and a tocodynamometer are applied to a patient's abdomen, and the fetal heart tracing is assessed for heart rate decelerations in response to uterine contractions. Three contractions in a 10-minute period are required for the test to be considered adequate; methods to induce contractions include nipple stimulation and administration of oxytocin.

A positive test result is defined as the presence of fetal heart rate decelerations after 50% or more of contractions, and a negative test result is defined as the absence of any decelerations. A negative test result is considered reassuring.

16. What is a fetal kick count?

A fetal kick count is the monitoring of fetal movements by the patient. Maternal perception of 10 fetal movements over a 2-hour period is considered reassuring; if this does not occur, additional evaluation is indicated (usually with an NST).

17. What is vibroacoustic stimulation (VAS), and how is it used?

VAS is the application of an electromechanical device that functions as an artificial larynx or "buzzer." Vibration sense is developed in the fetus as early as 22 weeks, and the fetus is sensitive to sounds surrounding it as early as 24 to 26 weeks. Healthy fetuses move in response to the stimulation. During an NST, the use of VAS can help distinguish between a normal fetal sleep cycle and a truly nonreactive test result.

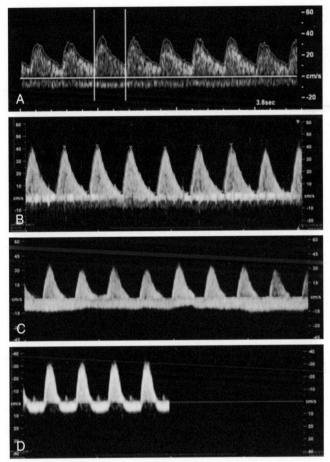

Figure 40-1. Progressive worsening of the umbilical artery Doppler pattern. A, Normal blood flow pattern.
B, Increased systolic-to-diastolic (S/D) ratio. **C,** Absent end-diastolic blood flow. **D,** Reversed end-diastolic blood flow.
(Modified from Bahtiyar MO, Copel JA: Doppler ultrasound: select fetal and maternal applications. In: Creasy RK, Resnik R, Iams JD, et al, eds. Creasy and Resnick's Maternal-Fetal Medicine: Principles and Practice, *7th ed. Philadelphia: Saunders; 2014:211-217.)*

18. In which patients should antepartum fetal surveillance be performed?
    Antepartum fetal surveillance should be initiated in pregnancies at increased risk for fetal demise.
    Risk factors can be categorized into maternal conditions, fetal conditions, and history-related indications. Although not exhaustive, examples include:
    - Maternal conditions: pregestational diabetes, hypertension, severe asthma, or cyanotic heart disease
    - Fetal conditions: intrauterine growth restriction, fetal anomalies, multifetal gestation, decreased fetal movement
    - History-related conditions: earlier stillbirth, teratogen exposure

19. When should antepartum fetal surveillance be initiated?
    In general, fetal surveillance is initiated at 32 weeks or when an indication is identified later in pregnancy. Surveillance may begin earlier in cases of severe maternal or fetal complications or risk factors. Additionally, some conditions carry a standardized surveillance start time.

KEY POINTS: ANTEPARTUM FETAL SURVEILLANCE

1. Antepartum fetal surveillance refers to the assessment of fetal well-being before the onset of labor. It is performed in pregnancies at increased risk for fetal demise.
2. In general, fetal surveillance is initiated at 32 weeks or when an indication is identified later in pregnancy.
3. An NST is the most commonly used test. It assesses the fetal heart rate for accelerations in response to fetal movement and is either reactive (i.e., reassuring) or nonreactive.
4. The BPP combines an NST with ultrasound evaluation to produce a score of fetal well-being.

BIBLIOGRAPHY

1. American College of Obstetricians and Gynecologists. Antepartum fetal surveillance. ACOG practice bulletin no. 145. *Obstet Gynecol.* 2014;124:182–192.
2. Beckmann CRB, Ling FW, Herbert WNP, et al. *Obstetrics and Gynecology.* 7th ed. Baltimore: Lippincott Williams & Wilkins; 2014.
3. Creasy RK, Resnik R, Iams JD, et al, eds. *Creasy and Resnick's Maternal-Fetal Medicine: Principles and Practice.* 7th ed. Philadelphia: Saunders; 2014.
4. Cunningham F, Leveno K, Bloom S, et al. *Williams Obstetrics.* 24th ed. New York: McGraw-Hill; 2014.
5. Magann EF, Chauhan SP, Doherty DA, et al. The evidence for abandoning the amniotic fluid index in favor of the single deepest pocket. *Am J Perinatol.* 2007;24:549–555.

GENETICS IN PREGNANCY

Isha Wadhawan, MD

1. **What are the basic components of genetic counseling, and when should it be offered?**
   As part of genetic counseling, detailed genetic history is taken that includes ethnic background, a pedigree with at least three generations is obtained, risk of heritable diseases is determined, and prenatal testing and reproductive options are discussed. The benefits, risks and limitations of genetic testing are also reviewed. Ideally, counselling should be offered prior to conception or early in pregnancy. Common indications are listed in Box 41-1.

Box 41-1. Common Indications for Genetic Counseling

- Advanced maternal age (>35 years at the time of estimated date of delivery)
- Parent with a known carrier state of genetic disorder
- Previous child or parent with chromosomal abnormality
- Pervious child, parent, or relative with a congenital malformation
- Previous child, parent, or relative with a single-gene disorder
- Recurrent miscarriages or stillbirth
- Teratogen exposure including diabetes (hyperglycemia)
- Consanguinity (e.g., first cousins)

---

2. **When should screening tests be offered to determine whether a patient is a carrier of a single-gene disorder?**
   The American College of Obstetricians and Gynecologists (ACOG) recommends that carrier screening for cystic fibrosis be offered to all pregnant women and women contemplating pregnancy. Screening tests for selected single-gene disorders are offered to individuals based on their ethnicity or family history (Table 41-1). Expanded screening is also available if desired.

Table 41-1. Recommendations for Carrier Screening

ETHNICITY	GENETIC DISEASE	CARRIER RISK	SCREENING TEST
African American	Sickle cell	1/10	Hemoglobin electrophoresis
Asian	α-Thalassemia	1/25	Mean corpuscular volume (MCV)
Mediterranean	β-Thalassemia	1/30	Mean corpuscular volume (MCV)
Ashkenazi Jewish	Tay-Sachs	1/30	Hexosaminidase A or DNA mutation testing
	Canavan	1/40	DNA mutation testing

3. **What is the percentage of children born with birth defects, and what causes these defects?**
   Two percent to 3% of liveborn infants have major malformations, and 5% have minor malformations. The etiology is heterogeneous and includes chromosomal abnormalities, single-gene disorders, teratogenic exposures, maternal diseases (e.g., diabetes, phenylketonuria), and infections (e.g., cytomegalovirus [CMV] infection, rubella). Most isolated malformations are presumed to be multifactorial.

4. **What screening tests are recommended during pregnancy to determine whether a fetus has a congenital malformation?**
   - **First trimester screening,** typically performed between 11 and 14 weeks, uses biochemical markers (pregnancy-associated plasma protein-A [PAPP-A] and free human chorionic gonadotropin [hCG]) and ultrasound assessment of **nuchal translucency (NT).** The NT is a sonolucent space behind the fetal neck and is present in all fetuses. In the setting of a normal karyotype, an abnormally large NT (>3.5 mm) is associated with congenital cardiac defects and an increased incidence of fetal loss.
   - **Second trimester screening** is performed between 15 and 22 weeks and uses four biochemical analytes to determine the risk of aneuploidy: α-fetoprotein (AFP), hCG, unconjugated estriol, and inhibin-A. An elevated AFP may be associated with neural tube or anterior abdominal wall defects (e.g., omphalocele, gastroschisis).
   - **Ultrasonography** at 18 to 22 weeks of gestation to perform a detailed anatomic survey and assess for congenital malformations is part of standard prenatal care.
   - **Fetal echocardiography** is indicated when a suspected cardiac defect is detected by ultrasonography, the fetus has a chromosomal abnormality or known malformation, or the woman has a family history of a cardiac defect in a first-degree relative (sibling or parent of the fetus). It may also be performed if the fetus is at risk for a genetic disorder associated with a cardiac defect, in cases affected by pregestational diabetes, or if exposure to a teratogen has occurred.
   - **Cell free fetal DNA** can also be obtained through sampling maternal blood; this allows for screening for aneuploidy and certain microdeletion disorders such as DiGeorge syndrome (22q11.2 deletion).

5. **Can a parental history of infertility affect the fetus?**
   Yes. Some causes of infertility can increase the risk of having a fetus with a chromosomal abnormality or a genetic disease. Approximately two thirds of boys and men with congenital bilateral absence of the vas deferens have at least one cystic fibrosis mutation. Severe oligospermia and azoospermia are associated with balanced translocations (3% to 5%), Klinefelter syndrome (47,XXY), and abnormalities and microdeletions of the Y chromosome. Individuals with sex chromosome abnormalities associated with subfertility—including XYY males, XXX females, and females with Turner syndrome mosaicism—have an increased risk for children with chromosomal abnormalities.

6. **How often do chromosomal abnormalities occur?**
   Chromosomal abnormalities can be numeric (aneuploidies) or structural, and they occur in autosomes or sex chromosomes. These abnormalities are present in approximately 1 in 160 newborns (0.6%), 5% of stillbirths, and 50% of first trimester spontaneous abortions. Major autosomal aneuploidies are listed in Table 41-2. The most common autosomal disorder is trisomy 21 (1 in 800); if only first trimester spontaneous abortions are considered, it is trisomy 16. Among sex chromosome aneuploidies (Table 41-3), Klinefelter syndrome (47,XXY) is the most common.

7. **What are risk factors for chromosomal abnormalities, and when should testing be offered?**
   Screening for chromosomal abnormalities should be offered to all pregnant women, and any patient who desires definitive diagnostic testing should be allowed to have it. Risk factors for a chromosomal abnormality include advanced maternal age, family history of malformations or intellectual disability, history of aneuploidy in a previous pregnancy, family history of a chromosomal abnormality, abnormal serum screening for aneuploidy, and known fetal malformation.

Table 41-2. Autosomal Chromosomal Disorders

CHROMOSOME ABNORMALITY	PREVALENCE AT BIRTH	CLINICAL FEATURES
Trisomy 21	1/800	Cardiac defects, duodenal atresia, characteristic facies, mental retardation
Trisomy 18	1/6000	Cardiac defects, omphalocele, IUGR, clenched fists with overlapping fingers, severe mental retardation, <10% survival to 1 year
Trisomy 13	1/10,000	Oral-facial clefts, ocular and CNS malformations, scalp defects, severe mental retardation, <10% survival to 1 year

CNS, Central nervous system; IUGR, intrauterine growth restriction.

Table 41-3. Sex Chromosome Abnormalities

CHROMOSOME ABNORMALITY	PREVALENCE AT BIRTH	CLINICAL FEATURES
45,X Turner syndrome	1/2500	Coarctation of aorta, renal abnormalities, webbed neck, shield chest, lymphedema hands and feet, short stature, streak gonads, primary amenorrhea, infertility usual
47,XXY Klinefelter syndrome	1/500	Taller stature than average, gynecomastia, infertility usual, IQ 10-15 points lower than siblings, predisposition to learning disabilities
47,XYY	1/1000	Taller stature than average, IQ 10-15 points lower than siblings, ADHD, learning disabilities
47,XXX	1/1000	Menstrual irregularities, infertility possible

ADHD, Attention deficit-hyperactivity disorder; *IQ*, intelligence quotient.

8. **What is the most common mechanism of numeric chromosomal abnormalities?**
   Nondisjunction during maternal meiosis I. This condition is most frequently associated with increased maternal age.

9. **What is chromosomal translocation?**
   Translocation occurs when segments of two or more chromosomes become interchanged. These changes are not associated with advanced parental age and occur sporadically. **Reciprocal translocations** occur when segments of two nonhomologous chromosomes are evenly exchanged and no genetic material is lost (i.e., the translocation is balanced). **Robertsonian translocations** comprise another type of balanced translocation in which two acrocentric chromosomes fuse near the centromere region and the short arms are lost. The genetic material in the lost pieces is not essential and does not affect phenotype; however, a risk of unbalanced gametes and fertility issues exists.

10. **What is mosaicism, How does it occur, and how does it manifest?**
    Mosaicism denotes the presence of two or more populations of cells with different genotypes in a single individual that may result in a mixed phenotype and variable features of the chromosomal abnormality.

11. **What are microdeletion or microduplication syndromes?**
    Microdeletion and microduplication syndromes are well-established disorders that result from submicroscopic (1 to 3 kilobase pairs) deletions or duplications of chromosomes; deletions (Table 41-4) are more common than duplications. These syndromes can be diagnosed only by techniques such as fluorescence in situ hybridization (FISH) or array comparative genomic hybridization (array CGH). Testing is recommended if sonographic markers are noted on prenatal imaging, if a parent is a known carrier, or if the woman has a history of a previously affected pregnancy.

Table 41-4. Microdeletion Syndromes

MICRODELETION SYNDROME	CHROMOSOME DELETION	CLINICAL FEATURES
Angelman	15q11-13	Severe mental retardation, seizures, ataxic gait
DiGeorge/velocardiofacial	22q11.2	Cardiac defects, hypocalcemia, immune deficiency, cleft palate, learning difficulties
Miller-Dieker	17p13.3	Lissencephaly, characteristic facies
Prader-Willi	15q11-13q	Mental retardation, short, hypotonia, obesity, characteristic facies, small feet
Williams	7q11.23	Supravalvular aortic stenosis, hypercalcemia, characteristic facies, mental retardation

12. **How are chromosomal abnormalities diagnosed?**
Definitive diagnostic tests are invasive and should be performed after thorough counseling regarding their risks, benefits, and limitations. They include chorionic villus sampling or amniocentesis to obtain fetal cells, which are then sent for cytogenetic analysis, to produce a karyotype, or molecular testing (e.g., FISH, array CGH/microarray). Molecular testing can detect small deletions or duplications that cannot be identified with a standard karyotype.

13. **What is FISH?**
FISH is a molecular technique used as an adjunct to standard cytogenetic testing. It can produce results more quickly than a karyotype and can be used to diagnose targeted deletions, duplications, and translocations. It can be performed on metaphase chromosome preparations from cultured lymphocytes, amniocytes, and chorionic villi, as well as interphase nuclei from blood, tissue, chorionic villi, and amniotic fluid. Evaluation of interphase cells is advantageous because neither time nor tissue viability for cell culture is necessary.

14. **What is array CGH?**
Array CGH, also known as microarray, can identify aneuploidy as well as diagnose small microdeletions or microduplications at the level of a few kilobase pairs. It cannot, however, identify triploidy or balanced translocations.

15. **How often do single-gene disorders occur?**
Single-gene disorders occur in 1% of neonates, with additional disorders manifested later in life. These disorders are uncommon, with incidences that rarely exceed 1 in 4000.

16. **What are autosomal dominant disorders?**
Autosomal dominant disorders require only a single copy of an allele to express a specific phenotype. Their overall incidence is approximately 1 in 200. The disease is usually transmitted to the child from an affected parent, and in these cases the recurrence risk is 50% in each pregnancy. Examples of autosomal dominant disorders include Huntington disease, Marfan syndrome, neurofibromatosis, achondroplasia, and familial polyposis.

17. **How can an autosomal dominant disorder appear in a newborn with unaffected parents?**
    - New mutation: Increased paternal age has been associated with autosomal dominant disorders such as achondroplasia, neurofibromatosis, and Apert syndrome. Recurrence risk in these cases is low.
    - Variable expression: A parent may have unrecognized mild or subclinical manifestations of the disorder.
    - Reduced penetrance: A parent may carry the gene but not exhibit clinical features associated with the disorder.
    - Nonpaternity

18. **What should be considered when two or more siblings have an autosomal dominant disorder in the absence of any family history?**
Germline mosaicism, which is when a mutation occurs only in a population of gonadal cells. In these cases, the parent is unaffected yet transmits the mutation to his or her children.

19. **What are autosomal recessive disorders?**
Autosomal recessive disorders occur in the children of couples who are both carriers, and the recurrence risk is 25% in each pregnancy. Examples include sickle cell disease, cystic fibrosis, and Tay-Sachs disease.

20. **Why do certain autosomal disorders appear with increased frequency in some populations?**
Reproductively isolated populations form the basis of differences now seen between various racial and ethnic groups. For example, Tay-Sachs, Canavan, Gaucher, and Niemann-Pick diseases are more common among individuals of Ashkenazi Jewish ancestry.

21. **What are X-linked disorders?**
X-linked recessive disorders are expressed in all boys and men with the allele, but only in homozygous girls and women. Examples are Duchenne muscular dystrophy and hemophilia A. Female carriers have a 50% risk of having an affected son.

X-linked dominant disorders are expressed in both men and women; only a single copy of the allele is necessary to display an affected phenotype. Affected mothers transmit the disorder to 50% of their sons and daughters. Affected fathers transmit the disease to all their daughters but to none of their sons. Examples are vitamin D–resistant rickets and hereditary hematuria.

22. **Can single-gene defects be identified antenatally in a fetus?**
Yes. The genes and mutations for many genetic disorders are well known. The fetus can be tested using invasive diagnostic testing (either chorionic villus sampling or amniocentesis) and molecular diagnosis.

23. **What is an unstable repeat expansion?**
Unstable repeat expansions occur when an affected gene lies within a segment of DNA with repeating tandem units of three or more nucleotides. The number of repeats increases from generation to generation and ultimately leads to abnormal function. Examples of disorders caused by this phenomenon include fragile X syndrome, myotonic dystrophy, and Huntington disease.

24. **What is fragile X syndrome, and what are indications for testing?**
Fragile X syndrome is the most common cause of familial mental retardation. The affected gene is on the X chromosome and contains the trinucleotide repeat CGG; normal persons have 6 to 50 repeats. Unaffected female carriers have a "permutation" of 50 to 200 repeats, which can expand during meiosis into a full mutation (defined as >200 repeats). In the full mutation, excessive methylation affects gene function and ultimately results in the syndrome's phenotype. Affected boys and men have large ears, prominent jaw, large testes, and mild to severe mental retardation, and they usually display autistic behavior. As a result of X inactivation that normally occurs in somatic cells of girls and women, carriers of the full mutation are less severely affected.
   Female carriers of the premutation have a 50% chance of transmitting the gene with a variable degree of expansion. When the gene is transmitted by male carriers, however, the number of repeats remains stable. Men with the premutation are normal, and all their daughters will be carriers of the premutation as well.
   Testing for fragile X syndrome is recommended in the following setting:
• Fetal testing if the mother is a known carrier
• Persons with mental retardation, developmental delay, or autism
• Persons with characteristic features of fragile X
• Persons with a family history of fragile X
• Persons with a history of a previous child with mental retardation of unknown origin

25. **What is genomic imprinting?**
Imprinting is a process in which activation of a gene preferentially occurs on either the maternal or paternal chromosome, but not both. The inactive gene is referred to as the **imprinted gene**; if the active gene (the one that is not imprinted) is deleted or abnormal, the fetus can be affected. Examples of conditions that result from imprinting are Angelman syndrome and Prader-Willi syndrome. Both disorders usually involve deletion of a region on chromosome 15 (15q11-13), but have differing phenotypes as a result of imprinting.

26. **What is uniparental disomy (UPD)?**
UPD occurs either by loss of a chromosome from an embryo with trisomy or by gain of a chromosome in an embryo with monosomy. The two chromosomes in question can be either genetically dissimilar (heterodisomy) or similar (isodisomy), depending on whether the event occurred during the first or second meiotic division, respectively. Examples of conditions that can arise from UPD include Prader-Willi and Angelman syndromes (a minority of cases) and Beckwith-Wiedemann syndrome.

27. **What is mitochondrial inheritance?**
Mitochondria exist in the cytoplasm of the ovum but not the sperm; their DNA is therefore transmitted from mother to child regardless of sex. Examples of genetic disorders caused by mutations in mitochondrial DNA include Leber hereditary optic neuropathy, Leigh disease, and myoclonic epilepsy with ragged red fibers. Because of **heteroplasmy**, in which cells contain variable amounts of affected mitochondria, expression of these disorders can also be variable.

28. **What are multifactorial disorders or conditions?**
Disorders that result from interactions between multiple genetic and environmental factors are referred to as **multifactorial.** They can demonstrate familial aggregation and recurrence without a clear mendelian pattern of gene transmission, and they are often limited to one organ system. Examples include hydrocephaly, anencephaly, neural tube defects, facial clefts (e.g., cleft lip or palate), cardiac defects, and club feet.

29. **What is the recurrence risk for a multifactorial disorder or condition?**
After the birth of an affected child, the recurrence risk is 1% to 5%. The recurrence risk in the children of the affected person is also 1% to 5%.

KEY POINTS: GENETICS IN PREGNANCY

1. The baseline rate of major congenital malformations is 2% to 3%.
2. Screening for congenital diseases includes first and second trimester maternal serum screening, nuchal translucency evaluation, second trimester anatomy evaluation, and fetal echocardiography when needed.
3. All women who are pregnant or are contemplating pregnancy should be screened for cystic fibrosis carrier status.
4. The most common autosomal disorders are trisomy 21 in live births and trisomy 16 in first trimester spontaneous abortions.
5. Microarray can be used to detect aneuploidy, as well as submicroscopic deletions and duplications, but it does not detect balanced translocations and triploidy.
6. Fragile X syndrome results from unstable repeat expansion of the trinucleotide CGG and is the most common heritable cause of mental retardation.

BIBLIOGRAPHY

1. American College of Obstetricians and Gynecologists. Screening for fetal chromosomal abnormalities. ACOG practice bulletin no. 77. *Obstet Gynecol.* 2007;109:217–227.
2. American College of Obstetricians and Gynecologists. Carrier screening for fragile X syndrome. ACOG committee opinion no. 469. *Obstet Gynecol.* 2010;116:1008–1010.
3. American College of Obstetricians and Gynecologists. The use of chromosomal microarray analysis in prenatal diagnosis. ACOG committee opinion no. 581. *Obstet Gynecol.* 2013;122:1374–1377.
4. Engel EM, DeLazier-Blanchet D. Uniparental disomy, isodisomy and imprinting: probable effects in man and strategies for their detections. *Am J Med Genet.* 1991;40:432–439.
5. Korf BR. Molecular diagnosis. *N Engl J Med.* 1995;332:1219–1220. 1489-1502.
6. Newton CR, Graham A, Heptinstall LE, et al. Analysis of any point mutation in DNA: the amplification refractory mutation system (ARMS). *Nucleic Acids Res.* 1989;17:2503.
7. Nussbaum RL, McInnes RR, Willard HF. *Thompson & Thompson Genetics in Medicine.* 7th ed. Philadelphia: Saunders; 2007.
8. Simson JL, Holzgreve W, Driscoll DA. Genetic counselling and genetic screening. In: Gabbe SG, Niebyl JR, Simpson JL, et al., eds. *Obstetrics: Normal and Problem Pregnancies.* 6th ed. Philadelphia: Saunders; 2012.
9. Simpson JL, Elias S. *Genetics in Obstetrics and Gynecology.* 3rd ed. Philadelphia: Saunders; 2003.

CERVICAL INSUFFICIENCY AND CERCLAGE

Erin Burnett, MD

CHAPTER 42

1. **What is cervical insufficiency?**
   Cervical insufficiency is defined as the inability of the uterine cervix to retain a pregnancy in the second trimester in the absence of uterine contractions. It causes painless cervical dilation.

2. **How common is cervical insufficiency?**
   The exact incidence of cervical insufficiency is not known; however, reports suggest that it affects 0.5% to 1% of pregnancies. The risk increases with each successive loss, although many women with a history of cervical insufficiency go on to have normal term pregnancies even without any intervention.

3. **How is cervical insufficiency diagnosed?**
   Cervical insufficiency is a diagnosis of exclusion. Women usually have a history of painless cervical dilation in the second trimester (usually before 24 weeks of gestation) during a previous pregnancy, with subsequent loss of the pregnancy. No other cause for the pregnancy loss and no signs of labor should be present.

4. **What are the risk factors for cervical insufficiency?**
   Risk factors are divided into acquired and congenital. Acquired risk factors include cervical laceration or obstetric injury, cervical instrumentation (dilation and curettage, elective abortion, cold knife cone, loop electrosurgical excision procedure, hysteroscopy), and earlier second trimester births. Congenital risk factors include collagen disorders (e.g., Ehlers-Danlos syndrome), uterine anomalies, and in utero exposure to diethylstilbestrol (DES).

5. **What is the association between elective termination of pregnancy and risk of preterm birth?**
   In a large meta-analysis, one elective termination increased the risk of preterm birth by approximately one third (odds ratio [OR]: 1.35). A history of more than one elective termination nearly doubled the risk (OR: 1.93). The pooled rate of preterm birth among included studies was 6.8%.

6. **How do women with cervical insufficiency present?**
   Many women with cervical insufficiency have no symptoms at all, or they may present with mild symptoms such as pelvic pressure, cramping, backaches, or increased vaginal discharge.

7. **Can women be screened for cervical insufficiency during pregnancy?**
   Yes. Women with a history of preterm delivery in a previous pregnancy should undergo cervical length screening with transvaginal ultrasound examination at 16 weeks of gestation, and they should have repeat measurements every 2 weeks. This frequency increases to a weekly basis if the length of the cervix falls to less than 30 mm. When cervical length is 25 mm or shorter, a cerclage is recommended.

8. **Should all women be screened for cervical insufficiency?**
   No set guidelines exist for universal cervical length screening. Providers who choose to screen all women should adhere to a set management protocol and ensure that ultrasonographers are properly trained.

9. **How is a cervical length measurement performed?**
   Cervical length is determined by transvaginal ultrasound examination. The distance of the closed portion of the cervix is measured (Fig. 42-1).

10. **What is the treatment for an incidental short cervix in a woman without a history of preterm delivery?**
    An incidental short cervix in the absence of an earlier preterm birth is not diagnostic of cervical insufficiency; in these cases, cerclage is not indicated. These women should be offered daily vaginal progesterone if their cervical length is less than 20 mm.

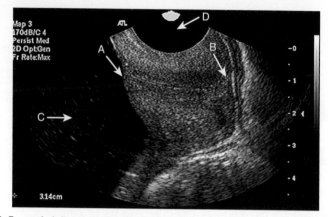

Figure 42-1. Transvaginal ultrasound and sagittal long-axis view of the endocervical canal. The cervical length is measured from the internal os to the external os along the endocervical canal. *A,* Internal os. *B,* External os. *C,* Amniotic fluid. *D,* Ultrasound probe. *(From Bahtiyar MO, Nayeri UA, Shaffer WK. Atlas of selected normal images. In: Copel JA, D'Alton ME, Gratacos E, et al, eds. Obstetric Imaging. 7th ed. Philadelphia: Saunders; 2012:1-12.)*

11. What is a cerclage?

A cerclage is a purse-string suture placed in the cervix to provide reinforcement at the level of the internal os and increase the functional length of the cervix (Fig. 42-2). Most cerclages are placed transvaginally.

12. What are the indications for a cerclage?
   - History-indicated cerclage: This occurs when a women has had one or more early preterm births (34 weeks of gestation) or second trimester losses or a history of cerclage placement for painless cervical dilation.
   - Ultrasound-indicated cerclage: This occurs when a short cervical length (≤25 mm) is noted on transvaginal ultrasound at less than 24 weeks in a woman with an earlier early preterm birth.
   - Physical examination–indicated cerclage: This occurs when cervical change (≥1 cm dilation or prolapsed membranes) is found on physical examination. These procedures are also known as "rescue" cerclages.

13. At what point in a pregnancy is a cerclage typically placed?

History-indicated cerclages are typically placed at 12 to 14 weeks. Ultrasound- and physical examination–indicated cerclages are placed later—anywhere from 16 to 23 weeks. It is not recommended to place a cerclage after fetal viability (24 weeks).

14. What are the two main types of cerclage?

Transvaginal and transabdominal. Transvaginal cerclages are performed using either the McDonald or Shirodkar technique.

15. What is the difference between a McDonald cerclage and a Shirodkar cerclage?
   - A McDonald cerclage involves placing a simple purse-string suture around the cervix at the level of the cervicovaginal junction by using nonresorbable material (Mersilene [polyethylene terephthalate] tape [Ethicon, Somerville, NJ], silk, or nylon).
   - A Shirodkar cerclage involves dissection of the vesicocervical mucosa to place the suture as close to the cervical internal os as possible. The bladder and rectum are dissected away from the uppermost portion of the cervix, and the mucosa is then replaced over the cerclage.

16. In which cases is a transabdominal cerclage performed?

A transabdominal cerclage is usually offered to women with a history of a failed transvaginal cerclage or when the patient has had a trachelectomy (removal of cervix) and a transvaginal cerclage is therefore impossible to place. This procedure carries a higher morbidity because it requires laparoscopy or laparotomy to place and subsequent cesarean delivery.

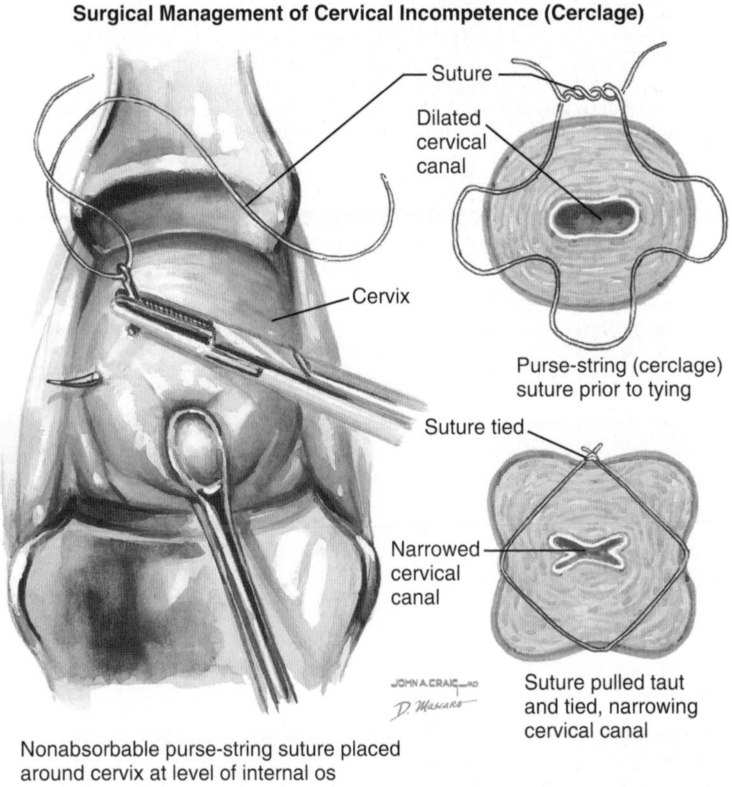
Surgical Management of Cervical Incompetence (Cerclage)
Suture
Dilated cervical canal
Cervix
Purse-string (cerclage) suture prior to tying
Suture tied
Narrowed cervical canal
Suture pulled taut and tied, narrowing cervical canal
Nonabsorbable purse-string suture placed around cervix at level of internal os

Figure 42-2. Cervical cerclage. *(From Smith RP.* Netter's Obstetrics and Gynecology. *2nd ed. Philadelphia: Elsevier; 2015. Copyright 2015 Elsevier Inc. All rights reserved. www.netterimages.com.)*

17. How effective are cerclages?
In a large trial of 302 women with an earlier spontaneous preterm birth between 16 and 34 weeks and a cervical length shorter than 25 mm, a cerclage significantly decreased the rate of perinatal death (8.8% vs. 16%), births at less than 24 weeks (6.1% vs. 14%), and births at less than 37 weeks (45% vs. 60%).

18. Is a cerclage effective in multiple gestations?
Evidence suggests that cerclage placement increases the rate of preterm birth in multiple gestations and should not be used.

19. What risks are involved with cerclage placement?
Although complication rates are low, cerclage placement increases the risk of membrane rupture, chorioamnionitis, bleeding, cervical lacerations, and fistulas. These risks are increased with physical examination–indicated cerclages.

20. What are the contraindications to cerclage placement?
Cerclages should be avoided in the presence of preterm labor or known infection. Up to 80% of asymptomatic women with a short cervix in the second trimester will have contractions on tocodynamometer monitoring. Women with four or more contractions per hour have twice the risk of preterm birth, and cerclage placement should be postponed in these cases. Additional contraindications include ruptured membranes, active bleeding, gestational age greater than 24 weeks, and major fetal anomalies.

21. **What are other treatment options for a short cervix during pregnancy?**
    Vaginal progesterone has been shown to be effective in reducing the rate of preterm birth in women with an incidental short cervix (<20 mm). A 2013 Cochrane Review on the use of pessaries in high-risk women demonstrated a reduction in preterm delivery at both less than 37 weeks and less than 34 weeks of gestation compared with expectant management (relative risk: 0.36 and 0.24, respectively). Pessaries alter the axis of the cervical canal and are thought to displace the weight of the uterus away from the cervix.

22. **Are activity restriction, bed rest, and pelvic rest effective in reducing preterm delivery in women with cervical insufficiency?**
    Nonsurgical treatment options such as bed rest, pelvic rest, and activity restrictions have not proven to be effective treatment for cervical insufficiency, and their use is discouraged.

23. **When is a cerclage removed?**
    In the absence of labor, ruptured membranes, or infection, cerclages should be removed at 36 to 37 weeks. Removal of a McDonald cerclage can often be done in the office.

KEY POINTS: CERVICAL INSUFFICIENCY AND CERCLAGE

1. Cervical insufficiency manifests with painless cervical dilation. This is in contrast to preterm labor, which manifests with painful contractions and cervical dilation.
2. A cerclage is a reinforcing suture that is placed at the level of the internal cervical os for women with a history of one or more preterm births, a short cervix (≤25 mm) and a history of one or more preterm births, or physical examination findings suggestive of cervical insufficiency.
3. Vaginal progesterone has been shown to be effective in reducing the rate of preterm birth in women with an incidental short cervix (<20 mm).

BIBLIOGRAPHY

1. Abdel-Aleem H, Shaaban OM, Abdel-Aleem MA. Cervical pessary for preventing preterm birth. *Cochrane Database Syst Rev.* 2013;5. CD007873.
2. American College of Obstetricians and Gynecologists. Cerclage for the management of cervical insufficiency. ACOG practice bulletin no. 142. *Obstet Gynecol.* 2014;123:372–379.
3. Berghella V, Iams JD. Cervical insufficiency. In: Creasy RK, Resnick R, Iams JD, et al., eds. *Creasy and Resnik's Maternal-Fetal Medicine: Principles and Practice.* 7th ed. Philadelphia: Saunders; 2014:654–662.
4. Schieve LA, Cohen B, Nannini A, et al. A population-based study of maternal and perinatal outcomes associated with assisted reproductive technology in Massachusetts. *Matern Child Health J.* 2007;11:517–525.
5. Shah P, Zao J, on behalf of Knowledge Synthesis Group of Determinants of Preterm/LBW Births. Induced termination of pregnancy and low birthweight and preterm birth: a systematic review and meta-analyses. *BJOG.* 2009;116:1425–1442.

NAUSEA AND VOMITING IN PREGNANCY

Alyssa Scott, MD

CHAPTER 43

1. **How common are nausea and vomiting in pregnancy (NVP)?**
   NVP are common manifestations of early pregnancy, with up to 80% of pregnant women report-ing nausea as a symptom and 50% reporting vomiting. The most severe form of NVP, hyperemesis gravidarum (HG), occurs in only 0.5% to 2% of pregnancies. Although NVP are commonly referred to as "morning sickness," symptoms often persist throughout the day. NVP usually resolve before the twentieth week of gestation but can persist until delivery.

2. **How are NVP differentiated from HG?**
   NVP and HG lie along a spectrum, with HG representing the most severe presentation. HG has no universally accepted definition; the most commonly used clinical definition requires all the following to be present:
   • Persistent vomiting without other cause
   • Evidence of dehydration (most commonly confirmed by ketonuria)
   • Weight loss of 5% of more from prepregnancy weight

3. **What are the risk factors for hyperemesis?**
   Women are found to be at increased risk if they have a multiple gestation, a molar pregnancy, a female fetus, a family history of HG, or a personal history of HG. In a large population-based study, women with HG in their first pregnancy were found to be more than 20 times more likely to have it in a later pregnancy as well.

4. **What causes NVP?**
   The etiology of NVP and HG is still largely unknown, but it is thought to be multifactorial. A strong association exists between human chorionic gonadotropin (hCG) and estrogen levels; the incidence of NVP and HG is higher in molar pregnancies and multiple gestations, which have higher than normal hCG levels.

5. **What is the differential diagnosis of NVP?**
   The differential diagnoses for nausea and vomiting in any adult—regardless of pregnancy status—is extensive. It includes numerous gastrointestinal, genitourinary, infectious, metabolic, and neurologic conditions. Given that healthy pregnant women who present with nausea and vomiting are most likely to have symptoms because of the pregnancy, NVP should be at the top of the list. However, another cause should be considered if nausea and vomiting are associated with significant headaches or abdominal pain, they acutely worsen or persist despite appropriate therapy, or they start after the first trimester.

6. **What laboratory abnormalities can be seen with NVP and HG?**
   Some of the more common laboratory abnormalities found with NVP and HG are abnormal electrolyte levels and hypochloremic metabolic alkalosis. Others are listed in Table 43-1.

7. **Do any fetal complications of NVP and HG exist?**
   In severe cases with poor maternal weight gain, an increased risk of low birth weight and preterm delivery exists. These risks return to baseline if women are able to gain a normal amount of weight during the pregnancy.

8. **What severe maternal complications are associated with NVP and HG?**
   Severe complications are rare but include Wernicke encephalopathy (secondary to thiamine deficiency from malnutrition), acute renal failure (secondary to dehydration), Mallory-Weiss tears, esophageal rupture, rhabdomyolysis, and coagulopathy (secondary to vitamin K deficiency).

Table 43-1. Common Laboratory Abnormalities With Nausea and Vomiting of Pregnancy and Hyperemesis Gravidarum

LABORATORY VALUE	CHANGE	COMMENTS
Bilirubin	↑	Usually <4 mg/dL
AST and ALT	↑	Usually <300 U/L
Lipase and amylase	↑	Up to five times normal levels
TSH	↓	Monitor thyroid levels without treatment unless other signs of thyroid dysfunction such as goiters are present or thyroid autoantibodies are found in further laboratory work
Thyroxine (T₄)	↑	
Ketones	↑	Serum or urine ketones
Urinary specific gravity	↑	Evidence of dehydration

↑, Increased; ↓, decreased, *ALT*, alanine aminotransferase; *AST*, aspartate aminotransferase; *TSH*, thyroid-stimulating hormone.

9. **How are NVG and HG treated?**
   All women should be counseled to avoid environmental and dietary triggers. They can eat many small meals every 1 to 2 hours and eliminate spicy, fatty, or strong-smelling foods from their diet. In general, treatment should progress in a stepwise fashion through increasingly aggressive regimens:
   1. **Pyridoxine** (vitamin B₆), 10 to 25 mg three to four times daily, is considered a first-line therapy. It has been shown to be efficacious and safe. If symptoms do not improve, **doxylamine,** 10 mg three to four times daily, can be added. Alternative antihistamines include diphenhydramine, meclizine, and dimenhydrinate.
   2. Dopamine antagonists include **promethazine**, prochlorperazine, and **metoclopramide.** No evidence of fetal side effects exists, but maternal tardive dyskinesia can occur.
   3. **Ondansetron**, a serotonin antagonist, can be given as an orally dissolving tablet or intravenously.
   4. **Methylprednisone** can be given in refractory cases, although results from studies have been equivocal. This drug should be avoided before 10 weeks of gestation because of the risk of oral clefts.
   5. **Total parenteral nutrition** is generally reserved as a last resort because of its associated risks.

10. **At what point do patients require admission to a hospital?**
    Patients should be admitted for treatment when outpatient management fails if signs of significant dehydration or electrolyte abnormalities are present. Initial intravenous fluids should contain thiamine to avoid Wernicke encephalopathy.

11. **Do alternative therapies have roles in NVG and HG?**
    Various supplements (e.g., ginger, peppermint, chamomile) have been used to decrease nausea. Multiple studies have found ginger to reduce symptoms significantly, with no proven side effects. Acupressure by wearing wristbands that stimulate the P6 acupressure site is occasionally used, although evidence of its efficacy has been inconclusive and equivocal.

KEY POINTS: NAUSEA AND VOMITING OF PREGNANCY

1. NVP usually resolve before 20 weeks of gestation.
2. NVP and HG lie along a spectrum, with HG representing the most severe form. HG has no universally accepted definition, although a widely accepted criterion is a weight loss from prepregnancy weight of 5% or more.
3. Women are at higher risk for hyperemesis if they have a history of it in an earlier pregnancy or if they have a multiple gestation or molar pregnancy.
4. Treatment should begin with dietary modification and proceed in a stepwise fashion.

BIBLIOGRAPHY

1. American College of Obstetricians and Gynecologists. Nausea and vomiting of pregnancy. ACOG practice bulletin no. 52. *Obstet Gynecol.* 2004;103:803–816.
2. Badell ML, Ramin SM, Smith JA. Treatment options for nausea and vomiting during pregnancy. *Pharmacotherapy.* 2006;26:1273–1287.
3. Gadsby R, Barnie-Adshead AM, Jagger C. Pregnancy nausea related to women's obstetric and personal histories. *Gynecol Obstet Invest.* 1997;43:108–111.
4. Goodwin TM. Nausea and vomiting of pregnancy: an obstetric syndrome. *Am J Obstet Gynecol.* 2002;186(Suppl): S184–S189.
5. Matthews A, Dowswell T, Haas DM, Doyle M, O'Mathúna DP. Interventions for nausea and vomiting in early pregnancy. *Cochrane Database Syst Rev.* 2010;9. CD007575.
6. Oliveira LG, Capp SM, You WB, Riffenburgh RH, Carstairs SD. Ondansetron compared with doxylamine and pyridoxine for treatment of nausea in pregnancy. *Obstet Gynecol.* 2014;124:735–742.
7. Trogstad LIS, Stoltenberg C, Magnus P, Skjaerven R, Irgens LM. Recurrence risk in hyperemesis gravidarum. *BJOG.* 2005;112:1641–1645.

CHAPTER 44

DISORDERS OF FETAL GROWTH

Maiuyen Nguyen, MD

1. **What is the definition of intrauterine growth restriction (IUGR)?**
   The term intrauterine growth restriction (or fetal growth restriction) is used to describe fetuses with an estimated fetal weight less than the 10th percentile for gestational age. It includes both normal, constitutionally small fetuses and pathologic, growth-restricted fetuses. Studies suggest that adverse perinatal outcomes are generally confined to those infants with weights lower than the 5th or perhaps even the 3rd percentile for gestational age.

2. **What is the difference between small for gestational age (SGA) and IUGR?**
   The term SGA describes **newborn infants** with birth weight less than the 10th percentile for gestational age. IUGR describes **fetuses** with the same condition. Even though the two terms address the same condition, they should not be used interchangeably.

3. **What are the causes of nonconstitutional IUGR?**
   Causes of IUGR can be divided into maternal, fetal, and placental. They all, however, share the same final common pathway of suboptimal uteroplacental perfusion (i.e., placental insufficiency) and fetal nutrition.

4. **How does the placenta play a role in IUGR?**
   IUGR occurs when the placenta cannot match fetal nutritional or respiratory demands. Early placental insufficiency is thought to affect all levels of fetal development and result in symmetric IUGR, in which both the head and the body of the fetus are smaller than expected. Late-onset placental diseases are thought to decrease fetal abdominal adipose stores and result in asymmetric (head-sparing) IUGR. However, there are multiple exceptions to the above rule.

5. **Which maternal medical conditions place the fetus at risk for IUGR?**
   Chronic vascular diseases such as diabetes, pregnancy-related hypertension, autoimmune disease, and antiphospholipid syndrome affect maternal microcirculation and can lead to reduced placental blood flow. In addition, poor maternal nutrition, obesity, infection, and low socioeconomic status have also been associated with poor fetal growth.

6. **What drugs are associated with abnormal fetal growth?**
   Antineoplastic agents, antiepileptics (valproic acid), antithrombotic drugs (warfarin), opioids, tobacco, and alcohol have all been associated with an increased risk of IUGR.

7. **What is the effect of maternal weight gain on birth weight?**
   Women who are underweight or who have poor weight gain during pregnancy are at increased risk for fetal growth restriction. Conversely, excessive weight gain during pregnancy can lead to a large for gestational age (LGA) fetus.

8. **Why are low birth weight and growth restriction more common in multifetal gestations?**
   Preterm delivery is a major cause of low birth weight in twins and higher-order multiples. Unequal placental sharing in monochorionic gestations can result in IUGR.

9. **Can viral infections cause IUGR?**
   Yes, although in only a minority of cases. Viral infections known to cause IUGR include cytomegalovirus (CMV) infection, rubella, toxoplasmosis, and varicella.

10. **Are genetic disorders a common cause of IUGR?**
    Yes. Chromosomal abnormalities account for up to 20% of IUGR cases and usually result in early, symmetric growth restriction.

11. **Are perinatal morbidity and mortality increased in fetuses with IUGR?**
    Absolutely. IUGR is associated with increased risk of perinatal mortality. Associated morbidities include delivery-associated hypoxemia, meconium aspiration, neonatal hypoglycemia, neonatal hypothermia, and abnormal neurologic development.

12. **Why do fetuses with IUGR have an increased risk of intrapartum complications?**
    The underlying cause of IUGR (uteroplacental insufficiency) is likely aggravated by labor, during which blood flow to the uterus is decreased by contractions. IUGR is also associated with diminished amniotic fluid volume, which increases the likelihood of umbilical cord compression. Up to 50% of fetuses with IUGR exhibit abnormal heart rate patterns in labor, and the risk of cesarean delivery is increased.

13. **How is the diagnosis of IUGR made, and what should be done following diagnosis?**
    Ultrasound measurements and calculation of estimated fetal weight are used to determine whether a fetus is at less than the 10th percentile for growth. After diagnosis, the patient should receive regular growth ultrasound examinations and be followed by an expert in high-risk pregnancies. Antepartum fetal surveillance should be performed, and potential genetic or infectious causes should be excluded. For more information on antepartum fetal surveillance, see Chapter 40.

14. **What is the role of umbilical artery Doppler velocimetry in evaluating fetuses with IUGR?**
    Umbilical artery Doppler velocimetry used in conjunction with fetal surveillance is associated with improved outcomes in fetuses with IUGR. Doppler assessment can be used to monitor fetal status and guide the timing of delivery. For more information on this topic, see Chapter 40.

15. **When should a growth-restricted fetus undergo delivery?**
    The optimal timing of delivery of IUGR fetus depends on the underlying cause and the estimated gestational age. Experts suggest delivery at 38 to 39 weeks in cases of isolated fetal growth restriction and delivery between 34 and 37 weeks in cases with additional risk factors (oligohydramnios, abnormal fetal testing or umbilical artery Doppler velocimetry, or maternal risk factors).

KEY POINTS: INTRAUTERINE GROWTH RESTRICTION

1. IUGR is a prenatal term, whereas SGA is used for neonates.
2. Although IUGR is defined as fetal weight less than 10th percentile, adverse perinatal outcomes increase at the 5th and 3rd percentiles.
3. IUGR may be caused by fetal, placental, or maternal factors. Karyotypic abnormalities account for up to 20% of all cases.
4. Fetuses with IUGR have high perinatal mortality and morbidity because of decreased placental reserve.

16. **What is the difference between LGA and macrosomia?**
    LGA refers to newborn infants with a birth weight greater than the 90th percentile for their gestational age. Macrosomia refers to growth beyond a specific threshold, usually 4000 or 4500 g.

17. **Is fetal macrosomia associated with an increased risk of perinatal complications?**
    Yes. Macrosomia is associated with risks to both the patient and her fetus. Maternal risks include higher rates of abnormal labor, cesarean delivery, postpartum hemorrhage, and severe vaginal lacerations. The most significant fetal risks are shoulder dystocia, decreased 5-minute Apgar scores, and admission to a neonatal intensive care unit.

18. **What are common risk factors for fetal macrosomia?**
    Large gestational weight gain, maternal diabetes, postterm pregnancy, genetic abnormalities, and male sex are all common risk factors.

19. **How do macrosomic infants of diabetic mothers differ from macrosomic infants without diabetes?**
    Macrosomic infants of diabetic mothers have larger shoulders, a greater amount of body fat, a decreased head-to-shoulder ratio, and increased skin folds in the upper extremities. These all act to increase the risk of shoulder dystocia.

20. **When is cesarean delivery recommended?**
The American College of Obstetricians and Gynecologists (ACOG) recommends cesarean delivery for fetuses with an estimated weight greater than 5000 g in women without diabetes and greater than 4500 g in women with diabetes.

21. **Does induction of labor have a role in cases of suspected or "impending" fetal macrosomia?**
No. Induction of labor has not been shown to reduce newborn morbidity or the rate of shoulder dystocia.

KEY POINTS: MACROSOMIA

1. Fetal macrosomia refers to growth beyond a specific threshold, usually 4000 or 4500 g.
2. Common risk factors for the development of fetal macrosomia include large gestational weight gain, maternal diabetes, and postterm pregnancy.
3. Important risks associated with fetal macrosomia include higher rates of shoulder dystocia, decreased 5-minute Apgar scores, postpartum hemorrhage, and severe vaginal lacerations.

BIBLIOGRAPHY

1. American College of Obstetrics and Gynecology. Fetal macrosomia. ACOG practice bulletin no. 22. *Obstet Gynecol.* 2000;96(5):707–713.
2. American College of Obstetrics and Gynecology. Fetal growth restriction. ACOG practice bulletin no. 134. *Obstet Gynecol.* 2013;121(5):1122–1133.
3. Baschat AA, Galn HL, Gabbe SG. Intrauterine growth restriction. In: Gabbe SG, Niebyl JR, Simpson JL, et al., eds. *Obstetrics: Normal and Problem Pregnancies.* 6th ed. Philadelphia: Saunders; 2012:706–741.
4. Berkley E, Chauhan SP, Abuhamad A. Doppler assessment of the fetus with intrauterine growth restriction. Society for Maternal-Fetal Medicine Publications Committee. [published erratum appears in *Am J Obstet Gynecol.* 2012;206:508] *Am J Obstet Gynecol.* 2012;206:300–308.
5. Creasy RK, Resnick R. Intrauterine growth restriction. In: Creasy RK, Resnik R, Iams JD, Lockwood CJ, Moore TR, eds. *Creasy and Resnik's Maternal-Fetal Medicine: Principles and Practice.* 6th ed. Philadelphia: Saunders; 2009:636–650.
6. Pallotto EK, Kilbride HW. Perinatal outcome and later implications of intrauterine growth restriction. *Clin Obstet Gynecol.* 2006;49:257–269.
7. Spong CY, Mercer BM, D'Alton M, Kilpatrick S, Blackwell S, Saade G. Timing of indicated late-preterm and early-term birth. *Obstet Gynecol.* 2011;118:323–333.

AMNIOTIC FLUID DISORDERS

CHAPTER 45

Jared Roeckner, MD

1. **What is the origin of amniotic fluid?**
   In the first trimester, amniotic fluid is a transudate of plasma from either the fetus or the mother, or both, although the exact mechanism is unknown. After the first trimester, the amniotic fluid is composed mainly of fetal urine. The fetal kidneys produce 1 to 1.2 L of urine per day at term. Fetal lungs also produce a small amount of liquid that contributes to the amniotic fluid volume.

2. **What prevents amniotic fluid from increasing indefinitely?**
   Amniotic homeostasis is achieved by mechanisms that remove fluid from the fetal compartment. Fetal swallowing removes approximately 500 to 1000 mL of amniotic fluid daily, and intramembranous absorption (consisting of the surface of the placenta and fetal vessels) contributes to the removal of 200 to 500 mL/day.

3. **How is amniotic fluid volume measured?**
   Ultrasound examination is used clinically to determine amniotic fluid volume. The amniotic fluid index (AFI) and deepest vertical pocket (DVP) are the two most commonly used methods. To obtain an AFI, the uterus is divided into four quadrants, and the depths (measured in centimeters) of the deepest pocket in each quadrant are added together. The patient should be in a supine position for ultrasound measurement.

4. **How long is an AFI valid?**
   Approximately 1 week.

5. **What is the significance of abnormal amniotic fluid?**
   Both oligohydramnios and polyhydramnios are associated with increased perinatal morbidity and mortality.

6. **What is oligohydramnios?**
   Oligohydramnios is defined as an AFI of less than 5 cm or a maximum DVP smaller than 2 cm.

7. **What is the first step in the evaluation of oligohydramnios?**
   Rupture of membranes should always be excluded. A detailed patient history should be obtained, with questions about fluid leakage and or increased vaginal discharge. A speculum examination should be performed to look for microscopic ferning (crystallization of amniotic fluid salts and proteins), pooling of fluid in the vagina, and visible leakage of fluid with the Valsalva maneuver or cough. Vaginal fluid pH should be assessed using nitrazine paper (color change from yellow to blue indicates a more neutral pH and suggests rupture). An ultrasound scan to examine fetal kidneys, bladder, and growth should also be performed.

8. **What is the differential diagnosis of oligohydramnios?**
   - Renal agenesis
   - Obstructive uropathy (e.g., posterior urethral valves)
   - Spontaneous rupture of membranes (SROM)
   - Premature rupture of membranes (PROM)
   - Severe uteroplacental insufficiency
   - Chromosomal abnormalities
   - Maternal dehydration/hypovolemia
   - TORCH (toxoplasmosis, other [syphilis, varicella-zoster, parvovirus B19], rubella, cytomegalovirus, herpes simplex) or other infections
   - Idiopathic conditions

9. **What is Potter syndrome?**
   Potter syndrome describes a set of findings that occur in association with bilateral renal agenesis. In the absence of urine production, severe oligohydramnios results in joint contractures, characteristic facies, club feet, and pulmonary hypoplasia.

10. **Why is oligohydramnios in the early second trimester often fatal?**
Fetal lung development requires a sufficient amount of amniotic fluid. The absence of amniotic fluid leads to pulmonary hypoplasia, which is not compatible with extrauterine life.

11. **What is the management of oligohydramnios at term?**
Oligohydramnios at term is widely considered to be an indication for delivery because of increased perinatal morbidity and mortality. This is especially true in prolonged pregnancies. This practice is not well supported by scientific literature, and some experts advocate expectant management.

12. **During labor, oligohydramnios is associated with what type of fetal heart rate deceleration?**
Variable decelerations are often seen in response to umbilical cord compression. Correction may be achieved with amnioinfusion (infusion of normal saline solution into the uterine cavity through a catheter), although this practice is not universal.

13. **What is polyhydramnios?**
Polyhydramnios is defined as an AFI greater than 24 cm or a single DVP larger than 8 cm.

14. **What is the differential diagnosis of polyhydramnios?**
   - Congenital abnormalities (impair fetal swallowing)
   - TORCH or other infection
   - Maternal diabetes
   - Idiopathic conditions

15. **What congenital abnormalities are associated with polyhydramnios?**
Upper gastrointestinal obstruction (esophageal, duodenal, or small bowel atresia), central nervous system abnormalities, and genetic conditions that cause hypotonia.

16. **What obstetric complications can be caused by polyhydramnios?**
Excess fluid distends the uterus, often leading to preterm labor, premature rupture of membranes, and discomfort for the patient. Polyhydramnios has been reported to increase the risk for placenta abruption, although this is rare. After delivery, uterine atony leading to postpartum hemorrhage can occur.

KEY POINTS: AMNIOTIC FLUID DISORDERS

1. After the first trimester, fetal urine is the major source of amniotic fluid production, and fetal swallowing is the major mode of resorption.
2. Oligohydramnios may be caused by fetal renal or urologic abnormalities, placental insufficiency, PROM, or maternal dehydration.
3. Fetal anomalies that cause polyhydramnios are those that interfere with swallowing, either neurologic or gastrointestinal.

BIBLIOGRAPHY

1. American College of Obstetricians and Gynecologists. Ultrasonography in pregnancy. ACOG practice bulletin no. 101. *Obstet Gynecol.* 2009;113:451–461.
2. Gabbe S, Niebyl J, Simpson J, et al., eds. *Obstetrics: Normal and Problem Pregnancies.* 6th ed. Philadelphia: Saunders; 2012.
3. Morris RK, Meller CH, Tamblyn J, et al. Association and prediction of amniotic fluid measurements for adverse pregnancy outcome: systematic review and meta-analysis. *BJOG.* 2014;121:686–699.
4. Zhou J, Wang D, Liang T, Guo Q, Zhang G. Amniotic fluid-derived mesenchymal stem cells: characteristics and therapeutic applications. *Arch Gynecol Obstet.* 2014;290:223–231.

CHAPTER 46

ALLOIMMUNIZATION

Debra Linker, MD

1. **What is alloimmunization, and why is it significant?**
   Alloimmunization is the formation of antibodies to red blood cell (RBC) surface antigens not present in the mother. These antibodies can cross the placenta and cause erythroblastosis fetalis (hemolytic disease of the fetus), a condition in which RBC destruction causes fetal anemia. In severe cases, hydrops fetalis and even fetal death can occur.

2. **How does alloimmunization occur?**
   Maternal exposure to nonself-antigens can occur if fetal RBCs carrying these antigens cross into maternal circulation. Fetomaternal hemorrhage occurs in up to 15% to 50% of births, most commonly during uncomplicated vaginal deliveries. Other clinical factors that can increase the risk of fetomaternal hemorrhage include multifetal gestation, cesarean delivery, manual extraction of the placenta, and placental abruption. Procedures such as amniocentesis, chorionic villus sampling, and external cephalic version can also cause exposure. Threatened abortion, subchorionic hemorrhage, and ectopic pregnancy have also been associated with alloimmunization. Some women are exposed through blood transfusions.

3. **What are the clinically significant RBC antigen groups?**
   The most commonly encountered RBC antigen group is the Rhesus (CDE) group, consisting of alleles C, c, D, E, and e. Most cases of alloimmunization involve Rh-D antigen incompatibility. The next most frequently encountered groups are the Lewis, Kell, and Duffy antigen groups.

4. **How do we manage women at risk for Rh alloimmunization?**
   Women should be screened for blood type and antibodies at their initial prenatal visit. In Rh(D)-negative women with a negative antibody screen, a standard (300 μg) dose of Rho-D immunoglobulin (anti-D globulin) is given at 28 weeks of gestation as long as a repeat antibody screen at that time is negative. At the time of delivery, if the infant is Rh(D) positive, the degree of fetomaternal hemorrhage should be determined (see later). If minimal fetomaternal hemorrhage occurred, a single 300-μg dose of Rho-D immunoglobulin can be administered post partum. Rho-D immunoglobulin should also be administered at the time of any event that places the woman at risk for fetomaternal hemorrhage (see earlier).

5. **What is Rho(D) immunoglobulin?**
   Rho(D) immunoglobulin is an anti-D immunoglobulin that binds to D antigens on fetal RBCs, thus preventing maternal sensitization to the fetal D antigen.

6. **If fetomaternal hemorrhage is suspected, how do we determine the dosage of Rho(D) immunoglobulin to prevent isoimmunization?**
   The Kleihauer-Betke (KB) test is used to quantify the amount of fetomaternal hemorrhage. A maternal peripheral blood smear is made, is then exposed to an acid bath to denature adult hemoglobin, and finally is stained. Intact fetal hemoglobin stains positive and allows for the percentage of fetal blood cells present in the sample to be calculated. Multiplying the KB percentage by the approximate maternal blood volume (assumed to be 5 L) will give the estimated volume of fetal RBCs in maternal circulation. Each 300-μg vial of Rho(D) immunoglobulin is able to neutralize 30 mL of whole fetal blood (15 mL of RBCs).
   Example: If the KB result is 0.6%, then 0.006×5000 mL $= 30$ mL fetal blood present.

7. **What if the screening antibody titer is positive?**
   Women without an earlier history of alloimmunization should be followed with monthly titers. A critical titer, generally considered to be 1:8 to 1:16, should prompt additional monitoring for hemolytic disease of the fetus. Titers vary among different laboratories; any change of more than one dilution is significant. Serial titers are not useful in women with a previously affected pregnancy; these women should always receive additional monitoring for signs of fetal hemolytic disease. This monitoring is performed by specialists in high-risk pregnancies.

8. **What is the first step in managing a pregnancy in which maternal alloimmuniza-tion has been identified?**

Paternity needs to be established to allow for testing of paternal RBC antigens. If the father of the fetus is negative for the antigen of concern (and paternity is certain), no further surveillance is necessary. If the father is heterozygous or his status is not known, fetal blood type can be determined by amniocentesis. With advances in noninvasive prenatal testing, cell free fetal DNA can also be extracted from maternal serum to determine fetal Rh(D) status, although this has not yet become the standard of care for determining fetal blood type.

When risk cannot be effectively ruled out for the fetus (i.e., the father carries the antigen of con-cern, cell free fetal DNA testing is not accessible, and the patient refuses amniocentesis), monitoring for signs of fetal hemolytic disease should be initiated if a critical titer is reached.

9. **How is a fetus monitored for hemolytic disease?**

Doppler velocimetry of the middle cerebral artery (MCA) is the preferred method and the standard of care for monitoring fetal anemia. As a fetus becomes more anemic, blood viscosity decreases, and the velocity of flow through the MCA increases. Peak systolic velocity (PSV) can be determined at 1- to 2-week intervals starting as early as 18 weeks. When results greater than 1.5 multiples of the expected mean (MoM) for the fetus's gestational age are obtained, cordocentesis is performed to determine the fetal hematocrit and administer a fetal blood transfusion if indicated. MCA velocimetry has a sensitivity of 88%, a specificity of 82%, and an accuracy of 85%, and it is reliable up to 35 weeks of gestation.

10. **What is the recommended timing of delivery for a pregnancy complicated by alloimmunization?**

Delivery requires a careful assessment of the degree of fetal anemia and weighing the risks of prema-turity. Patients with cases of mild fetal hemolysis are generally delivered between 37 and 38 weeks; earlier delivery can be considered if amniocentesis confirms fetal lung maturity. In cases of severe hemolysis requiring multiple invasive procedures and transfusions, delivery at 32 to 34 weeks after maternal steroid administration (to promote fetal lung maturity) can be considered.

11. **What are fetal alloimmune thrombocytopenia and neonatal alloimmune thrombo-cytopenia (NAIT)?**

Fetal and neonatal alloimmune thrombocytopenia is the most common cause of severe thrombocyto-penia in fetuses and neonates and of intracranial hemorrhage in term newborns. It occurs in 1 in 1000 live births and is caused by incompatibility between parents for platelet-specific antigens. Unlike Rh-associated alloimmunization, severe fetal thrombocytopenia can occur during the same pregnancy in which the alloimmunization develops. Unfortunately, screening is not cost effective, and the diagnosis is usually made after an affected pregnancy. Patients with known or suspected fetal and neonatal alloimmune thrombocytopenia in a previous pregnancy should be referred for specialist care.

KEY POINTS: ALLOIMMUNIZATION

1. Fetal hemolytic disease can occur if the mother produces antibodies against fetal RBC antigens.
2. Common RBC antigens associated with this disease are Rh antigens D, C, c, E, e, Kell, Kidd, and Duffy.
3. RhoGAM, which is anti-D immunoglobulin, is given to Rh-negative women at 28 weeks, at other times when fetomaternal hemorrhage may occur, and after delivery if the newborn is Rh positive.
4. Doppler velocimetry of the MCA is the preferred method and standard of care for monitoring fetal anemia.

BIBLIOGRAPHY

1. American College of Obstetrics and Gynecology. Management of alloimmunization during pregnancy. ACOG practice bulletin no. 75. *Obstet Gynecol.* 2006;108:457–464.
2. Gabbe SG, Niebyl JR, Simpson JL, et al., eds. *Obstetrics: Normal and Problem Pregnancies.* 6th ed. Philadelphia: Saunders; 2012.
3. Moise Jr KJ. Management of rhesus alloimmunization in pregnancy. *Obstet Gynecol.* 2008;112:164–175.
4. Pacheco LD, Berkowitz RL, Moise Jr KJ, Bussel JB, McFarland JG, Saade GR. Fetal and neonatal alloimmune thrombocytopenia: a management algorithm based on risk stratification. *Obstet Gynecol.* 2011;118:1157–1163.

CHAPTER 47

RENAL DISEASE IN PREGNANCY

Rebecca M. Geer, MD

1. **What anatomic changes take place in the urinary system during pregnancy?**
   During normal pregnancy, the kidneys increase in size, weight, and volume. Dilation of the ureter and renal pelvis can be seen as early as 6 weeks of gestation, and physiologic hydronephrosis can be seen in most patients (90% of right kidneys and 67% of left kidneys). Ureteral or calyceal dilation is thought to be secondary to uterine expansion and dextrorotation with advancing gestational age. However, dilation is also influenced by progesterone-mediated smooth muscle relaxation.

2. **What physiologic changes take place in the urinary system during pregnancy?**
   Increased glomerular filtration rate (GFR) and renal plasma flow result from increased cardiac output as well as decreased renal vascular resistance. By the second trimester, GFR increases by more than 40% to 65%. Creatinine (Cr) clearance increases by up to 50%. Serum Cr decreases to 0.4 to 0.6mg/dL as a result of both increased GFR and increased plasma volume; a level of 1 mg/dL is abnormally high and indicates potential renal disease.

3. **Is glucosuria an abnormal finding in pregnancy?**
   No. The higher GFR of pregnancy can result in glucose filtration exceeding the reabsorptive capacity for glucose in the renal tubules.

4. **How is sodium balance maintained in normal pregnancy?**
   Total body sodium increases by 950 mg by the end of pregnancy. This increase results from shifting balances in GFR, atrial natriuretic peptide, progesterone (salt wasting), aldosterone, and deoxycortico-sterone (salt conserving).

5. **Why are pregnant women at increased risk for pyelonephritis?**
   Increased risk is thought to reflect anatomic changes in the urinary system during pregnancy. These changes result in urinary stasis, which allows for ascending infection. Five percent to 6% of sexually active women have asymptomatic bacteriuria, and urinary tract infections can be seen in up to 20% of pregnancies. Pyelonephritis occurs in 1% to 2% of pregnant women, and it is one of the most common serious complications of pregnancy.

6. **Do patients with pyelonephritis require hospital admission?**
   Traditionally, pregnant women with pyelonephritis have been admitted for intravenous antibiotics and close observation; outpatient management is controversial. If outpatient management is attempted, the patient should have no other complicating factors, be able to tolerate oral medication, and demonstrate compliance with follow-up visits.

7. **Does pregnancy increase the incidence of urolithiasis?**
   No. Pregnant women have an incidence of urolithiasis similar to that of nonpregnant women. Along with increased filtration of calcium and uric acid, stone formation inhibitors such as citrate, magnesium, and glycosaminoglycans are also increasingly filtered. The incidence of symptomatic nephrolithiasis ranges from 1 in 244 to 1 in 2000 pregnancies.

8. **How does urolithiasis manifest, and what should be included in the initial evaluation?**
   The most common presenting symptom is abdominal flank pain, occurring in 85% to 100% of patients. Frank hematuria can be seen in up to 30% of patients. Initial evaluation should include urinalysis to evaluate for hematuria, pyuria, and alterations in pH; up to 95% to 100% of patients will have microscopic hematuria, and pyuria may suggest concomitant infection. Urine pH greater than 7 may indicate the presence of urea-splitting organisms, and pH lower than 5 may indicate uric acid stones. The imaging modality of choice in pregnant women with signs or symptoms of urolithiasis is ultrasound.

9. **How is chronic renal disease diagnosed in pregnancy?**
   In the nonpregnant state, the severity of chronic renal disease is determined by calculated GFR. Given the significant anatomic and physiologic changes in the urinary system in pregnancy, GFR can prove challenging to calculate, and serum Cr levels are more often used, with 0.6 mg/dL the normal expected value. Values higher than 0.8 to 0.9 mg/dL should prompt further evaluation with urinalysis, serum electrolytes, and 24-hour urine collection for protein. Renal ultrasound examination may also be considered, and patients should be referred to appropriate subspecialists.

10. **What are the effects of pregnancy on chronic renal disease?**
    Women with mild disease tend to have little risk of disease progression. Once Cr rises to more than 2.0 mg/dL, the risk of disease progression is 33%.
    Obstetric complications of preterm delivery (often secondary to maternal indications) and pre-eclampsia are increased for women with chronic renal disease. Mild disease, Cr levels of 1.4 mg/dL or higher, and Cr levels of 2.5 mg/dL or higher are associated with preterm birth rates of 20%, 59%, and 86%, respectively. For preeclampsia, rates are 10% for women with mild disease and 40% for those with Cr levels higher than 2.5 mg/dL.

11. **What are the causes of nephrotic syndrome in pregnancy?**
    The most common cause of nephrotic-range proteinuria in pregnancy (3.5 g/day) is preeclampsia. Other causes include diabetic nephropathy, systemic lupus erythematosus, minimal change disease, membranous glomerulonephritis, and chronic renal disease.
    Differentiating preeclampsia from chronic renal disease may be difficult because hypertension with proteinuria can exist in both diseases, although preeclampsia has additional symptoms such as transaminitis, azotemia, coagulopathy, oliguria, pulmonary edema, and persistent headache or vision changes. For more information on this topic, see Chapter 49.

12. **What complications can be seen in pregnant patients undergoing dialysis?**
    Dialysis dramatically increases the risk of miscarriage, fetal growth restriction, preterm delivery, and perinatal demise. The median gestational age at delivery is 33.8 weeks, and the median birth weight is 1750 g. Perinatal survival has increased greatly over the past several decades, however, from 23% in 1980 to more than 90% at present. Hypertension occurs in 80% of pregnancies in women undergoing dialysis, and preeclampsia and severe-range blood pressures are frequent indications for preterm delivery.

13. **What are the risks in pregnancy for women who have received a renal transplant?**
    Neonatal outcomes tend to depend on baseline renal function after transplantation, with a Cr level of 1.5 mg/dL or less leading to better outcomes. Moderate or severe disease is associated with higher rates of preterm birth and perinatal mortality. Women are recommended to wait at least 1 year to conceive after receiving a transplant, and waiting 2 years has been shown to optimize graft survival. Comorbidities that are often present in these patients (e.g., hypertension and diabetes) can add additional risk to a pregnancy.

14. **Should women who have had a renal transplant stop or change their medications when they become pregnant?**
    Ideally, women with a transplant should receive preconception counseling and have their immunosuppressive medications switched to agents with the best safety profiles before they become pregnant. Cyclosporine, tacrolimus, azathioprine, and steroids are considered relatively safe in pregnancy. Mycophenolate mofetil has been shown to cause malformations and fetal demise; women should transition to another agent at least 6 weeks before conception.

KEY POINTS: RENAL DISEASE IN PREGNANCY

1. During pregnancy, increased renal plasma flow and increased glomerular filtration rate lead to decreased serum blood urea nitrogen and Cr level.
2. Pregnancy increases the risk of pyelonephritis because of anatomic changes that promote urinary stasis, but it does not increase the rate of urolithiasis.
3. The most common cause of nephrotic-range proteinuria in pregnancy is preeclampsia.
4. Maternal chronic renal disease increases the risk of miscarriage, perinatal demise, preterm delivery, and preeclampsia.

BIBLIOGRAPHY

1. Castellano G, Losappio V, Gesualdo L. Update on pregnancy in chronic kidney disease. *Kidney Blood Press Res.* 2011;34:253–260.
2. Davison JM, Dunlop W. Renal hemodynamics and tubular function normal human pregnancy. *Kidney Int.* 1980;18:152–161.
3. Deshpande NA, Coscia LA, Gomez-Lobo V, et al. Pregnancy after solid organ transplantation: a guide for obstetric management. *Rev Obstet Gynecol.* 2013;6:116–125.
4. Hooten TM. Uncomplicated urinary tract infection. *N Engl J Med.* 2012;366:1028–1037.
5. Manisco G, Poti' M, Maggiulli G, Di Tullio M, Losappio V, Vernaglione L. Pregnancy in end-stage renal disease patients on dialysis: how to achieve a successful delivery. *Clin Kidney J.* 2015;8:293–299.
6. Maynard SE, Thadhani R. Pregnancy and the kidney. *J Am Soc Nephrol.* 2009;20:14–22.
7. Odutayo A, Hladunewich M. Obstetric nephrology: renal hemodynamic and metabolic physiology in normal pregnancy. *Clin J Am Soc Nephrol.* 2012;7:2073–2080.
8. Sheffield JS, Cunningham FG. Urinary tract infection in women. *Obstet Gynecol.* 2005;106:1085–1092.
9. Sheikh F, Venyo A. Proteinuria in pregnancy: a review of the literature. WebmedCentral, category: Obstetrics and Gynaecology, 2012;3(11):WMC003814. Available at webmedcentral.com/article_view/3814.
10. Srirangam SJ, Hickerton B, Cleynenbreugel BV. Management of urinary calculi in pregnancy: a review. *J Endourol.* 2008;22:867–875.

CHAPTER 48

PREGESTATIONAL AND GESTATIONAL DIABETES

Kristen M. McMaster, MD

1. **What is the incidence of pregestational diabetes?**
   Pregestational diabetes complicates 1% of all pregnancies.

2. **What is the White classification of diabetes in pregnancy?**
   Historically, the White classification system has been used to help stratify women with diabetes (Table 48-1). Its use is declining in favor of categorizing diabetes simply as either gestational or pregestational and mentioning the presence of vascular compromise when applicable.

Table 48-1. White Classification of Diabetes in Pregnancy

DM CLASS	DEFINITION
A1	Gestational diabetes: diet controlled
A2	Gestational diabetes: on medication
B	Age of onset >20 years, duration <10 years
C	Age of onset 10-19 years, duration 10-19 years
D	Age of onset <10 years, duration >20 years
F	Renal disease
H	Cardiac disease
R	Proliferative retinopathy

DM, Diabetes mellitus.

3. **What type of testing should a pregnant woman with pregestational diabetes undergo to determine baseline end-organ damage?**
   - Comprehensive eye examination
   - Baseline renal function; assessed using serum creatinine level and 24-hour urine collection for protein
   - Electrocardiogram

4. **What are the findings in diabetic retinopathy?**
   - Background retinopathy: retinal microaneurysms and dot-blot hemorrhages
   - Proliferative retinopathy: neovascularization; needs treatment with laser therapy

   Acute, rigorous metabolic control during pregnancy has been linked to acute worsening of retinopathy, but it ultimately slows the process of long-term deterioration. Regression of retinopathy after delivery is common.

5. **What is the relationship between pregestational diabetes and thyroid function?**
   Approximately 30% of women with type 1 diabetes also have thyroid dysfunction; this number is lower for type 2 diabetes but is still higher compared with the general population. Because of the risks of thyroid disease in pregnancy (see Chapter 50), thyroid-stimulating hormone (TSH) levels should be checked in all patients with pregestational diabetes.

6. **What obstetric complications are associated with pregestational diabetes?**
   Spontaneous abortion, congenital anomalies, fetal macrosomia, intrauterine fetal death, polyhydramnios, preeclampsia, preterm delivery, and primary cesarean delivery.

7. **What is the incidence of congenital anomalies in patients with pregestational diabetes?**

   Overall, major congenital anomalies occur in 6% to 12% of infants of women with pregestational diabetes. Glycosylated hemoglobin (HbA1c) levels correlate directly with the rate of anomalies—as high as 20% to 25% in women with HbA1c 10% or greater. If HbA1C levels are 5% to 6%, the rate returns to baseline (2% to 3%).

8. **What are the effects of pregnancy on insulin and glucose metabolism?**

   Pregnancy causes generalized insulin resistance and hyperglycemia. This effect is less pronounced in the first trimester, possibly because of high levels of estrogen (which can increase insulin sensitivity). Later in pregnancy, insulin resistance predominates secondary to the effects of human placental lactogen, progesterone, prolactin, placental growth hormone, and cortisol.

9. **What is the pathophysiology of abnormal fetal growth in pregnancies complicated by diabetes?**

   In cases of long-standing diabetes and significant vascular disease, fetal growth can be diminished. More often, however, maternal hyperglycemia stimulates fetal hyperinsulinemia, which in turn stimulates fetal growth. Infants born to diabetic mothers have increased subcutaneous fat and a higher risk of shoulder dystocia. For more information on fetal macrosomia, see Chapter 44.

10. **How should fetal assessment be performed in women with pregestational diabetes?**

    A fetal anatomic survey should be performed at 18 to 20 weeks of gestation, followed by careful fetal cardiac evaluation. Patients should then receive serial ultrasound examinations to monitor fetal growth. Antepartum fetal surveillance should begin at 32 weeks of gestation. For more information on this topic, see Chapter 40.

11. **When is delivery indicated in pregnancies complicated by pregestational diabetes?**

    Patients with well-controlled diabetes may be allowed to reach 39 weeks of gestation as long as antenatal testing results remain reassuring. Continuation of pregnancy beyond 40 weeks is not recommended. Patients with vasculopathy, nephropathy, poor glycemic control, or earlier stillbirth should be managed in consultation with a subspecialist, and delivery timing is generally earlier.

12. **What are the neonatal consequences of poorly controlled pregestational diabetes?**

    Neonatal complications include hypoglycemia, respiratory distress syndrome, polycythemia, and hyperbilirubinemia. Infants are also at risk for cognitive developmental delay and diabetes in later in life.

13. **What is the pathophysiology of neonatal hypoglycemia in infants born to diabetic mothers?**

    Elevated maternal glucose levels are transported through the placenta to the fetus. Maternal insulin does not cross the placenta, so fetal insulin production increases to compensate for maternal glucose levels. Immediately after delivery, transport of glucose to the infant ceases but hyperinsulinemia remains, resulting in neonatal hypoglycemia.

14. **What are the incidence and pathogenesis of diabetic ketoacidosis (DKA) in pregnancy?**

    DKA occurs in 5% to 10% of all pregnancies with pregestational diabetes. Although DKA is more commonly seen in patients with type 1 diabetes, it can also been seen in those with type 2 diabetes. The mean glucose level needed to enter into DKA is lower in pregnancy compared with the nonpregnant state.

15. **What is the typical presentation of DKA in pregnancy?**

    Abdominal pain, nausea and vomiting, altered sensorium, low arterial pH, low serum bicarbonate, elevated anion gap, positive serum ketones, and continuous fetal monitoring showing repetitive late decelerations.

16. **How should DKA in pregnancy be managed?**

    Similarly to nonpregnant patients. Patients should be monitored in a critical care unit, and a continuous insulin infusion should be started, with careful attention paid to blood glucose and electrolyte levels. As glucose levels normalize, a regular diet and subcutaneous insulin can be resumed. These patients should be managed in consultation with critical care and high-risk pregnancy specialists. Continuous fetal heart rate monitoring should be used in viable pregnancies until the patient's status normalizes.

17. **What is the fetal mortality rate in DKA?**
Ten percent to 35% of cases.

KEY POINTS: PREGESTATIONAL DIABETES

1. The risk of congenital anomalies increases as HbA1c rises; to minimize this risk, it is important to achieve good glycemic control before conception occurs.
2. Antenatal management should include screening for maternal end-organ damage and preexisting thyroid disease, fetal anatomy and growth ultrasound examinations, fetal echocardiogram, and antepartum fetal surveillance.
3. Obstetric complications in women with pregestational diabetes include spontaneous abortion, congenital anomalies, fetal macrosomia, intrauterine fetal death, polyhydramnios, preeclampsia, preterm delivery, and primary cesarean delivery.

18. **What is the definition of gestational diabetes mellitus (GDM)?**
Diabetes mellitus that develops for the first time during pregnancy.

19. **What is the prevalence of GDM?**
The prevalence varies with ethnicity and region. In general, 5% to 7% of all pregnancies are complicated by diabetes, and 90% of those cases are gestational.

20. **Who should be screened for GDM, and how is it done?**
Trying to identify and exclude "low-risk" women reduces the number screened by only 10%, so most providers screen all women. The most commonly used method is a two-step process, which begins with a 1-hour, 50-g oral glucose challenge test (GCT) performed at 24 to 28 weeks of gestation. If results are abnormal, a confirmatory 3-hour, 100-g glucose tolerance test (GTT) is done. It is estimated that approximately 95% of all obstetric practices use this screening technique. Various cutoff values have been proposed, resulting in varying levels of sensitivity and specificity. Most recommended threshold values for the 1-hour GCT range between 130 and 140 mg/dL.

21. **How is the 1-hour GCT administered?**
The patient (who does not need to be fasting) is given a 50-g glucose drink. One hour later, a blood sample is drawn, and the glucose level is assessed. Because of the potential variation in capillary glucose values, a glucometer should not be used for this test.

22. **How is the 3-hour GTT administered?**
Patients should fast for at least 8 hours before this test. A fasting serum sample is obtained, and then the patient is given a 100-g glucose solution. Additional serum samples are collected 1, 2, and 3 hours afterward. If two or more of the four values are abnormal, gestational diabetes is diagnosed.

23. **Are other screening test options available?**
Yes. Another option is the 75-g, 2-hour GTT. The diagnosis of GDM would be made based on a single glucose value meeting or exceeding established cutoff values (fasting value, ≥ 92 mg/dL; 1-hour value, ≥ 180 mg/dL; 2-hour value, ≥ 153 mg/dL). This method is not currently endorsed by the American College of Obstetricians and Gynecologists (ACOG), and as many as 18% of women test positive for GDM with it.

24. **Which patients should be screened before 24 to 28 weeks of gestation?**
Early screening should be performed on women with a previous history of GDM, known insulin insensitivity, obesity (body mass index ≥ 30), or a strong family history of type 2 diabetes.

25. **If results of screening before 24 to 28 weeks of gestation are normal, does screening have to be repeated?**
Yes. A normal early screening result excludes only pregestational diabetes. Patients should be rescreened for GDM at 24 to 28 weeks.

26. **What are the potential complications of GDM?**
GDM is associated with increased rates of gestational hypertension, preeclampsia, cesarean delivery, operative delivery, more severe vaginal lacerations, and development of overt diabetes later in life. Fetal complications include macrosomia, neonatal hypoglycemia and hyperbilirubinemia, shoulder dystocia, and birth trauma.

27. **What is the risk that a woman with GDM will develop type 2 diabetes later in life?**
One third of women with GDM will have either persistent diabetes or insulin insensitivity diagnosed post partum, and up to 50% of women with GDM will develop type 2 diabetes within 22 to 28 years. This risk is exacerbated by certain factors such as ethnicity; for example, 60% of Hispanic women develop type 2 diabetes within 5 years after a pregnancy complicated by GDM.

28. **Does an increased risk of congenital malformations in GDM exist?**
No. GDM develops long after organogenesis is complete. However, a positive early screening test result indicates the possibility of undiagnosed pregestational diabetes. An HbA1c level can be used in these cases to assess the degree of chronic hyperglycemia and the possibility of congenital anomalies.

29. **What nutritional recommendations can be made for patients with GDM?**
Diet should consist of 33% to 40% carbohydrates, with the remaining 20% protein and 40% fat. Complex carbohydrates are preferred over simple carbohydrates, and three meals and two snacks per day are recommended to prevent large fluctuations in glucose levels. Moderate exercise is also beneficial. For more information on exercise in pregnancy, see Chapter 37.

30. **What is the best pharmacologic treatment for GDM?**
Depending on the severity of insulin resistance, either insulin or oral medications can be used.

31. **What are the recommendations for fetal testing in pregnancies complicated by GDM?**
Antepartum fetal surveillance is recommended in women with poorly controlled GDM, but no evidence supports this testing in patients with well-controlled GDM.

32. **Should women with GDM be delivered early?**
Women with good glycemic control can be managed expectantly up to 39 to 40 weeks of gestation. Patients with poor glycemic control should be managed in consultation with a subspecialist, and delivery timing should be adjusted on a case-by-case basis.

33. **How should women with GDM be managed after delivery?**
In general, patients with true GDM do not need to continue treatment after delivery. However, they should all be screened for diabetes 6 to 12 weeks post partum by using the 75-g, 2-hour GTT.

KEY POINTS: GESTATIONAL DIABETES

1. GDM is diabetes that develops for the first time during pregnancy.
2. Screening for GDM is done with the 1-hour, 50-g glucose challenge test between 24 and 28 weeks of gestation, and diagnosis is made with the 3-hour, 100-g glucose tolerance test if the 1-hour screen test result is positive.
3. Women with GDM should be tested for persistent diabetes with a 2-hour, 75-g glucose tolerance test 6 to 12 weeks post partum.

34. **How should blood glucose levels be monitored in pregnancy?**
In general, blood glucose is recorded four times a day: one fasting value and three 1- or 2-hour postprandial values. Postprandial values are preferred over preprandial values because they are more predictive of fetal morbidity and macrosomia.

35. **What are target glucose levels in pregnancy?**
Fasting glucose levels should be lower than 95 mg/dL, 1-hour postprandial values lower than 140 mg/dL, and 2-hour values lower than 120 mg/dL. Overnight glucose levels should never drop to less than 60 mg/dL, and HbA1c values should not be greater than 6%.

36. **What are the principles of insulin use in pregnancy?**
Insulin does not cross the placenta and is classically thought of as the gold standard pharmacologic therapy for GDM. Typical starting doses are 0.7 to 1.0 units/kg daily, divided into doses of both intermediate and short-acting insulin analogues. Insulin requirements increase over the course of a pregnancy, reaching 1.2 units/kg/day (or higher) in the third trimester.

37. **What is the action profile of commonly used insulin analogues in pregnancy?**
    • Lispro: onset of action within 1 to 15 minutes, peak action at 1 to 2 hours, duration of action 4 to 5 hours
    • Regular: onset of action within 30 to 60 minutes, peak action in 2 to 4 hours, duration of action 6 to 8 hours
    • NPH: onset of action within 1 to 3 hours, peak action in 5 to 7 hours, duration of action 13 to 18 hours

38. **Which oral hypoglycemic agents are used in pregnancy?**
Although glyburide and metformin are frequently used in pregnancy, neither agent is approved by the Food and Drug Administration (FDA) for this purpose. These medications have both been demonstrated to cross the placenta, although no adverse fetal effects have been established. Metformin inhibits hepatic gluconeogenesis and glucose absorption, which increases insulin sensitivity in peripheral tissues. Glyburide increases pancreatic insulin secretion, as well as insulin sensitivity in peripheral tissues. Women treated with glyburide are less likely to require insulin supplementation than are those treated with metformin.

39. **What are target glucose levels in labor?**
Strict intrapartum glycemic control is encouraged to prevent fetal hyperglycemia and subsequent neonatal hypoglycemia. A target level of less than 110 mg/dL is recommended, and continuous insulin infusions may be required to achieve this goal.

40. **What happens to insulin requirements after delivery?**
Insulin requirements decrease rapidly after delivery. In the postpartum period, patients should be started on an insulin regimen using approximately one half the amount of their earlier doses.

BIBLIOGRAPHY

1. American College of Obstetricians and Gynecologists. Gestational diabetes mellitus. ACOG practice bulletin no 137. *Obstet Gynecol.* 2013;122:406–416.
2. American College of Obstetricians and Gynecologists. Pregestational diabetes mellitus. ACOG practice bulletin no. 60. *Obstet Gynecol.* 2005;105:675–685.
3. Buchanan TA. *Pregnancy in preexisting diabetes.* In: *Diabetes in America.* 2nd ed. Bethesda, MD: National Institutes of Health; 1995.
4. Cunningham F, Leveno KJ, Bloom SL, et al. *Diabetes mellitus.* In: *Williams Obstetrics.* 24th ed. New York: McGraw-Hill; 2013.
5. Perros P, McCrimmon RJ, Shaw G, Frier BM. Frequency of thyroid dysfunction in diabetic patients: value of annual screening. *Diabet Med.* 1995;12:622–627.
6. Ryan EA, Enns L. Role of gestational hormones in the induction of insulin resistance. *J Clin Endocrinol Metab.* 1998;67:341–347.

CHAPTER 49

HYPERTENSION IN PREGNANCY

Erin Burnett, MD

1. **What is the definition of hypertension?**
   Hypertension is defined as systolic blood pressure 140 mm Hg or higher or diastolic blood pressure 90 mm Hg or higher.

2. **What are the various types of hypertension that can occur in pregnancy?**
   The National Institutes of Health (NIH) Working Group on Hypertension in Pregnancy has classified hypertension into four categories: chronic hypertension (CHTN), gestational hypertension (GHTN), preeclampsia, and CHTN with superimposed preeclampsia (SIPE).

3. **What is the definition of CHTN?**
   CHTN is defined as elevated blood pressure (≥140 systolic or ≥90 diastolic) on two separate occasions before pregnancy, in the first 20 weeks of pregnancy, or persisting past 12 weeks post partum.

4. **What is the definition of GHTN?**
   GHTN is defined as the presence of new-onset blood pressure (≥140 mm Hg systolic or ≥90 mm Hg diastolic) after 20 weeks of gestation in the absence of proteinuria or other signs of preeclampsia.

5. **What is the definition of preeclampsia?**
   Preeclampsia is characterized by the dysfunction of multiple organs and is considered a systemic disease. Clinically, it is defined as new-onset elevated blood pressure (≥140 mm Hg systolic or ≥90 mm Hg diastolic) accompanied by proteinuria. It can also be diagnosed in the absence of proteinuria if the patient has new-onset hypertension and any sign of severe preeclampsia (thrombocytopenia, elevated creatinine, elevated liver function test results, neurologic symptoms, or pulmonary edema).

6. **What is the definition of SIPE?**
   An abrupt increase in blood pressures from baseline in a woman with known CHTN, along with proteinuria or any sign of severe preeclampsia.

7. **How is proteinuria defined?**
   Proteinuria is defined as the presence of 300 mg or more of protein in a 24-hour urine collection or a urine protein/creatinine ratio of 0.3 or greater. Although not ideal, a random urine sample can also be used if other tests are not feasible or obtainable; 30 mg/dL (1+ dipstick) is considered positive.

8. **What are the diagnostic criteria for preeclampsia with severe features?**
   Systolic blood pressure 160 mm Hg or higher or diastolic blood pressure 110 mm Hg or higher on two occasions 4 hours apart while on bed rest or elevated blood pressures (≥140 mm Hg systolic or ≥90 mm Hg diastolic) and any of the following: platelet count lower than 100,000/μL, serum creatinine level higher than 1.1 mg/dL or a doubling from baseline, increased liver function test results to twice the normal concentration, pulmonary edema, neurologic symptoms, or severe right upper quadrant or epigastric pain unrelieved by medication.
   Proteinuria greater than 5 g and intrauterine growth restriction are no longer considered criteria for preeclampsia with severe features.

9. **What causes the right upper quadrant or epigastric pain associated with preeclampsia?**
   Hepatic involvement can cause distention of the liver capsule that often causes pain, nausea, and vomiting. In the most severe cases, rupture and massive hemorrhage can occur.

10. **What are risk factors for preeclampsia?**
    - Nulliparity
    - Extremes of age (<15 and >35 years)
    - African-American ethnicity
    - Personal or family history of preeclampsia

- Multiple gestation
- Obesity
- Molar pregnancy
- Other medical conditions (e.g., diabetes, lupus, CHTN, antiphospholipid syndrome)

11. **How common is preeclampsia?**
   In general, preeclampsia occurs in 4% of all pregnancies that extend beyond the first trimester. The rate for nulliparous patients is approximately 7%.

12. **What is the incidence of preeclampsia among women with pregestational diabetes?**
   Rates increase with duration of diabetes and the presence of any associated vascular complications. The incidence of preeclampsia is 11% to 12% in class B diabetes, 21% to 23% in class C or D diabetes, and 36% to 54% in class F or R diabetes. For more information on diabetes in pregnancy, see Chapter 48.

13. **What causes preeclampsia?**
   The true cause of preeclampsia is unknown. It is hypothesized that incomplete trophoblastic invasion into maternal spiral arteries results in poor placental perfusion and hypoxia, which in turn result in the release of free radicals and oxidative stress.

14. **Can preeclampsia be prevented?**
   No true preventive measures exist, but studies have shown a rate reduction in women with risk factors who take low-dose aspirin. The magnitude of risk reduction is greatest among women with a history of preeclampsia before 34 weeks of gestation.

15. **What is the effectiveness of aspirin in reducing the risk of preeclampsia?**
   A meta-analysis of 34 randomized control trials found that starting low-dose aspirin before 16 weeks in women at increased risk for preeclampsia was associated with significant decreases in rates of preeclampsia (53%), severe preeclampsia (90%), intrauterine growth restriction (54%), and preterm birth (78%). Aspirin must be started by 16 weeks (before the placental changes that can precipitate preeclampsia take place), and it should be stopped by 37 to 38 weeks in anticipation of delivery.

16. **What fetal and maternal risks are associated with preeclampsia?**
   - Maternal risks
     - HELLP (hemolysis, elevated liver enzymes, and low platelets; 20%)
     - Disseminated intravascular coagulation (DIC) (10%)
     - Placental abruption (1% to 4%)
     - Renal failure (1% to 2%)
     - Seizures (1%)
     - Cerebral hemorrhage (<1%)
     - Liver hemorrhage (<1%)
     - Death (rare)
   - Fetal risks
     - Preterm birth (15% to 60%)
     - Intrauterine growth restriction (10% to 25%)
     - Perinatal death (1% to 2%)
     - Hypoxemia-associated neurological injury (<1%)

17. **Does preeclampsia recur in subsequent pregnancies?**
   One earlier episode of preeclampsia imparts a 15% to 25% risk of recurrence; two earlier episodes increase that risk to at least 30%. These rates change based on paternity, maternal age at the time of the next pregnancy, gestational age and severity of preeclampsia in the past, and the presence of underlying medical diseases. Women who were multiparous at the time of a previous case are at even higher risk in subsequent pregnancies.

18. **Does preeclampsia have any long-term effects?**
   Yes. Studies have shown that these women are at increased risk for cardiovascular disease in the future, even before menopause. The risk is highest for women who had preeclampsia at an early gestational age or were multiparous.

19. **How is preeclampsia treated?**
    The only "cure" for preeclampsia is delivery. In the absence of severe features, women with preeclampsia may be closely monitored until 37 weeks of gestation. These patients require close blood pressure monitoring, weekly laboratory tests, and twice weekly fetal testing. This testing may be done in the hospital or on an outpatient basis if the patient is reliable and compliant. Although growth restriction is no longer a criterion for severe preeclampsia, fetal growth assessment is prudent.
    Women diagnosed with preeclampsia before 34 weeks should receive a course of steroids (betamethasone or dexamethasone) in anticipation of iatrogenic preterm delivery. Steroids have been shown to decrease respiratory distress syndromes, intraventricular hemorrhage, necrotizing enterocolitis, and overall morbidity and mortality in the first year of life. In a few situations, delivery should occur after maternal stabilization without delay for antenatal steroids. These include uncontrolled severe-range blood pressures (≥160 mm Hg systolic or ≥110 mm Hg diastolic), pulmonary edema, placental abruption, DIC, eclampsia, or a persistent category 3 fetal heart rate tracing.
    In certain cases, preeclampsia with severe features diagnosed before 34 weeks may be expectantly managed in conjunction with subspecialist consultation.

20. **Which women are candidates for expectant management in the setting of preeclampsia with severe features?**
    Some data suggest that some women can be expectantly managed with oral antihypertensive medication if they are at less than 34 weeks of gestation and their only symptom of severity is elevated blood pressure. These patients require hospital admission for frequent blood pressure and symptom evaluations, daily laboratory tests, and daily fetal surveillance. On average, 85% of these women will be delivered because of worsening disease or fetal status within 1 week of diagnosis. Delivery should be planned for no later than 34 weeks.

21. **How should preeclampsia with severe features diagnosed before pregnancy viability be managed?**
    These women should be stabilized and delivered, even though that means termination of the pregnancy.

22. **How are preeclamptic patients managed during labor and delivery?**
    To decrease the risk of seizures, continuous intravenous (IV) infusion of magnesium sulfate is given in cases of preeclampsia with severe features. Magnesium is usually given at a rate of 1 to 2 g/hour after a 4 g loading dose and is continued for 12 to 24 hours post partum. Patients without severe features should be closely monitored, and magnesium should be initiated if severe features develop.

23. **What medications can be used to control blood pressure acutely?**
    Severe-range blood pressures (≥160 mm Hg systolic or ≥110 mm Hg diastolic) should be treated with IV medication; hydralazine and labetalol are the most common agents used. If IV access has not yet been obtained, oral nifedipine can be used as an alternative. Because preeclampsia is a state of vasoconstriction and intravascular depletion, diuretics can exacerbate this problem and are not used for this purpose.

24. **What is the best route of delivery for a preeclamptic patient?**
    Cesarean delivery has no advantage over vaginal delivery for women with preeclampsia, and the route of delivery should be based on obstetric indications.

25. **How is a patient with eclampsia managed?**
    An eclamptic patient should first be stabilized (airway, breathing, circulation) and given IV magnesium sulfate (4-6 g) to try to stop the seizure. If magnesium is not readily available, alternative medications include lorazepam and phenytoin. Once stabilized, the mother should be delivered, and a continuous magnesium infusion should be started.

26. **What is the best route of delivery for an eclamptic patient?**
    The presence of eclampsia alone does not require a mother to have a cesarean delivery. Once the woman is stabilized, labor can be induced, and vaginal delivery can be anticipated. This decision should be made on a case-by-case basis, taking all obstetric factors into consideration.

27. **What is HELLP syndrome?**
    HELLP syndrome is a poorly understood variant of severe preeclampsia. The acronym represents the abnormalities that characterize this syndrome—hemolysis, elevated liver enzymes, and low

platelets. It is associated with increased morbidity and mortality for both woman and fetus and is treated by immediate delivery (or delivery after the administration of antenatal corticosteroids if <34 weeks of gestation). Either the vaginal or cesarean route is appropriate based on the clinical situation.

28. **How are patients with CHTN managed during pregnancy?**
Women with CHTN should be evaluated for underlying end-organ damage that may have occurred before conception. This should include a 24-hour urine collection for protein, electrocardiogram, and echocardiogram (if indicated). Baseline platelet count, serum creatinine, and liver function tests should be drawn at the first prenatal visit. Establishing the presence of proteinuria or baseline laboratory abnormalities can be of great use later in pregnancy to help diagnose SIPE.

    Medications should be reviewed and angiotensin-converting enzyme (ACE) inhibitors and angiotensin receptor blockers (ARBs) stopped. Methyldopa, labetalol, and nifedipine are the oral antihypertensives recommended during pregnancy because of their safety profiles and long history of use. Doses are usually titrated to maintain blood pressures between 120 mm Hg and 160 systolic and 80 and 105 mm Hg diastolic.

    Blood pressure and dipstick urine analysis for protein should be performed at every visit, and the patient should be asked whether she has experienced any recent signs and symptoms of preeclampsia. Fetal ultrasound examinations to assess growth and antepartum fetal surveillance should also be performed.

29. **How are patients with GHTN managed during pregnancy?**
Women with gestational hypertension should have blood pressure checks at least twice a week, weekly urine dips for protein, antepartum fetal surveillance, fetal ultrasound examinations to assess growth, and monitoring for signs and symptoms of preeclampsia.

30. **When should patients with CHTN and GHTN hypertension be delivered?**
    - Well-controlled CHTN not requiring medication: 38 to 39 weeks
    - Well-controlled CHTN requiring medication: 37 to 39 weeks
    - Poorly controlled CHTN requiring frequent medication or dose changes: 36 to 37 weeks
    - GHTN: 37 to 38 weeks

31. **How long should women with GHTN, preeclampsia, eclampsia, or HELLP be monitored after delivery?**
These women should be monitored in the hospital or with the equivalent outpatient surveillance for 72 hours following delivery and again at 7 to 10 days or earlier in women with symptoms.

32. **Can preeclampsia or eclampsia occur after delivery?**
Yes. Although most cases occur in the immediate postpartum period, cases of eclampsia as late as 23 days post partum have been reported.

KEY POINTS: HYPERTENSION

1. Gestational hypertension is hypertension that develops during pregnancy after 20 weeks of gestation.
2. Preeclampsia is a systemic disease diagnosed by hypertension and proteinuria. Evidence of neurologic, hepatic, hematologic, or renal dysfunction is also diagnostic.
3. Treatment of preeclampsia is delivery. In the absence of severe features, women may be closely monitored until 37 weeks of gestation.
4. Intrapartum magnesium sulfate is given for seizure prophylaxis and treatment of eclamptic seizures.

BIBLIOGRAPHY

1. American College of Obstetricians and Gynecologists. Hypertension in pregnancy. ACOG executive summary. *Obstet Gynecol.* 2013;122:1122–1131.
2. American College of Obstetricians and Gynecologists. Cerclage for the management of cervical insufficiency. ACOG practice bulletin no. 142. *Obstet Gynecol.* 2014;123:372–379.
3. Magnussen EB, Vatten LJ, Smith GD, Romundstad PR. Hypertensive disorders in pregnancy and subsequently measured cardiovascular factors. *Obstet Gynecol.* 2009;114:961–970.

4. Markham KB, Funai EF. Pregnancy related hypertension. In: Creasy R, Resnik R, Iams JD, Lockwood CJ, Moore TR, eds. *Creasy and Resnik's Maternal Fetal Medicine: Principles and Practice*. 7th ed. Philadelphia: Saunders; 2014: 756–781.
5. Servalli V, Baxter JK. Hypertensive disorders. In: Berghella V, ed. *Maternal Fetal Evidence Based Guidelines*. 2nd ed. New York: Informa Healthcare; 2012:1–19.
6. Sibai BM. Diagnosis, prevention, and management of eclampsia. *Obstet Gynecol*. 2005;105:402–410.
7. Spong CY, Mercer BM, D'alton M, Kilpatrick S, Blackwell S, Saade G. Timing of indicated late-preterm and early-term birth. *Obstet Gynecol*. 2011;118:323–333.

CHAPTER 50

THYROID DISEASE IN PREGNANCY

Kristen M. McMaster, MD

1. **What are the normal changes in the thyroid gland in pregnancy?**
   Fifteen percent of women will experience a noticeable increase in the size of their thyroid gland. This growth is mediated by a physiologic decrease in plasma iodine levels during pregnancy in response to fetal uptake of iodine, as well as increased maternal renal clearance. The thyroid returns to normal size in the postpartum period.

2. **What are the normal physiologic changes in thyroid function during pregnancy?**
   Table 50-1 is an overview of thyroid function changes in pregnancy.

Table 50-1. Normal Physiologic Changes in Thyroid Function During Pregnancy

TEST	CHANGES IN PREGNANCY	COMMENTS
Thyroid-stimulating hormone (TSH)	No change	Transient suppression in first trimester from hCG
Thyroid-binding globulin (TBG)	Increase	From reduced hepatic clearance and estrogenic stimulation of TBG synthesis
Total thyroxine (TT_4)	Increase	From increased TBG
Total triiodothyronine (TT_3)	Increase	From increased TBG
Resin triiodothyronine uptake (RT_3U)	Decrease	From increased TBG
Free thyroxine (FT_4) and free triiodothyronine (FT_3)	No change (possible transient early increase)	Transient increase in first trimester from hCG stimulation
Free thyroxine index (FTI)	No change (possible transient early increase)	Transient increase in first trimester from hCG stimulation

*h*CG, Human chorionic gonadotropin.

3. **What laboratory tests are used to diagnose thyroid disease in pregnancy?**
   Thyroid-stimulating hormone (TSH) and free thyroxine (FT_4) should be measured. The free portion of T_4 is biologically active and not subject to changes in the amount of thyroid-binding globulin that occur in pregnancy. Free triiodothyronine (FT_3) is useful only in patients with suppressed TSH and normal FT_4 levels.

4. **What is the relationship between hyperemesis gravidarum and hyperthyroidism?**
   Nausea and vomiting of pregnancy have been associated with high human chorionic gonadotropin (hCG) levels, which have also been linked to hyperthyroidism; several studies have documented an inverse relationship between hCG with TSH levels. However, patients with hyperemesis rarely present with clinical symptoms of hyperthyroidism; the disorder is considered biochemical and does not require treatment. For more information on hyperemesis gravidarum, see Chapter 43.

5. **Which patients should be screened for thyroid disease?**
   Women with a personal history of thyroid disorder or symptoms of thyroid disease. Testing of an asymptomatic patient with a mildly enlarged thyroid gland as the only finding is *not* warranted.

6. **What is the normal function of the fetal thyroid?**
   The fetal thyroid begins concentrating iodine at 10 to 12 weeks and responds to TSH from its own pituitary at 20 weeks. Fetal serum hormone levels reach adult levels at 36 weeks.

7. **Which modulators of thyroid function can cross the placenta?**
   Thyroid hormones (T_3, T_4, thyrotropin-releasing hormone), TSH receptor immunoglobulins, and thioamide medications (propylthiouracil [PTU], methimazole) all cross the placenta. TSH does *not* cross the placenta.

8. **What are common symptoms of hyperthyroidism?**
   Nervousness, tremors, palpitations, tachycardia, hypertension, frequent stools, sweating, heat intolerance, weight loss, goiter, and insomnia. Symptoms more specific to Graves disease include ophthalmopathy (lid lag), exophthalmos, and dermopathy (pretibial myxedema).

9. **What are the definition and differential diagnosis of thyrotoxicosis of pregnancy?**
   Thyrotoxicosis is exposure to excess thyroid hormone of any cause. The differential diagnosis includes Graves disease, excessive production of TSH, gestational trophoblastic disease (e.g., molar pregnancy), hyperfunctioning thyroid adenoma, toxic multinodular goiter, subacute thyroiditis, extrathyroid source of thyroid hormone (e.g., struma ovarii), and ingestion of T_4.

10. **What are the obstetric risks of untreated hyperthyroidism?**
    Preterm delivery, preeclampsia, heart failure, nonimmune hydrops, low birth weight, and fetal demise.

11. **What is the incidence of hyperthyroidism in pregnancy, and what is the most common cause?**
    Hyperthyroidism affects 0.2% of pregnancies, and 95% of these cases are caused by Graves disease.

12. **What is Graves disease?**
    An autoimmune disorder leading to production of thyroid-stimulating immunoglobulins (TSIs) and TSH-binding inhibitory immunoglobulins (TBIIs), which either stimulate or inhibit the thyroid gland through the TSH receptor.

13. **How is Graves disease diagnosed?**
    Suppressed TSH, with elevated FT_4 or FT_4 index (FTI), in the absence of thyroid nodules. The presence of antibodies is not required; very high levels of thyroid-stimulating antibodies, however, correlate with perinatal thyrotoxicosis.

14. **What are the effects of Graves disease on the fetus?**
    Autoantibodies can cross the placenta and either stimulate or inhibit the fetal thyroid. TSIs lead to neonatal hyperthyroidism or Graves disease. TBIIs can cross the placenta and cause transient neonatal hypothyroidism.

15. **Can a woman with well-controlled Graves disease and normal thyroid function tests still have an affected infant?**
    Yes. The incidence of neonatal disease cannot be predicted by maternal thyroid function. Women who have been treated surgically or with radioactive iodine ablation may be at increased risk because of transplacental passage of antibodies in the setting of no suppressive treatment. In women treated with medication, the overall incidence of neonatal thyroid dysfunction is low (1% to 5%) because these medications also cross the placenta. Because antibodies are cleared slowly after birth, infants born to these women should be evaluated for delayed neonatal Graves disease.

16. **What medications can be used to treat hyperthyroidism?**
    The thioamides PTU and methimazole function by blocking the organification of iodide. PTU also blocks peripheral conversion of T_4 to T_3 and has a shorter response time. Out of concern for teratogenicity associated with methimazole, PTU is preferred in the first trimester. PTU, however, has been associated with hepatotoxicity, and methimazole is the recommended agent during the second and third trimesters. β-Blockers can be offered at any time in pregnancy to provide symptomatic relief until thyroid hormone levels respond to thioamide treatment.

17. **What are the fetal risks of maternal thioamide treatment?**
    Thioamides can suppress fetal and neonatal thyroid function and can be associated with transient fetal goiter. Some studies have linked first trimester methimazole use with embryopathy that includes esophageal or choanal atresia and aplasia cutis, which is a defect of the scalp. PTU use can cause hepatotoxicity, although this complication is rare.

18. **Can women taking thioamides breastfeed?**
    Yes. Only small amounts of PTU cross into breast milk, and studies have found normal thyroid hormone levels in neonates breastfed by mothers taking PTU. Methimazole is also safe but is excreted in slightly higher amounts.

19. **How is treatment of hyperthyroidism in pregnancy monitored?**
    The goal is to use the lowest possible dose of medication required to maintain FT_4 in the high-normal range. Hormone levels are generally assessed every 2 to 4 weeks after initiation of therapy until normalized and then every 4 to 6 weeks or once per trimester.

20. **Should pregnant or breastfeeding women receive diagnostic or therapeutic iodine treatments?**
    No. These treatments involve radioactive iodine, which can cross the placenta and cause iatrogenic fetal hypothyroidism. The fetus is at risk from this effect at any time after 10 weeks of gestation, when the fetal thyroid begins concentrating iodine. Breastfeeding should be postponed for at least 120 days following radioactive iodine treatment.

21. **What is thyroid storm, and how is it treated?**
    Thyroid storm is a rare medical emergency that occurs in 1% of pregnant women with hyperthyroidism. It is a hypermetabolic state manifested by fever, tachycardia, altered mental status, restlessness, nervousness, confusion, seizures, vomiting, diarrhea, cardiac arrhythmias, shock, coma, and heart failure. Patients should be treated in an intensive care setting with PTU or methimazole, with PTU having the added benefit of blocking peripheral conversion of T_4 to T_3. Saturated iodide solutions are also administered to block the release of thyroid hormone, and propranolol is given to inhibit the adrenergic effects of the hyperthyroid state. These patients should receive continuous cardiac monitoring and supportive care with intravenous fluids, oxygen, and antipyretics.

22. **What are the signs and symptoms of hypothyroidism?**
    Fatigue, constipation, cold intolerance, muscle cramps, hair loss, dry skin, diminished deep tendon reflexes, carpal tunnel syndrome, weight gain, and intellectual slowness. In severe cases, these symptoms can progress to myxedema and myxedema coma.

23. **What are the definition and differential diagnosis of hypothyroidism?**
    Hypothyroidism is characterized by elevated TSH and low T_4 and T_3 levels. The differential diagnosis includes Hashimoto disease (chronic autoimmune thyroiditis), subacute thyroiditis, radioactive iodine treatment, iodine deficiency, and thyroidectomy.

24. **What are the most common causes of hypothyroidism?**
    Iodine deficiency is the most common cause worldwide. In developed countries, Hashimoto disease is the most common.

25. **What is the incidence of hypothyroidism in pregnancy?**
    Overt hypothyroidism complicates 0.2% to 1% of all pregnancies, and most of these cases are mild.

26. **What is subclinical hypothyroidism?**
    Subclinical hypothyroidism is the presence of elevated TSH in the setting of normal T_4 levels in an asymptomatic patient. Although some studies have suggested that subclinical hypothyroidism may be associated with adverse pregnancy outcomes, this is controversial. The American College of Obstetricians and Gynecologists (ACOG) currently recommends against the universal screening of asymptomatic patients.

27. **What are the obstetric risks of maternal hypothyroidism?**
    Preeclampsia, low birth weight, preterm delivery, and placental abruption. Infants of untreated mothers can also develop congenital cretinism, which is associated with growth failure, mental retardation, and other neuropsychological deficits.

28. **How is hypothyroidism in pregnancy treated?**
    Levothyroxine supplementation is required to normalize TSH levels. In patients with newly diagnosed hypothyroidism, TSH levels should be monitored every 4 weeks until stable. TSH monitoring every trimester is appropriate in patients with stable levels.

29. **What are the incidence and presentation of postpartum thyroiditis?**
Postpartum thyroiditis is autoimmune inflammation of the thyroid gland occurring within the first year after childbirth. It develops in 5% to 10% of women without a history of thyroid disease and manifests as new-onset, painless alteration of thyroid function. It is fairly evenly split among hypothyroidism, hyperthyroidism, and transient hyperthyroidism followed by hypothyroidism.

30. **How is postpartum thyroiditis diagnosed?**
Postpartum thyroiditis is diagnosed by new-onset abnormal values of TSH, FT_4, or both. The diagnosis can be supported by the detection of antimicrosomal, antithyroglobulin, or antithyroid peroxidase antibodies.

31. **What is the prognosis for patients with postpartum thyroiditis?**
Approximately 30% of women with postpartum thyroiditis will develop permanent hypothyroidism. Patients most likely to develop permanent sequelae are those with markedly elevated TSH and antithyroid peroxidase antibodies. Among women who recover normal thyroid function, postpartum thyroiditis tends to recur in subsequent pregnancies.

32. **How should a thyroid nodule be assessed during pregnancy?**
Ultrasound examination should be performed to evaluate nodule size and determine whether the mass is solid or cystic (solid lesions are more likely to be malignant). If concern for malignancy exists, fine-needle aspiration (FNA) is an appropriate next step. Radioiodine scanning in pregnancy is contraindicated because of the risk of iatrogenic fetal thyroid injury.

33. **What is the risk of thyroid cancer in pregnancy?**
Thyroid cancer is found in up to 40% of thyroid nodules in pregnancy, at an incidence of 1 in 1000 women. Prognosis is not affected by pregnancy.

KEY POINTS: THYROID DISEASE IN PREGNANCY

1. Although total circulating T_4 and T_3 increase in pregnancy because of an increase in thyroid-binding globulin, free levels are unchanged.
2. Even in well-controlled hyperthyroidism, thyroid-stimulating antibodies can cross the placenta and cause fetal or neonatal hyperthyroidism.
3. Out of concern for teratogenicity associated with methimazole, PTU is preferred in the first trimester. However, methimazole is the recommended agent during the second and third trimesters out of concern for PTU-associated hepatotoxicity.
4. When untreated, maternal hyperthyroidism and hypothyroidism are both associated with obstetric complications.

BIBLIOGRAPHY

1. American College of Obstetricians and Gynecologists. Thyroid disease in pregnancy. ACOG practice bulletin no. 37. *Obstet Gynecol.* 2015;125:996–1005.
2. Cunningham F, Leveno KJ, Bloom SL, et al. *Endocrine disorders.* In: *Williams Obstetrics.* 24th ed. New York: McGraw-Hill; 2013.
3. Food and Drug Administration and American Thyroid Association. *Propylthiouracil-related liver toxicity.* Washington, DC: Public Workshop; April 19, 2009.

CHAPTER 51

AUTOIMMUNE DISEASES IN PREGNANCY

Anna Karina Celaya, MD

1. **What are autoimmune diseases?**

   Autoimmune diseases are caused by the production of antibodies directed at the body's own tissues. Referred to as autoantibodies, these antiself antibodies can be organ specific or non–organ specific. Examples of organ-specific antibodies include antithyroid and anti–smooth muscle antibodies. Non–organ-specific antibodies include antiphospholipid antibodies (anticardiolipin antibody, lupus anticoagulant, and anti–β_2-glycoprotein antibody), antinuclear antibodies (ANAs), and antihistone antibodies (Table 51-1). Major autoimmune diseases include antiphospholipid syndrome (APS or APLS, systemic lupus erythematosus (SLE), rheumatoid arthritis (RA), myasthenia gravis, and idiopathic thrombocytopenic purpura (ITP). Thyroid disease and diabetes are discussed in Chapters 50 and 48, respectively.

Table 51-1. Autoimmune Diseases and Associated Autoantibodies

AUTOIMMUNE DISEASE	ASSOCIATED AUTOANTIBODIES
Antiphospholipid syndrome	ACA, LA
Systemic lupus erythematosus	ANA, anti-DNA, anti-SSA, anti-SSB, ACA, anti-Sm
Myasthenia gravis	Anti–acetylcholine receptor antibodies
Rheumatoid arthritis	Rheumatoid factor
ITP	Antibody to antigens on platelet glycoproteins (IIb-IIIa or Ib-IX)

ACA, Anticardiolipin antibody; *ANA,* antinuclear antibody; *ITP,* idiopathic thrombocytopenic purpura; *LA,* lupus anticoagulant; *Sm,* Smith.

2. **What are lupus anticoagulant, anticardiolipin antibodies, and anti–β_2-glycoprotein antibodies?**

   Lupus anticoagulant and anticardiolipin antibodies are antiphospholipid antibodies that bind to negatively charged phospholipids found in all cell membranes. Both have been associated with thrombosis and adverse pregnancy outcomes. Lupus anticoagulant is measured as either present or absent, whereas anticardiolipin antibodies are measured in immunoglobulin G (IgG) and IgM isotypes. β_2-Glycoprotein I is an abundant plasma protein that enhances the binding of antiphospholipid antibodies to phospholipid; anti–β_2-glycoprotein is also measured in IgG and IgM isotypes.

3. **What are the medical implications of antiphospholipid antibodies?**

   Antiphospholipid antibodies have been associated with arterial and venous thrombosis, autoimmune thrombocytopenia, recurrent embryonic and fetal loss, intrauterine growth restriction, and preeclampsia.

4. **What are the diagnostic criteria for antiphospholipid syndrome?**

   The diagnosis requires the presence of at least one clinical criterion and one laboratory criterion (see questions 5 and 6).

5. **What are the clinical criteria for diagnosis of antiphospholipid syndrome?**
   - One or more episodes of arterial, venous, or small vessel thrombosis (excluding superficial venous thrombosis)
   - One or more unexplained death of a normal-appearing fetus at 10 or more weeks of gestation
   - One or more premature births of a normal-appearing neonate at less than 34 weeks of gestation as a result of preeclampsia with severe features, eclampsia, or placental insufficiency
   - Three or more unexplained, consecutive, spontaneous pregnancy losses at less than 10 weeks of gestation; maternal and paternal chromosomal abnormalities should be excluded

6. **What are the laboratory criteria for antiphospholipid syndrome?**
   - Lupus anticoagulant present on two or more occasions at least 12 weeks apart
   - Anticardiolipin antibody, either IgG or IgM, present in a medium or high titer on two or more occasions at least 12 weeks apart
   - Anti-β_2-glycoprotein I antibody, either IgG or IgM, present on two or more occasions at least 12 weeks apart

7. **How is lupus anticoagulant detected in plasma?**
   Lupus anticoagulant is detected in the plasma by using a combination of clotting assays (e.g., lupus anticoagulant–sensitive activated partial thromboplastin time and dilute Russell viper venom time). Lupus anticoagulant disrupts the formation of the prothrombin complex and prolongs the time for clot formation.

   If the presence of lupus anticoagulant is suspected, a mixing study should be performed for confirmation. In this test, the suspected plasma is mixed with normal plasma; the addition of normal plasma corrects the clotting time in the setting of a factor deficiency. If lupus anticoagulant is present, the clotting time will remain prolonged.

8. **How is antiphospholipid syndrome treated during pregnancy and the postpartum period?**
   Treatment can be categorized into two groups: women with and without a history of a thrombotic event.
   - For women with an earlier thrombotic event, prophylactic anticoagulation with heparin is recommended throughout pregnancy and until 6 weeks post partum.
   - For women without an earlier thrombotic event, expert consensus suggests that either close clinical surveillance or prophylactic heparin use throughout pregnancy and 6 weeks post partum can be offered.
   For women with sporadic or recurrent pregnancy loss and no earlier thrombotic event, prophylactic use of heparin and low-dose aspirin may reduce pregnancy loss by 50%. The benefits of prednisone or intravenous immune globulin (IVIG) are unclear, and their use is not recommended.

9. **How is SLE diagnosed?**
   Revised criteria of the American Rheumatism Association for the diagnosis of lupus require four or more of the following criteria at any time:
   1. Malar rash
   2. Discoid rash
   3. Photosensitivity
   4. Oral ulcers
   5. Arthritis
   6. Serositis
   7. Renal disorder (proteinuria >0.5 g/day)
   8. Neurologic disorders (seizures, psychosis)
   9. Hematologic disorders (hemolytic anemia, thrombocytopenia)
   10. Immunologic disorders (anti-dsDNA [anti–double-stranded DNA] or anti-Sm [ant—Smith] antibodies, false-positive Venereal Disease Research Laboratories [VDRL] test result, abnormal anticardiolipin or lupus anticoagulant results)
   11. Antinuclear antibodies

   Several drugs are known to cause drug-induced lupus, which is characterized by the presence of antihistone antibodies. These drugs include procainamide, quinidine, hydralazine, methyldopa, phenytoin, and phenobarbital. Most symptoms resolve on discontinuation of the medication.

10. **How does SLE affect pregnancy?**
    SLE occurs more often in women, and the prevalence among women of childbearing age is approximately 1 in 500. The course of SLE during pregnancy is variable; outcomes are best for patients who are in remission for at least 6 months before conception occurs. For women with active disease, morbidity and mortality can be significant, particularly in the setting of renal involvement. Rates of stillbirth, preeclampsia, growth restriction, and indicated preterm delivery are all increased. Fetal well-being should be closely monitored with antepartum surveillance and regular ultrasound examinations for fetal growth assessment. (For more information on this topic, see Chapter 40). Ro is one of three different proteins that constitute an heterogenous antigentic complex commonly seen in autoimmune diseases such as Lupus. If anti-Ro/SSA (anti–Ro/skin-sensitizing antibody) or anti-LA/SSB (anti–lupus anticoagulant/SSB) antibodies are present, infants are also at risk for neonatal lupus, which can include hematologic or hepatobiliary abnormalities, rash, and congenital heart block.

11. **What is RA, and how does it affect pregnancy?**

    RA is a chronic, multisystem disease of unknown etiology that creates an inflammatory response in joints—particularly in the hands, feet, knees, and wrists, and usually in a symmetric distribution. Synovial inflammation can lead to cartilage destruction and bone erosions, which can result in joint deformities. Women are affected three times more often than men, and there appears to be a genetic predisposition.

    The American College of Rheumatology requires at least four of the following seven criteria for diagnosis:
    1. Morning joint stiffness
    2. Arthritis of three or more joints
    3. Arthritis of the wrist, metacarpophalangeal joint, or proximal interphalangeal joint
    4. Symmetric distribution of symptoms
    5. Rheumatoid nodules
    6. Serum rheumatoid factor
    7. Radiographic changes

    RA improves in up to 90% of women during pregnancy, although an increased risk of flares exists in the postpartum period. Nonsteroidal antiinflammatory drugs (NSAIDs) including aspirin are frequently used for management in pregnancy, with regular ultrasound examinations and antepartum testing because of the potential for oligohydramnios and premature closure of the ductus arteriosus. Immunosuppression is generally avoided, although azathioprine may be considered for severe cases. Screening for anti-Rho/SSA and anti-LA/SSB antibodies should be performed because of their associated risk of neonatal lupus.

12. **What is myasthenia gravis, and what considerations should be made during pregnancy?**

    Myasthenia gravis is an autoimmune disease caused by antibodies that block acetylcholine receptors at the postsynaptic neuromuscular junction, with resulting muscular weakness and fatigue. The disease course in pregnancy is variable. Delivery requires special considerations; the uterus is smooth muscle, but the second stage of labor requires the use of skeletal muscles. Vaginal delivery is possible, but assistance with a vacuum or forceps may be needed. If cesarean delivery occurs, regional anesthesia is preferred over general anesthesia to avoid use of muscle relaxants. Magnesium sulfate can precipitate a myasthenic crisis and should never be given. Infants are at risk of neonatal myasthenia, which can cause respiratory distress and poor feeding.

13. **What is multiple sclerosis, and how does pregnancy affect it?**

    Multiple sclerosis is a chronic disease of the central nervous system that involves the autoimmune destruction of myelin. Symptoms vary widely, ranging from benign to disabling. Multiple sclerosis frequently relapses during pregnancy, although the rate of flares increases during the postpartum period. Immunologic medications are generally discontinued because of unknown fetal effects, but IVIG and steroids can be used in symptomatic women. Multiple sclerosis has no known direct effects on the fetus, and pregnancy does not significantly affect the long-term course of the disease.

14. **What is ITP?**

    ITP is characterized by immune-mediated platelet destruction secondary to antiplatelet antibodies. Typical clinical manifestations include easy bleeding and bruising; rare hemorrhagic symptoms generally do not appear until the platelet count is lower than 20,000/μL. Although ITP is a diagnosis of exclusion, it has four common findings:
    1. Persistent thrombocytopenia (platelets <100,000/μL)
    2. Normal or increased numbers of megakaryocytes in the bone marrow
    3. Exclusion of other disorders or drugs associated with thrombocytopenia (e.g., SLE, human immunodeficiency virus [HIV] infection, sulfonamide drugs, β-lactams, and pseudothrombocytopenia or laboratory error)
    4. Absence of splenomegaly

15. **How is ITP differentiated from gestational thrombocytopenia?**

    Gestational thrombocytopenia affects as many as 8% of all pregnancies. Most women have no earlier history of thrombocytopenia, unless during a previous pregnancy. Platelet counts are typically higher than 70,000/μL, and most cases resolve within 2 to 12 weeks post partum. It is important to exclude other causes such as HELLP (hemolysis, elevated liver enzymes, and low platelets) and preeclampsia. Gestational thrombocytopenia is generally a benign, self-limiting process with no major effects on maternal or fetal health.

16. **How is ITP managed during pregnancy?**
    Before delivery, asymptomatic women with platelet counts higher than 20,000/μL do not require treatment. As delivery approaches, treatment is usually considered to prepare for procedures such as regional anesthesia and cesarean delivery. The ideal platelet count for regional anesthesia is variable and provider specific, but a count of more than 50,000/μL is desirable for surgical treatment.
    First-line treatment is with prednisone (1 to 2 mg/kg/day) until platelets reach an acceptable level, which can take 3 to 7 days. The dosage can then be tapered. IVIG can be used in refractory cases, when platelets are lower than 10,000/μL in the third trimester, when platelets are lower than 30,000/μL in the presence of bleeding, or when platelets are lower than 30,000/μL before delivery. Splenectomy is reserved for patients in whom both steroid and IVIG treatments fail and who have platelet counts lower than 10,000/μL. Transfusion of platelets should be performed only to treat bleeding or before a procedure; survival time of the donor platelets is decreased by autoimmune destruction. Immunosuppression with drugs such as azathioprine is reserved for rare situations because of the potential of adverse fetal effects.

17. **Do any fetal considerations exist in a patient with ITP?**
    Yes. Although uncommon, a risk of fetal thrombocytopenia caused by transplacental passage of maternal antiplatelet antibodies exists. This complication does not correlate with maternal platelet counts or antibody titers, and cesarean delivery has not been shown to prevent bleeding complications such as intracranial or internal hemorrhage. A platelet count is generally obtained from the newborn at birth.

KEY POINTS: AUTOIMMUNE DISEASES

1. Antiphospholipid antibodies have been associated with arterial and venous thrombosis, autoimmune thrombocytopenia, recurrent embryonic and fetal loss, intrauterine growth restriction, and preeclampsia.
2. The course of SLE during pregnancy is variable; outcomes are best for patients who are in remission for at least 6 months before conception occurs.
3. Congenital heart block is associated with the presence of maternal anti-Rho/SSA or anti-LA/SSB antibodies.
4. Magnesium sulfate is contraindicated in patients with myasthenia gravis.
5. Multiple sclerosis usually improves during pregnancy.

BIBLIOGRAPHY

American College of Obstetricians and Gynecologists. Antiphospholipid syndrome. ACOG practice bulletin no. 132. *Obstet Gynecol.* 2012;120:1514–1521.
American College of Obstetricians and Gynecologists. Thrombocytopenia in pregnancy. ACOG practice bulletin no. 6. *Obstet Gynecol.* 1999;67(2):117–128. Reaffirmed 2014.
Bove R, Alwan S, Friedman JM, et al. Management of multiple sclerosis during pregnancy and the reproductive years: a systematic review. *Obstet Gynecol.* 2014;124:1157–1168.
Cunningham F, Leveno KJ, Bloom SL, et al. Connective-tissue disorders. In: *Williams Obstetrics.* 23rd ed. New York: McGraw-Hill; 2010:1145–1163.
Miyakis S, Lockshin MD, Atsumi T, et al. International consensus statement on an update of the classification criteria for definite antiphospholipid syndrome (APS). *J Thromb Haemost.* 2006;4:295–306.
Practice Committee of the American Society for Reproductive Medicine. Evaluation and treatment of recurrent pregnancy loss: a committee opinion. *Fertil Steril.* 2012;98:1103–1111.

CHAPTER 52

NEUROLOGIC ISSUES IN PREGNANCY

Stephanie G. Valderramos, MD, PhD

1. **What is the most frequent neurologic complication in pregnant women?**
   Epilepsy, which affects between 0.3% and 0.6% of pregnant women.

2. **How does pregnancy affect seizure disorders?**
   The frequency of seizures increases in 30% to 50% of patients, most commonly in the first trimester. Patients with infrequent attacks (less than one every 9 months) are less likely to experience exacerbation of seizure frequency during pregnancies.

3. **What is the etiology of increased seizure frequency in pregnancy?**
   Although the exact cause is unknown, it may be related to metabolic, hormonal, or hematologic changes in pregnancy, fatigue or sleep deprivation, or decreased antiepileptic drug concentrations.

4. **How do seizures affect the course of pregnancy?**
   Patients with seizure disorder may have a higher risk of preeclampsia, preterm labor, congenital malformations, and stillbirth. An increased risk of clinical or subclinical coagulopathy is also noted in neonates of mothers taking antiepileptic drugs.

5. **What is the therapeutic approach to epilepsy in pregnancy?**
   Uncontrolled seizures are dangerous to the fetus because of the resulting hypoxia and acidemia. Ideally, monotherapy with a single agent is preferred at the lowest dose protective against seizures. Folic acid supplementation of 4 mg daily should also be provided.

6. **How does pregnancy change the levels of antiepileptic medications?**
   The total levels—and to a lesser extent the free levels—of most antiepileptic agents are decreased in pregnancy, and an adjustment of dose is sometimes required. The reason for these changes may be related to the dilutional effect of increased plasma volume, poor compliance with drug regimen, decreased absorption resulting from nausea and vomiting, and changes in the metabolism and excretion of the drugs. Folic acid may lower plasma levels of phenytoin during pregnancy. Drug levels of antiepileptics should be measured periodically throughout pregnancy and adjusted as needed.

7. **What are the teratogenic effects of antiepileptics?**
   The use of antiepileptic drugs has been associated with a 4% to 6% risk of major and minor congenital malformations, compared with the baseline population risk of 2% to 3%. Phenytoin, carbamazepine, phenobarbital, and valproic acid have been associated with higher malformation rates (Table 52-1). Limited information on teratogenicity is available for newer antiepileptics such as gabapentin, lamotrigine, levetiracetam, or topiramate.

8. **Which antiepileptic drugs are contraindicated in pregnancy?**
   Valproic acid has a 1% to 2% rate of neural tube defects (NTDs) and is also associated with urogenital, craniofacial, and cardiac abnormalities. Fetuses exposed to valproic acid have a 10- to 20-fold increase in major malformations. This drug should be avoided in pregnancy, particularly in the first trimester.

9. **Should patients with epilepsy stop their medication when they become pregnant?**
   No. Ideally, antiepileptic therapy should be optimized before pregnancy to minimize fetal exposure to potentially teratogenic medications. With the possible exception of valproic acid, the patient should continue her antiepileptic regimen. The benefit of changing medications solely to reduce teratogenic risk is limited once the pregnancy has been established for several weeks because this change may precipitate seizures and expose the fetus to additional antiepileptic drugs.

Table 52-1. Rates of Congenital Malformations With Common Antiepileptic Drugs

DRUG	OVERALL RISK OF MALFORMATIONS	ASSOCIATED MALFORMATIONS
Valproic acid	10.7%	Neural tube defects, urogenital malformations, craniofacial defects, cardiac malformations, neurocognitive delay
Phenytoin	7.4%	Fetal hydantoin syndrome (digital hypoplasia, cleft lip or palate, microcephaly, cardiac malformations, urogenital malformations)
Phenobarbital	4.9%	Cardiac malformations, cleft lip or palate, urogenital malformations
Carbamazepine	4.6%	Spina bifida, genitourinary malformations

10. **Is it safe to breastfeed while taking antiepileptic medication?**
    Antiepileptics are minimally secreted into breastmilk and are thought to pose minimal risk to the infant. Notable exceptions are carbamazepine and lamotrigine, which can be detected in infant serum (although at less than therapeutic levels). Limited data are available for newer drugs. Although antiepileptic therapy is not a reason to stop breastfeeding, all infants—especially those younger than 2 months of age—should be monitored for drowsiness, adequate weight gain, and developmental milestones. Updated information on lactation and specific medications can be found at LactMed (see the Bibliography).

11. **How is status epilepticus treated in pregnancy?**
    Although status epilepticus is rare, it may lead to maternal or fetal death. Seizure activity should be controlled as rapidly as possible while maintaining control of the airway. Treating glucose and electrolyte abnormalities is critical. Intravenous (IV) diazepam or lorazepam usually provides initial control, and IV phenytoin (or fosphenytoin) can be administered to prevent recurrence. Other anticonvulsants such as phenobarbital or midazolam may be used.

12. **How is status epilepticus differentiated from an eclamptic seizure?**
    Eclamptic seizures are associated with hypertension, proteinuria, or other laboratory signs of preeclampsia or HELLP (hemolysis, elevated liver enzymes, low platelets) syndrome. Eclamptic seizures are also usually self-limited. IV magnesium should be administered to prevent recurrence of eclamptic seizures.

13. **What is the approach to headaches in the pregnant patient?**
    Headache is a common complaint in pregnancy and requires evaluation. Preeclampsia must always be considered and is usually distinguished from more benign causes by elevated blood pressure, proteinuria, and other laboratory abnormalities. The most common types of headache are tension headaches, which are typically chronic, worsen throughout the day, and are most intense in the back of the head. Migraine headaches are episodic and may be preceded by visual, sensory, or motor symptoms. They are commonly lateralized and may be accompanied by nausea, vomiting, photophobia, and visual disturbances. The sudden development of severe headache associated with other neurologic symptoms should trigger an evaluation for an acute intracranial cause.

14. **How does pregnancy affect women with migraines?**
    Migraines occasionally worsen during the first 3 months of pregnancy and often improve after the first trimester. Women with severe migraines during pregnancy have a higher risk of preeclampsia and severe hyperemesis gravidarum.

15. **How are migraines managed in pregnancy?**
    First-line treatments are acetaminophen, metoclopramide, and caffeine. For severe pain, opioids can be given. For recurrent migraines unresponsive to other drugs, triptan medications can be considered. Sumatriptan is the most commonly used medication in this class; at present, no increased risk of significant adverse pregnancy outcomes has been associated with this medication.

KEY POINTS: NEUROLOGIC ISSUES IN PREGNANCY

1. Anticonvulsant therapy should be optimized before conception occurs, ideally by using monotherapy at the lowest doses.
2. Folic acid, 4 mg/day, has been shown to decrease the risk of NTDs in women at high risk and should be given to women taking anticonvulsant medications.
3. The risk of major and minor congenital anomalies in women taking anticonvulsants is 4% to 6%, compared with the baseline population risk of 2% to 3%.

BIBLIOGRAPHY

1. Aminoff MJ, Douglas VC. Neurologic disorders. In: Creasy R, Resnik R, Iams JD, Lockwood CJ, Moore TR, eds. *Creasy and Resnick's Maternal-Fetal Medicine: Principles and Practice*. 7th ed. Philadelphia: Saunders; 2014:1100–1120.
2. Hill DS, Wlodarczyk BJ, Palacios AM, Finnell RH. Teratogenic effect of antiepileptic drugs. *Expert Rev Neurother*. 2010;10:943–959.
3. National Library of Medicine, National Institutes of Health. LactMed drugs and lactation database. Available at toxnet.nlm.nih.gov/cgi-bin/sis/htmlgen?LACTMED. Accessed November 7, 2015.

CHAPTER 53

PULMONARY DISEASE IN PREGNANCY

Antonio Bonet, MD

1. **How does pregnancy change pulmonary mechanics?**
   Hormonal changes of pregnancy affect the upper respiratory tract and airway mucosa and produce hyperemia, mucosal edema, hypersecretion, and increased mucosal friability.

   Hormonal changes and the growing uterus change the dimensions of the thoracic cage. The thoracic circumference enlarges as both the anteroposterior and transverse diameters of the thorax increase, and the diaphragm shifts up to 4 cm cephalad. Diaphragmatic function and excursion, however, remain unchanged.

2. **How does pregnancy change lung volumes and pulmonary physiology?**
   - **Functional residual capacity (FRC):** Changes to the dimensions of the thorax result in a progressive decrease of approximately 10% to 20%.
   - **Vital capacity** is unchanged.
   - **Total lung capacity** decreases slightly at term.
   - **Expiratory reserve volume** decreases
   - **Residual volume** may decrease slightly, although this change is inconsistent (Fig. 53-1). Pregnancy does not appear to change lung compliance, but chest wall and total respiratory system compliance are reduced at term. Airway function is preserved; airflow measurements such as forced vital capacity (FVC) and forced expiratory volume in 1 second (FEV_1) normally remain stable.

3. **What are the changes in gas exchange associated with pregnancy?**
   Oxygen consumption increases by 20% to 30% because of fetal demands and increased maternal metabolism. A rise in tidal volume by approximately 30% to 35% also occurs, resulting in increased minute ventilation (20% to 40% higher than baseline at term) and alveolar ventilation. The respiratory rate does not significantly change. Higher levels of progesterone stimulate the respiratory center; production of carbon dioxide is increased, and respiratory drive is enhanced. Physiologic hyperventilation results in compensated respiratory alkalosis; plasma carbon dioxide tension drops to 28 to 32 mm Hg, but pH remains unchanged because of renal excretion of bicarbonate.

4. **What is dyspnea of pregnancy?**
   Dyspnea during pregnancy is also known as physiologic dyspnea. It is a common complaint, occurring in approximately 20% of women at rest and 60% with exertion. Although the origin is unclear, it is thought that progesterone-induced hyperventilation is the most important driving mechanism. Distinguishing physiologic dyspnea from pathologic causes is crucial.

5. **Does pregnancy affect asthma?**
   Asthma is a common medical condition that complicates approximately 4% to 8% of pregnancies. The effects of pregnancy on asthma are variable; approximately 23% of women report an improvement in symptoms, whereas 30% of women report worsening. The goal of asthma therapy during pregnancy is to ensure adequate oxygenation of the fetus by minimizing episodic hypoxemia. The risks of untreated asthma to the patient and fetus far outweigh those associated with asthma medications.

6. **Does asthma affect pregnancy?**
   Prospective studies have consistently shown good outcomes with mild or moderate asthma in pregnant patients. However, substandard control of asthma may be associated with maternal and fetal risk. Data show a correlation between decreased FEV_1 and low birth weight and prematurity.

7. **How should pregnant women with asthma be managed?**
   Pregnant women with asthma should have routine evaluation of their asthma symptoms as well as their pulmonary function with either peak flow measurements or spirometry. Treatment of asthma during pregnancy is similar to that in nonpregnant patients and proceeds in a stepwise fashion.

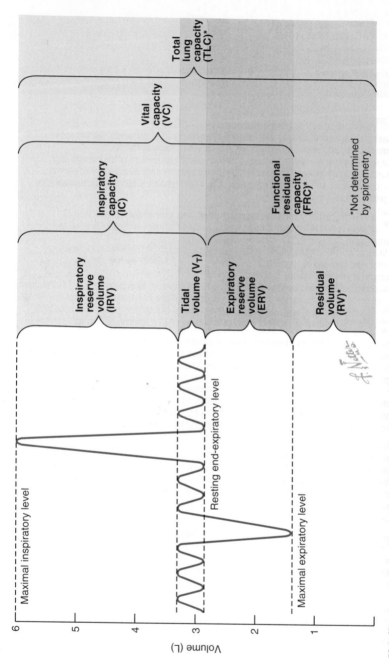

Figure 53-1. Measurement of lung volumes and capacities by spirometry.

For mild intermittent asthma, no controller therapy is indicated; short-acting β_2-agonists (SABA) such as albuterol should suffice.

For persistent asthma, inhaled corticosteroids (ICSs) comprise the mainstay therapy. In mild persistent asthma, a low-dose ICS combined with SABA is recommended, and moderate persistent asthma or asthma that does not respond should be treated with either a medium-dose ICS or low-dose ICS in addition to a long-acting β-agonist (LABA). Leukotriene receptor antagonists (LTRAs) and theophylline are alternative options, although they are less effective than LABAs. If these regimens fail to control asthma symptoms, a high-dose ICS should be used. Some patients with severe, difficult-to-control symptoms may require systemic steroids.

Among ICSs, budesonide is recommended (category B), although no data suggest that the other ICS formulations are unsafe.

8. **What is status asthmaticus, and how is it treated in pregnancy?**
Status asthmaticus is a severe form of acute asthma that affects or threatens oxygenation. Management requires immediate administration of supplemental oxygen, inhaled SABAs, and intravenous or oral corticosteroids. Depending on the severity, subcutaneous catecholamines such as terbutaline or epinephrine may be necessary. If these measures fail and oxygenation is compromised, endotracheal intubation should be performed. The fetus should be monitored during treatment, and subspecialists with expertise in high-risk pregnancies and critical care should be immediately available.

9. **Does pregnancy increase the risk of pulmonary embolism?**
Yes. Venous thromboembolism (VTE) is five times more common in pregnant women compared with age-matched controls. It is a leading cause of maternal morbidity and nonobstetric mortality. Venous stasis, cesarean delivery, advanced maternal age, multiparity, prolonged bed rest, hemorrhage, sepsis, obesity, and inherited or acquired thrombophilias have all been identified as risk factors.

10. **How is venous thromboembolic disease diagnosed?**
Lower extremity edema and discomfort are common during pregnancy and are unreliable in diagnosing deep vein thrombosis. At present, the recommended first test is real-time B-mode ultrasonography; the most reliable diagnostic criterion is an inability to compress the venous lumen fully. The sensitivity and specificity for identifying proximal thrombi are 95% and 99%, respectively. Impedance plethysmography is an alternative diagnostic modality. D-dimer should not be used to rule out VTE in pregnant women.

Diagnostic evaluation for pulmonary embolism should also include a chest radiograph and an electrocardiogram, which may be abnormal in 70% of positive cases. If results of lower extremity compression ultrasound examination are negative and clinical suspicion remains high, additional imaging can be performed using ventilation-perfusion lung scanning or pulmonary angiography.

11. **How should thromboembolic disease in pregnancy be treated?**
When VTE is strongly suspected or diagnosed, treatment with either intravenous unfractionated heparin (UFH) or subcutaneous low-molecular-weight heparin (LMWH) should be started immediately. Neither drug crosses the placenta. Warfarin is teratogenic, however; its use in pregnancy is generally restricted to women with mechanical heart valves. Anticoagulation should be continued for at least 6 weeks post partum or until at least 3 months have been completed. Warfarin is compatible with breastfeeding and is not contraindicated for postpartum women.

12. **What organisms are associated with pneumonia in pregnancy?**
Virtually any organism can cause pneumonia during pregnancy. *Streptococcus pneumoniae* is the most common pathogen; other causative bacteria include *Haemophilus influenzae*, *Mycoplasma pneumoniae*, *Legionella*, and *Klebsiella* species. Viruses such as influenza and varicella can cause atypical pneumonia and are associated with higher mortality rates compared with nonpregnant women. Pneumonia can occur any time during gestation, and infection in the third trimester is associated with preterm labor. Maternal comorbidities—especially chronic lung diseases—increase the risk of poor outcomes.

13. **How is tuberculosis (TB) diagnosed in pregnancy?**
In the United States, most cases of TB occur in immigrants or foreign-born residents from TB-endemic countries. Patients at risk should be screened by skin testing using the purified protein derivative (PPD), which is both safe and valid in pregnancy. The QuantiFERON-TB Gold (QFT; Cellestis; distributed by Qiagen, Valencia, Calif) test is a more recently developed test that measures the release of

interferon-γ in blood in response to peptide antigens that simulate mycobacterial proteins. This test has been found to have comparable results to those in nonpregnant women. The gold standard for diagnosis of active TB is culture, and susceptibility testing is important to ensure adequate treatment.

14. **How is active TB treated in pregnancy?**
Because of the risk of low-birth-weight in infants of women with untreated TB, treatment should be initiated whenever the probability of disease is moderate to high. The recommended initial treatment regimen consists of isoniazid (INH), rifampin (RIF), and ethambutol (EMB) daily for 2 months, followed by INH and RIF daily, or twice weekly for 7 months (9 months total). INH treatment should be given in conjunction with pyridoxine to decrease the risk of peripheral neuropathy. The effects of pyrazinamide (PZA) on the fetus are unknown, and this drug is not recommended in most cases. Streptomycin is contraindicated because of teratogenicity.

15. **What is sarcoidosis, and how does it affect pregnancy?**
Sarcoidosis is an idiopathic, inflammatory, multisystem granulomatous disease that can affect virtually any organ, although the lungs and intrathoracic lymph nodes are predominantly involved. It is characterized by the formation of noncaseating granulomas that may impair organ function. The diagnosis relies on the combination of physical findings, imaging studies, and confirmation of granulomas on tissue biopsy.
    The overall prevalence of sarcoidosis in pregnancy is estimated at 9.6 cases per 100,000 births. Women with sarcoidosis are more likely to have pre-eclampsia, eclampsia, VTE, preterm delivery, cesarean delivery, and postpartum hemorrhage. In spite of these risks, women with sarcoidosis can have successful pregnancies.

16. **What is cystic fibrosis (CF), and how does it affect pregnancy?**
CF is an autosomal recessive genetic disorder that affects exocrine gland function in several organs and results in chronic respiratory failure and pancreatic insufficiency. It is caused by caused by loss-of-function mutations in the CF transmembrane conductance regulator (CFTR) protein, a cyclic adenosine monophosphate (cAMP)–regulated chloride channel. Persons with CF are more susceptible to contracting respiratory infections. Pregnant women with CF need frequent pulmonary and cardiac assessment throughout the gestational period, and special attention should be devoted to nutritional status. With intensive monitoring by a multidisciplinary team of physicians, women with CF are now more likely to carry out successful pregnancies.

17. **What is amniotic fluid embolism, and how is it treated?**
Amniotic fluid embolism (AFE) is a rare obstetric emergency characterized by cardiovascular collapse. In addition to profound hypotension, hypoxemia, coagulopathy, and altered mental status are frequently present. Mortality approaches 80%. AFE is thought to be caused by the entrance of amniotic fluid, fetal cells, or other debris into the maternal circulation, and this may precipitate an anaphylactic reaction. AFE typically occurs during labor, but it has also been described during abortions and after abdominal trauma. The diagnosis has traditionally been made post mortem by finding fetal cells in the maternal pulmonary circulation, although this finding is nonspecific; fetal squamous cells can also be found in the circulation of nonaffected laboring women.
    Treatment is supportive. Vascular support and maintenance of adequate oxygenation are crucial, and anemia and coagulopathy can be treated with blood products. In women with a viable fetus of 24 weeks of gestation or greater, fetal status should also be assessed, and emergency delivery should be performed if necessary. For more information on the resuscitation of a pregnant patient, see Chapter 64.

KEY POINTS: PULMONARY DISEASE IN PREGNANCY

1. Pregnancy causes decreases in FRC, total lung capacity, and expiratory reserve volume; vital capacity remains unchanged.
2. The effects of pregnancy on asthma are variable, and treatment is similar to that in nonpregnant women.
3. VTE is five times more common in pregnant women compared with age-matched controls.
4. Active tuberculosis in pregnancy should be treated.

BIBLIOGRAPHY

1. American Thoracic Society. Centers for Disease Control and Prevention, Infectious Diseases Society of America. Treatment of tuberculosis. *MMWR Recomm Rep.* 2003;52(RR-11):1–77.
2. Clark SL. New concepts of amniotic fluid embolism: a review. *Obstet Gynecol Surv.* 1990;45:360–368.
3. Dombrowski MP, Schatz M. ACOG Committee on Practice Bulletins-Obstetrics. ACOG practice bulletin #90, Feb. 2008: asthma in pregnancy. *Obstet Gynecol.* 2008 Feb;111(2 Pt 1):457–464.
4. Elkus R, Popovich Jr J. Respiratory physiology in pregnancy. *Clin Chest Med.* 1992;13:555–565.
5. Hadid V, Patenaude V, Oddy L, Abenhaim HA. Sarcoidosis and pregnancy: obstetrical and neonatal outcomes in a population-based cohort of 7 million births. *J Perinat Med.* 2015 Mar;43(2):201–207.
6. Leung A, Bull TM, Jaeschke R, et al. An official American Thoracic Society/Society of Thoracic Radiology clinical practice guideline: evaluation of suspected pulmonary embolism in pregnancy. *Am J Respir Crit Care Med.* 2011;184:1200–1208.
7. Lighter-Fisher J, Surette AM. Performance of an interferon-gamma release assay to diagnose latent tuberculosis infection during pregnancy. *Obstet Gynecol.* 2012;119:1088–1095.
8. McColgin SW, Glee L, Brian BA. Pulmonary disorders complicating pregnancy. *Obstet Gynecol Clin North Am.* 1992;19: 697–717.

CHAPTER 54

CARDIOVASCULAR DISEASE IN PREGNANCY

Bao Tran, MD

1. **What are the normal changes in cardiac physiology that occur during pregnancy?**
   Normal cardiac physiologic changes include increased blood volume (preload) associated with hemodilution, decreased systemic vascular resistance (afterload) and blood pressure, and increased heart rate. These changes lead to a 30% to 50% increase in cardiac output.

2. **What are the normal changes in cardiac physiology that occur during labor and delivery?**
   The maximum increase in cardiac output occurs around this time. With each uterine contraction, 300 to 500 mL of blood is shifted from the uterus to the maternal systemic circulation. This "autotransfusion" leads to increased systemic venous return (increased preload). Maternal pain and anxiety can result in increased adrenaline, which increases blood pressure and heart rate. Immediately after delivery, cardiac output is further increased from relief of vena caval compression and an additional autotransfusion of blood from the contracted uterus.

3. **What are the hemodynamic effects of regional anesthesia?**
   Both spinal anesthesia and epidural anesthesia cause peripheral vasodilation, which can produce a significant decrease in preload. This in turn can cause decreased cardiac output and blood pressure. To diminish these changes, maternal hydration is routine. If hydration is insufficient, use of phenylephrine may be considered.

4. **What are the most common cardiovascular diseases during pregnancy?**
   In the Western world, congenital heart disease is the most frequent cardiovascular disease present during pregnancy. Most cases involve intracardiac shunts. In non-Western countries, rheumatic valvular disease is the most common cardiovascular disease encountered in pregnancy.

5. **What common cardiac medications convey risk to the fetus?**
   - Category D (evidence of fetal risk): amiodarone, atenolol, angiotensin-converting enzyme (ACE) inhibitors, angiotensin receptor blockers (ARBs), and warfarin in women with a mechanical heart valve
   - Category X (not to be taken in pregnancy): statins, warfarin in women without a mechanical heart valve

6. **What cardiovascular conditions convey the highest risk for maternal morbidity and mortality?**
   - Significant pulmonary arterial hypertension
   - Systemic ventricular dysfunction (left ventricular ejection fraction [LVEF] <30%) with significant symptoms (New York Heart Association functional class III or IV)
   - History of peripartum cardiomyopathy (PPCM) with residual left ventricular dysfunction
   - Severe mitral stenosis
   - Severe aortic stenosis
   - Severe coarctation of the aorta
   - Unrepaired complex cyanotic congenital heart disease
   - Marfan syndrome with aortic root dilation greater than 4.5 cm

   Pregnancy is contraindicated in patients with these conditions, and termination may be considered if it occurs.

7. **What is pulmonary hypertension (PH)?**
   PH encompasses a group of diseases that ultimately result in increased pressure in the pulmonary vasculature. If progressive, PH will eventually result in right-sided heart failure. The World Health Organization (WHO) separates PH into five groups:
   1. Primary pulmonary arterial hypertension (PAH)
   2. PH caused by left-sided heart disease

3. PH caused by lung disease
4. Chronic thromboembolic PH (CTEPH)
5. PH with unclear multifactorial mechanisms

Regardless of origin, even moderate PH increases risk of maternal mortality, and severe PH is a contraindication to pregnancy.

8. **What is Eisenmenger syndrome?**
Eisenmenger syndrome describes the process in which a left-to-right intracardiac shunt (most commonly a large ventricular septal defect) becomes reversed. This results from irreversible PH caused by increased flow through the pulmonary vasculature; once pulmonary arterial pressure approaches systemic pressure, the shunt reverses. Entry of nonoxygenated blood into the systemic circulation results in hypoxemia and cyanosis. Pregnant women with Eisenmenger syndrome have extremely high mortality and fetal mortality rates (up to 50% in some series).

9. **What is Marfan syndrome?**
Marfan syndrome is the most common cause of pregnancy-related aortic dissection. It is an autosomal dominant genetic disorder that causes abnormal fibrillin, which results in connective tissue abnormalities throughout the body. Patients can have long limbs, scoliosis, joint laxity, aortic root dilation, and optic lens dislocation. Mortality during pregnancy is caused by aortic dissection or rupture; the risk of dissection increases when the aortic root grows larger than 4.0 cm, and pregnancy is contraindicated when it reaches 4.5 cm or more.
   Other conditions that increase the risk of aortic dissection during pregnancy include Loeys-Dietz syndrome, Ehlers-Danlos syndrome (type IV), Turner syndrome, and bicuspid aortic valves.

10. **How should pregnant women with Marfan syndrome be managed?**
These women should receive regular echocardiograms to assess aortic root size, and β-blockers are used to protect the aortic root from the increased hemodynamic forces of pregnancy. Hypertension should be aggressively controlled. Although losartan has been shown to be beneficial in patients with Marfan and aortic root dilatation, ARBs are relatively contraindicated in pregnancy.

11. **What is the most common cause of mitral stenosis in pregnancy?**
The most common cause of mitral stenosis in pregnancy is rheumatic heart disease.

12. **Why is mitral stenosis problematic during pregnancy?**
Women with severe mitral stenosis do not tolerate the hemodynamic burden of pregnancy. A stenotic mitral valve impedes blood flow from the left atrium to the left ventricle during diastole. The increased preload (associated with pregnancy) that normally increases cardiac output backs up into the left atrium instead, resulting in pulmonary congestion and an increased risk of pulmonary edema. Atrial distention can cause atrial fibrillation, which increases the risk of stroke and requires anticoagulation. The increased heart rate associated with pregnancy also decreases left ventricular filling (and therefore cardiac output) by shortening diastole.

13. **How are patients with mitral stenosis managed during pregnancy?**
β-Blocker therapy decreases heart rate and consequently increases diastolic filling time and maximizes cardiac output. Diuretics can also be used to decrease preload and pulmonary congestion. In severely symptomatic patients, percutaneous mitral valvuloplasty (expands the narrowed valve using a balloon) can be considered. This procedure is generally deferred until after 20 weeks of gestation because of the unavoidable radiation exposure.
   During labor, adequate control of pain and anxiety is important to maintain a normal maternal heart rate. Regional anesthesia is usually well tolerated. Autotransfusion at the time of delivery (see question 2) can cause pulmonary edema, and a diuretic may be required.

14. **What is the most common cause of aortic stenosis in pregnancy?**
The most common cause of aortic stenosis in pregnancy is congenital bicuspid valve.

15. **Why is aortic stenosis problematic during pregnancy?**
As aortic stenosis progresses, the left ventricle initially hypertrophies in response to the increased pressure gradient. Eventually, it dilates and fails. Women with severe aortic stenosis have a narrow window of appropriate fluid balance; excessive preload can cause pulmonary congestion, and decreased preload can lead to hypotension and sudden death. The classic symptoms of aortic stenosis are angina, syncope, and congestive heart failure. Because the presence of symptoms significantly increases the risk of maternal mortality, it is reasonable to perform exercise stress testing in asymptomatic patients.

16. **How are patients with aortic stenosis managed during pregnancy?**
   As with mitral stenosis, percutaneous valvuloplasty may be considered in severely symptomatic or decompensated patients who do not respond to medical therapy. Careful fluid management should take place during labor. Regional anesthesia is possible, but it must be titrated slowly to avoid hypotension. At the time of delivery, the threshold for volume resuscitation in response to postpartum blood loss should be low. Invasive hemodynamic monitoring may be helpful in complicated cases.

17. **How are patients with mitral and aortic regurgitation managed during pregnancy?**
   In general, regurgitant valve lesions carry a lower risk than stenotic lesions. The decreased systemic vascular resistance of pregnancy is favorable to the hemodynamics associated with regurgitant lesions, and even women with severe mitral or aortic regurgitation can tolerate pregnancy if left ventricular function is preserved and they are asymptomatic. If these conditions are not met, however, the risk of worsening heart failure is high. In these patients, surgical intervention to address the valve may be indicated before delivery.

18. **What are the most common causes of acute coronary syndrome during pregnancy?**
   Coronary atherosclerosis is still a common cause of acute myocardial infarction (MI) in pregnant women, although it is less prevalent compared with the general population. Other common causes of MI during pregnancy include spontaneous coronary artery dissection, coronary vasospasm, and embolization of clots into coronary arteries. In pregnant women with ST-segment elevation MI (STEMI) or non–ST-segment elevation MI (NSTEMI) with high-risk features, coronary angiography and possible percutaneous coronary intervention (PCI) should be performed. Data on the use of thrombolytics in pregnancy are minimal.

19. **What is peripartum cardiomyopathy (PPCM)?**
   PPCM is defined as development of systolic heart failure (LVEF <45%) toward the end of pregnancy or in the first few months following delivery. Although several risk factors have been identified (advanced maternal age, African descent, multiparity, and preeclampsia), the origin is unknown and likely multifactorial. Presentation is similar to that of other forms of systolic heart failure: dyspnea, pedal edema, orthopnea, and paroxysmal nocturnal dyspnea. Treatment is also similar; β-blockers, digoxin, and diuretics can be used, and ACE inhibitors and ARBs are avoided. Hydralazine and nitrates may be used instead of ACE inhibitors or ARBs.
   Approximately 50% of women with PPCM eventually recover left ventricular function, 25% do not improve, and 25% worsen. Women with persistent left ventricular dysfunction should be counseled against subsequent pregnancies because of the risk of heart failure progression. Women whose left ventricular size and function normalize after delivery have an overall good prognosis, although the risk of recurrence during subsequent pregnancies is high.

20. **What is hypertrophic cardiomyopathy (HCM)?**
   HCM is characterized by abnormal left ventricular wall thickening; it is the most common genetic cardiac disease. Symptoms of heart failure result from to diastolic dysfunction and increased end-diastolic pressure from outflow tract obstruction. Pregnancy is generally well tolerated, although risk is increased in patients who are symptomatic or have marked outflow tract obstruction (assessed with an echocardiogram). As in aortic stenosis, neither hypovolemia nor volume overload is well tolerated. Careful fluid management is required during labor and delivery, and regional anesthesia is usually avoided. A β-blocker can be useful to control heart rate and improve symptoms.

21. **How are arrhythmias managed during pregnancy?**
   Women with a documented arrhythmia should be evaluated for structural heart disease with an electrocardiogram and echocardiogram. Atrioventricular (AV) nodal reentrant tachycardia (AVNRT) and AV reciprocating tachycardia (AVRT) are the most common arrhythmias in pregnancy. Management can often be successful with vagal maneuvers or AV-nodal blocking agents; in the setting of hemodynamic compromise, immediate direct-current cardioversion should be performed.
   Idiopathic right ventricular outflow tract tachycardia is a common type of ventricular tachycardia in this population and can be managed with either verapamil or β-blockers.

KEY POINTS: CARDIOVASCULAR DISEASE IN PREGNANCY

1. Cardiac output increases in pregnancy, first by increased stroke volume then by increased heart rate. Systemic vascular resistance decreases during pregnancy and causes decreased blood pressure.
2. Labor and delivery are critical times for women with cardiac disease because of dramatic fluctuation in hemodynamics and volume status.
3. Eisenmenger syndrome, severe mitral stenosis or aortic stenosis, pulmonary hypertension, and Marfan syndrome with a dilated aortic root carry the greatest risk of maternal mortality during pregnancy.
4. Stenotic valvular lesions carry higher pregnancy risk than regurgitant valvular lesions. Left-sided valve diseases carry higher risk than right-sided valve diseases.
5. Be aware that some major cardiac drug classes are relatively contraindicated in pregnancy.

BIBLIOGRAPHY

1. Amsterdam EA, Wenger NK, Brindis RG, et al. 2014 AHA/ACC Guideline for the management of patients with non–ST-elevation acute coronary syndromes: a report of the American College of Cardiology/American Heart Association Task Force on Practice Guidelines. *Circulation.* 2014;130:e344–e426.
2. European Society of Gynecology, Association for European Paediatric Cardiology, German Society for Gender Medicine, et al. ESC guidelines on the management of cardiovascular diseases during pregnancy: the Task Force on the Management of Cardiovascular Diseases During Pregnancy of the European Society of Cardiology (ESC). *Eur Heart J.* 2011;32:3147–3197.
3. Nishimura RA, Otto CM, Bonow RO, et al. 2014 AHA/ACC guideline for the management of patients with valvular heart disease: a report of the American College of Cardiology/American Heart Association Task Force on Practice Guidelines. *Circulation.* 2014;129:e521–e643.
4. Yancy CW, Jessup M, Bozkurt B, et al. 2013 ACCF/AHA guideline for the management of heart failure: a report of the American College of Cardiology Foundation/American Heart Association Task Force on Practice Guidelines. *J Am Coll Cardiol.* 2013;62:e147–e239.

CHAPTER 55

INFECTIONS IN PREGNANCY

Kristina Galyon, DO

1. **Why should pregnant women be screened for group B *Streptococcus* (GBS), and how is screening performed?**

   In the United States, GBS is the leading cause of infection-related neonatal morbidity and mortality in the first week of life. It can be prevented by identifying women at risk for transmitting it to their newborns and giving them intravenous antibiotics during labor. The Centers for Disease Control and Prevention (CDC) and the American College of Obstetricians and Gynecologists (ACOG) recommend that all pregnant women should be screened for GBS colonization between 35 and 37 weeks of gestation. This includes women in whom cesarean delivery is planned because labor may occur before the scheduled date. Women with symptoms of preterm labor before 35 weeks or with preterm premature rupture of membranes should also be screened. The only exceptions to universal screening are in women who have previously given birth to a neonate with early-onset GBS disease or who have had GBS bacteriuria during the current pregnancy; these women are considered to be at highest risk and should be treated during labor without being screened.

   Collection of a specimen for GBS culture involves swabbing the lower vagina and rectum (through the anal sphincter). These prevention methods have decreased the incidence of early invasive GBS disease (i.e., within the first week of life) from 1.7 cases per 1000 live births in the early 1990s to 0.34 to 0.37 cases per 1000 live births at present.

2. **When should intrapartum antibiotic prophylaxis be given for the prevention of early-onset GBS disease?**

   Intrapartum prophylaxis should be given in all the following women:
   - Previous infant with invasive GBS disease
   - History of GBS bacteriuria in the current pregnancy
   - Positive GBS screening in the current pregnancy
   - Unknown GBS status during labor and any of the following:
     - Gestational age less than 37 weeks
     - Amniotic membrane rupture greater than or equal to 18 hours
     - Intrapartum temperature greater than or equal to 38° C

3. **What antibiotic should be given for GBS prophylaxis?**

   Penicillin G, 5 million units intravenously [IV], followed by 2.5 to 3 million units every 4 hours until delivery, should be given. An acceptable alternative regimen is **ampicillin,** 2 g IV, followed by 1 g IV every 4 hours until delivery.

   If a patient has had an allergic reaction to penicillin that *did not* include anaphylaxis, angioedema, respiratory distress, or urticaria, **cefazolin,** 2 g IV followed by 1 g IV every 8 hours, should be given.

   If a patient has had an allergic reaction to penicillin or a cephalosporin that *did* include anaphylaxis, angioedema, respiratory distress, or urticaria, **vancomycin,** 1 g IV every 12 hours until delivery, should be given unless sensitivity testing was performed and the bacteria isolated is known to be sensitive to *both* clindamycin and erythromycin. In these cases, **clindamycin,** 900 mg IV every 8 hours until delivery, should be given.

4. **What is chorioamnionitis, and how is it treated?**

   Chorioamnionitis is a polymicrobial infection of the amniotic fluid, membranes, or placenta. It is diagnosed clinically, based on the presence of a fever of 38° C or higher and two or more of the following:
   1. Maternal tachycardia (>100 beats/minute)
   2. Fetal tachycardia (>160 beats/minute)
   3. Uterine tenderness
   4. Foul-smelling amniotic fluid
   5. Maternal leukocytosis (>15,000 white blood cells/μL)

Once chorioamnionitis is diagnosed, antipyretics should be given and cooling measures applied. The patient should be promptly started on broad-spectrum antibiotics with coverage for β-lactamase–producing aerobes and anaerobes. A common first-line regimen is ampicillin, 2 g IV every 6 hours, and gentamicin, 1.5 mg/kg every 8 hours or 5 mg/kg every 24 hours. An increased association exists between chorioamnionitis and postcesarean endometritis related to anaerobic colonization, so consideration should be given to adding clindamycin, 900 mg, if an affected patient has a cesarean delivery.

5. **What are risk factors for chorioamnionitis?**
   Risk factors include prolonged labor, prolonged rupture of membranes, internal fetal or uterine monitoring, GBS colonization, and the presence of genital tract infections such as *Chlamydia* infection, gonorrhea, and bacterial vaginosis.

6. **What is postpartum endometritis, and how is it treated?**
   Postpartum endometritis is a polymicrobial infection of the endometrium or myometrium, or both, after delivery of the fetus and placenta or membranes. As with chorioamnionitis, endometritis is diagnosed clinically; signs include a postpartum fever in the presence of lower abdominal pain, uterine tenderness, or purulent or malodorous lochia. Treatment should include broad-spectrum antibiotics, with coverage for both aerobes and anaerobes. A common regimen is clindamycin, 900 mg IV every 8 hours, and gentamicin, 1.5 mg/kg every 8 hours or 5 mg/kg every 24 hours.

7. **What are risk factors for endometritis?**
   Risk factors are similar to those for chorioamnionitis and include prolonged labor, prolonged rupture of membranes, internal fetal and uterine monitoring, and the presence of genital tract infections. Additional risk factors include chorioamnionitis in labor, manual removal of the placenta, and cesarean delivery.

8. **What is the risk for vertical transmission of human immunodeficiency virus (HIV) in pregnancy without treatment, and how can this risk be reduced?**
   In the absence of any intervention, the rate of perinatal HIV transmission is approximately 25%. The single most important interventions are the initiation and continuation of highly active antiretroviral therapy (HAART) regardless of viral load; treatment with zidovudine (former name, azathioprine; AZT) alone can reduce this rate to 8%, and combination therapy reduces it to less than 2%.
   If the viral load is lower than 1000 copies/mL, vaginal delivery can be safely attempted. For viral loads higher than 1000 copies/mL, cesarean delivery is recommended. These latter women should be delivered at 38 weeks and receive preoperative AZT IV for at least 3 hours before delivery. Interventions that increase exposure to contaminated maternal blood and vaginal secretions should be avoided, and these women should not breastfeed.

9. **Who should be tested for HIV infection in pregnancy?**
   All pregnant women should be screened for HIV infection as early as possible. Additionally, rescreening should take place in the third trimester for high-risk patients—women who use illicit drugs, have sexually transmitted infections diagnosed during pregnancy, have multiple sex partners, or live in areas with a high prevalence of HIV.

10. **Who should be tested for hepatitis B in pregnancy?**
    All pregnant women. The rate of vertical transmission during or after delivery in women who are chronic carriers of the hepatitis B virus is high. Additionally, a large proportion of infected infants will become chronic carriers, thus placing them at risk for cirrhosis and hepatocellular carcinoma. The CDC recommends that all pregnant women be screened for the hepatitis B surface antigen and that all newborn infants receive vaccination against hepatitis B. Infants of antigen-positive mothers should be given hepatitis B immune globulin within the first 12 hours of life as well as the vaccine.

11. **Who should be tested for gonorrhea and *Chlamydia* infection in pregnancy?**
    Pregnant women younger than 25 years of age or at increased risk for infection should be screened for gonorrhea and *Chlamydia* infection at the first prenatal visit; many authorities recommend routine testing in all pregnant women. Neonatal chlamydial infection occurs in 60% to 70% of infants passing through an infected birth canal; conjunctivitis develops in 25% to 50% of exposed infants, and chronic pneumonia occurs in 10% to 20%. Before the mandatory use of ophthalmic antibiotic prophylaxis after delivery, gonorrheal transmission at birth caused blindness in many newborn infants **(gonococcal ophthalmia neonatorum).** Gonococci can also cause chorioamnionitis and preterm premature rupture of membranes (PPROM), resulting in a high rate of prematurity and infant morbidity.

12. **How are gonorrhea and *Chlamydia* infection treated during pregnancy?**
During pregnancy, treatment of *Chlamydia* infection consists of a single oral dose of azithromycin (1 g). Treatment of gonorrhea consists of a single oral dose of azithromycin (1 g) and one intramuscular dose of ceftriaxone (250 mg). Sexual partners should be referred for evaluation and treatment at the time of diagnosis, and a test of cure should be obtained 3 to 4 weeks after treatment for either infection. Repeat testing should also be performed 3 months after diagnosis and at 36 weeks of gestation.

13. **How are primary and recurrent herpes simplex virus infections managed during pregnancy?**
If a primary outbreak occurs at the time of vaginal delivery, the risk for neonatal infection is as high as 30% to 60%; in the setting of recurrent lesions, the transmission rate is 3%. If active genital lesions or prodromal symptoms are present at the onset of labor, cesarean delivery should be performed to minimize the risk of vertical transmission. Women with a known history of genital herpes simplex can be treated with suppressive viral therapy (acyclovir or valacyclovir) starting at 36 weeks to reduce the need for cesarean delivery resulting from active lesions.

14. **What are the maternal and fetal risks of parvovirus infection?**
Although parvovirus infection is rare in pregnancy, it can be extremely dangerous for the fetus. Maternal infection manifests as erythema infectiosum or fifth disease, which is characterized by low-grade fever, malaise, arthralgia, and a "slapped cheek" facial appearance. Parvovirus can cross the placenta and infect fetal red blood stem cells, which can result in severe fetal anemia and fetal hydrops. The risk for fetal hydrops is greatest when infection occurs in the first trimester and decreases with advancing gestational age. The infection can be treated with intrauterine fetal blood transfusion. Patients with a recognized infection during pregnancy should be referred to a specialist in high-risk pregnancies for surveillance and further management.

15. **What is the significance of congenital rubella infection, and how can it be prevented?**
Most rubella infections are subclinical. If maternal infection does manifest, it is characterized by a disseminated, nonerythematous, maculopapular rash. The frequency of congenital infection largely depends on gestational age at time of exposure; 50% to 80% of fetuses exposed in the first trimester will develop congenital rubella syndrome, with the most common sequela including hearing impairment, visual impairment, central nervous system defects, and cardiac malformations. Primary prevention has been successful because of vaccination programs, although immunity can wane over time and require repeat vaccination.

16. **How is maternal syphilis infection detected and managed?**
All pregnant women should be screened for syphilis, which is caused by the spirochete *Treponema pallidum*. Screening should be repeated early in the third trimester for high-risk women and at delivery. A nonspecific antibody test (Venereal Disease Research Laboratories [VDRL] or rapid plasma reagin [RPR]) is used for screening, followed by a confirmatory *Treponema*-specific test (fluorescent Treponema antibody absorption test [FTA-ABS] or *Treponema pallidum* particle agglutination assay [TPPA]) in women who screen positive. Penicillin is the only approved treatment for syphilis in pregnancy; if a patient is allergic, desensitization must be performed. Treatment during the second half of pregnancy carries a risk of preterm labor or fetal distress if the Jarisch-Herxheimer reaction occurs (see Chapter 10), and women should be cautioned to seek medical care if they have any symptoms. Nontreponemal test antibody titers can be used to monitor response to treatment, with a fourfold titer change considered clinically significant. These titers should be checked early in the third trimester and at delivery, or on a monthly basis for women at high risk for reinfection or who live in an area of high disease prevalence.

17. **What are the manifestations of congenital syphilis?**
Congenital syphilis can be associated with severe fetal sequelae including stillbirth, hydrops, maculopapular rash, snuffles, splenomegaly, eighth nerve deafness, Hutchinson teeth, mulberry molars, saddle nose, saber shins, and neurologic manifestations.

18. **How is toxoplasmosis transmitted, and what are the potential consequences of infection during pregnancy?**
Toxoplasma is a protozoan that can infect humans through ingestion of infected meat or exposure to infected cat feces; approximately half of all adults in the United States have immunity

because of previous infection. Although testing for immunity in pregnancy is not indicated, precautions should be taken by all pregnant women when handling raw meat or around cat feces. If maternal infection is identified during pregnancy, treatment with antiparasitic therapy can reduce the risk for congenital infection. The risk for fetal injury is greatest when infection occurs in the first trimester, but vertical transmission is most likely to develop when infection occurs in the third trimester. Clinical manifestations of congenital toxoplasmosis include hepatosplenomegaly, purpuric rash, chorioretinitis, periventricular calcifications, ventriculomegaly, and developmental delay.

19. **What are the potential consequences of maternal cytomegalovirus (CMV) infection during pregnancy?**
Most women in the United States have had previous CMV infection; reactivation or infection with a different strain, however, can still occur. Congenital infection is more common with primary infection, but it can occur with recurrent infection. As in toxoplasmosis, the risk for severe fetal injury is greatest in the first trimester, and vertical transmission most likely in the third. Complications include growth restriction, intracranial calcifications, microcephaly, hepatosplenomegaly, sensorineural hearing loss, developmental delay, chorioretinitis, and jaundice. At present, maternal treatment of affected pregnancies with ganciclovir or CMV hyperimmune globulin is still considered experimental.

20. **What are the risks of maternal varicella infection in pregnancy?**
Varicella is caused by the varicella-zoster virus. Many women have immunity from earlier infection or vaccination; nonimmune women of reproductive age should be vaccinated. Maternal infection during pregnancy has an increased risk of morbidity and mortality, and varicella-zoster immunoglobulin or antiviral therapy should be given within 72 to 96 hours of exposure in at-risk women. The absolute risk of congenital varicella infection is very low. The risk for neonatal varicella, however, is much higher; it can occur in infants of women who develop varicella in the period of 5 days before delivery to 2 days after delivery. Neonatal varicella is characterized by mucocutaneous lesions, pneumonia, and encephalitis.

21. **What is listeriosis, and what are the consequences of infection during pregnancy?**
Listeria monocytogenes is a Gram-positive, rod-shaped bacterium commonly found in soil and water. It is resistant to diverse environmental conditions and is able to grow at very low temperatures, thus making it resistant to refrigeration. It can be killed by pasteurization and cooking; however, contamination may occur after factory cooking but before packaging. Common sources that should be avoided in pregnancy are uncooked meats and vegetables, unpasteurized milk and "raw" cheeses, processed meats (hot dogs, deli meat), and smoked seafood.

Listeriosis primarily affects older or immunocompromised adults, pregnant women, and newborns. Maternal infection can be asymptomatic or may cause an influenza-like illness, with fever, chills, fatigue, headache, and myalgia. Vertical transmission can occur even if a pregnant woman shows no signs of illness, and complications include spontaneous abortion, stillbirth, chorioamnionitis, preterm labor, and neonatal septicemia and meningitis. The diagnosis is confirmed on isolation of *Listeria monocytogenes* from a normally sterile source such as blood, amniotic fluid, or the placenta. Treatment is generally with ampicillin and gentamicin and is continued for at least 14 days.

KEY POINTS: INFECTIONS

1. Pregnant women should be screened for GBS infection between 35 and 37 weeks of gestation unless they have tested positive earlier in the pregnancy, have GBS bacteriuria, or have a history of an infant affected by GBS.
2. Chorioamnionitis and endometritis are polymicrobial and should be treated with broad-spectrum antibiotics.
3. All pregnant women should be screened for HIV infection, syphilis, and hepatitis B virus infection.
4. In women with HIV infection, treatment with HAART significantly reduces vertical transmission rates.
5. The risk of listeriosis in pregnancy can be minimized by avoiding uncooked meats and vegetables, unpasteurized milk and "raw" cheeses, processed meats, and smoked seafood.

BIBLIOGRAPHY

1. American College of Obstetricians and Gynecologists. Perinatal viral and parasitic infections. ACOG practice bulletin no. 20. Washington, DC: American College of Obstetricians and Gynecologists; 2000.
2. American College of Obstetricians and Gynecologists. Scheduled cesarean delivery and the prevention of vertical transmission of HIV infection. ACOG committee opinion no. 234. Washington, DC: American College of Obstetricians and Gynecologists; 2000.
3. American College of Obstetricians and Gynecologists. Management of herpes in pregnancy. ACOG practice bulletin no. 82. Washington, DC: American College of Obstetricians and Gynecologists; 2007.
4. American College of Obstetricians and Gynecologists. Prevention of early-onset group B streptococcal infection in newborns. ACOG committee opinion no. 485. Washington, DC: American College of Obstetricians and Gynecologists; 2011.
5. American College of Obstetricians and Gynecologists. Use of prophylactic antibiotics in labor and delivery. ACOG practice bulletin no. 120. Washington, DC: American College of Obstetricians and Gynecologists; 2011.
6. Centers for Disease Control and Prevention. Prevention of perinatal group B streptococcal disease. *MMWR Recomm Rep.* 2010;59:1–36.
7. Centers for Disease Control and Prevention. Listeria (listeriosis). Available at www.cdc.gov/listeria.
8. Centers for Disease Control and Prevention. Sexually transmitted diseases treatment guidelines, 2015. *MMWR Recomm Rep.* 2015;64:1–137.
9. Creasy RK, Resnik RI, Iams JD, Lockwood CJ, Moore TR, eds. *Creasy and Resnik's Maternal-Fetal Medicine: Principles and Practice.* 6th ed. Philadelphia: Saunders; 2009.
10. Mitra AG, Whitten MK, Laurent SL, et al. A randomized prospective study comparing once daily gentamicin versus thrice daily gentamicin in the treatment of puerperal infection. *Am J Obstet Gynecol.* 1997;177:786–792.
11. Nigro G, Adler SP, La Torre R, et al. Passive immunization during pregnancy for congenital cytomegalovirus infection. *N Engl J Med.* 2005;353:1350–1362.
12. Panel on Treatment of HIV-1–Infected Women and Prevention of Perinatal Transmission. Recommendations for Use of Antiretroviral Drugs in Pregnant HIV-1–Infected Women for Maternal Health and Interventions to Reduce Perinatal HIV Transmission in the United States. Available at http://aidsinfo.nih.gov/contentfiles/lvguidelines/perinatalgl.pdf.
13. Silk BJ, Date KA, Jackson KA, et al. Invasive listeriosis in the Foodborne Diseases Active Surveillance Network (FoodNet), 2004-2009: further targeted prevention needed for higher-risk groups. *Clin Infect Dis.* 2012;54 (Suppl 5):S396–S404.
14. Tita AT, William AW. Diagnosis and management of clinical chorioamnionitis. *Clin Perinatol.* 2010;37:339–354.
15. Von Kaisenberg CS, Jonat W. Fetal parvovirus B19 infection. *Ultrasound Obstet Gynecol.* 2001;18:280–288.

CHAPTER 56

SURGERY DURING PREGNANCY

Ella Speichinger, MD

1. **How often are surgical procedures performed in pregnancy?**
   Approximately 1.5% to 2% of pregnant women undergo nonobstetric surgical procedures.

2. **What is the best time to perform surgical procedures in pregnancy?**
   The second trimester is the preferred time for nonurgent surgical procedures because the risk of miscarriage is decreased and few concerns exist regarding preterm labor. However, surgical treatment should not be delayed if systemic infection or severe disease is suspected; these are associated with higher risks to both mother and fetus.

3. **What are the recommendations for venous thromboembolism (VTE) prophylaxis?**
   Although pregnancy increases the risk of VTE, no firm recommendation is available regarding the preferred prophylaxis for pregnant patients undergoing surgical procedures; both mechanical and pharmacologic methods have been shown to reduce the incidence of VTE. Pneumatic compression devices have few contraindications and should be considered for all pregnant women undergoing surgical intervention. Pharmacologic thromboprophylaxis should be weighed against the patient's individual risk of thrombosis versus the risk of perioperative bleeding.

4. **What are the risks of general anesthesia in pregnancy?**
   All general anesthetics cross the placenta but are not considered teratogenic. Physiologic changes in pregnancy such as increased oropharyngeal swelling, decreased glottis opening, and delayed gastric emptying can complicate intubation and ventilation. This situation can lead to aspiration, failed intubation and subsequent maternal and fetal hypoxia. Regional anesthesia minimizes fetal exposure but may not be appropriate for all procedures. For more information on this topic, see Chapter 64.

5. **What pregnancy-specific intraoperative measures should take place during surgical procedures?**
   To decrease compression of the inferior vena cava and optimize uterine perfusion, care should be taken to place the patient in a lateral leftward tilt. Maternal oxygen and fluid status should be closely monitored, and continuous fetal monitoring should be employed if the fetus is viable and doing so will not interfere with the procedure. If the procedure prevents continuous fetal monitoring of a viable fetus, a nonstress test should be performed immediately preoperatively and postoperatively. For more information on the nonstress test, see Chapter 40. For pregnancies that are not yet viable, obtaining fetal heart tones immediately before and after the surgical procedure is generally sufficient.

6. **Are perioperative prophylactic tocolytics recommended?**
   Although many providers use them, no evidence supports the use of perioperative tocolytics. Premature labor appears to be uncommon unless visceral perforation or peritonitis is present or significant uterine manipulation occurs.

7. **Is laparoscopy safe in pregnancy?**
   Laparoscopy is considered safe for most procedures in the first and second trimester. Advantages are decreased postoperative pain and recovery time, as well as the potential of less uterine manipulation. Possible drawbacks include the risk of injury to the gravid uterus, decreased surgical exposure because of the enlarged uterus, and excessive intraabdominal pressure causing increased carbon dioxide absorption and decreased uterine blood flow.

8. **What are the most common surgical diseases in pregnancy?**
   - Appendicitis
   - Cholecystitis
   - Intestinal obstruction
   - Adnexal torsion
   - Trauma

- Cervical disease
- Breast disease

9. **Is appendicitis more common in pregnancy?**
No. However, the rate of rupture in pregnancy is two to three times more common because of delays in both diagnosis and making the decision to operate.

10. **What makes the diagnosis of appendicitis in pregnancy difficult?**
Signs and symptoms of pregnancy overlap with those of appendicitis, namely nausea, anorexia, and mild leukocytosis. Although the appendix is usually found near its normal location, the growing uterus displaces the anterior peritoneum and leads to less obvious peritoneal signs.

11. **What other conditions are in the differential diagnosis of appendicitis?**
- Gastrointestinal conditions: gastroenteritis, small bowel obstruction, diverticulitis, pancreatitis, cancer
- Gynecologic conditions: ruptured corpus luteum cyst, adnexal torsion, degenerating fibroids, ectopic pregnancy, pelvic inflammatory disease
- Obstetric conditions: placental abruption, early labor, round ligament pain, chorioamnionitis

12. **Why are pregnant women more likely to suffer from cholecystitis?**
Pregnant women share many of the risk factors normally associated with cholecystitis: female sex, fertility, and obesity. Both progesterone and estrogen increase bile lithogenicity, and progesterone decreases gallbladder contractility.

13. **What signs and symptoms of cholecystitis overlap with pregnancy?**
Both pregnant women and patients with cholecystitis can present with anorexia, nausea, vomiting, dyspepsia, and intolerance of fatty foods.

14. **What is the best imaging test to detect gallstones?**
The diagnostic accuracy of ultrasound for detecting gallstones is 95%, thus making it the most accurate and safest choice.

15. **How should patients with gallbladder disease be treated?**
The initial management of symptomatic cholelithiasis and cholecystitis in pregnancy is nonoperative. Patients should be placed on bowel rest, and intravenous hydration and analgesics should be given. Antibiotics should be administered if no improvement is seen within 12 to 24 hours or if systemic symptoms develop. Most acute symptoms resolve with this treatment.
   Surgical intervention is indicated if symptoms fail to improve with medical management, for recurrent episodes of biliary colic, and for complications such as recurrent cholecystitis, choledocholithiasis, and gallstone pancreatitis. Surgical treatment has become more common because recurrence rates for symptomatic biliary disease during pregnancy are high, especially in the second trimester.
   Endoscopic retrograde cholangiopancreatography (ERCP) may be an alternative for selected patients with common bile duct stones.

16. **How do pregnant patients with acute intestinal obstruction present, and when is it most likely to occur?**
Symptoms are similar to those seen in nonpregnant patients: abdominal pain, vomiting, and obstipation. Acute intestinal obstruction occurs most commonly in the third trimester.

17. **What are the most common causes of acute intestinal obstruction in pregnancy?**
Adhesions (60%) and volvulus (25%), followed by intussusception, hernia, and neoplasms.

18. **How is acute intestinal obstruction managed in pregnancy?**
The management is the same as for nonpregnant patients. The core principles are bowel decompression, intravenous hydration, correction of electrolyte imbalances, and timely surgical intervention when indicated.

19. **What two rare conditions manifest with left upper quadrant pain and occur more frequently during pregnancy?**
   1. **Splenic rupture:** The hypervolemia and relative anemia associated with pregnancy contribute to hypersplenism, which increases the risk for spontaneous rupture.
   2. **Splenic artery aneurysm rupture:** Twenty-five percent of cases of this rare but catastrophic event occur in pregnant women. Diseased vessels are further compromised by pregnancy-induced hypersplenism and moderate displacement of the spleen by the gravid uterus. Immediate laparotomy is warranted, and the mortality rate is high.

20. Which two surgical conditions are more likely to occur during periods of rapid change in uterine size (second trimester and postpartum period)?
    1. **Adnexal torsion:** The presence of an adnexal mass increases this risk. Cystectomy by laparoscopy or laparotomy is often necessary.
    2. **Intestinal obstruction:** Adhesions (usually related to earlier surgical procedures) may incarcerate loops of bowel as the intraabdominal contents shift.

21. What are the most common causes of an adnexal mass in pregnancy?
    Most adnexal masses are functional or corpus luteum cysts and spontaneously resolve by 16 weeks, unlike pathologic ovarian neoplasms. (Of the masses that persist, 1% to 10% will be malignant.) The most common ovarian neoplasms during pregnancy are benign cystic teratomas and serous or mucinous cystadenomas.

22. When should an adnexal mass be managed surgically during pregnancy?
    Surgical intervention is advised if concern exists for rupture, torsion, or malignancy. It is estimated that only approximately 2% of masses rupture during pregnancy, and torsion occurs in 0% to 15% of cases.

23. What is the incidence of cancer in pregnancy?
    The incidence of cancer in pregnancy is approximately 1 in 1000. The most common malignant diseases diagnosed during pregnancy are cervical cancer (26%), breast cancer (26%), leukemia (15%), lymphoma (10%), and malignant melanoma (8%).

24. Can chemotherapy be used during pregnancy?
    Chemotherapy is avoided (if possible) during the first trimester because of the risks of miscarriage and fetal malformations. When it is used during the second and third trimesters, higher rates of abnormal fetal growth and preterm delivery are observed for many agents.

25. How is cervical cancer diagnosed in pregnancy?
    The diagnosis of cervical cancer is usually made on the basis of a cervical biopsy after an abnormal Papanicolaou (Pap) smear or visualization of a mass. Pregnancy is not a contraindication to colposcopy, although endocervical curettage is avoided.

26. How is cervical cancer managed in pregnancy?
    Management is dictated by the stage of the cancer, the gestational age, and the patient's desires regarding the pregnancy. The fetus is not affected by the maternal disease process but may suffer morbidity from iatrogenic preterm delivery. Pregnancy does not appear to affect the prognosis for women with cervical cancer, and cisplatin use in the second and third trimesters has not been found to be associated with increased risk to the fetus.

27. How is breast cancer diagnosed and managed during pregnancy?
    Breast cancer is diagnosed on biopsy of a suspicious mass. In general, treatment during pregnancy is affected by the need to avoid ionizing radiation or chemotherapy in the first trimester. A multidisciplinary team including high-risk pregnancy specialists and oncologists is required, and management should be tailored to each specific case.

28. What are the risks of imaging studies to a pregnancy?
    - **Ionizing radiation** is both a teratogen and a carcinogen, although the risk of structural or developmental problems in fetuses at doses lower than 5 cGy does not appear to be increased (Table 56-1). The most common malformations seen are microcephaly, intrauterine growth restriction, and eye abnormalities. Fetal exposure to 2 to 5 cGy is estimated to increase the relative risk for fatal childhood cancer by a factor of 1.5 to 2, but the absolute risk is still very low (2 in 2000 exposures at this level).
    - **Magnetic resonance imaging (MRI):** Most studies show no harm from MRI during pregnancy, although theoretic concerns for teratogenesis and acoustic damage exist. The safety of both iodine and gadolinium contrast agents is unclear; they should be avoided unless information obtained with their use would be vital to management decisions.
    - **Ultrasound** is routinely used in pregnancy. It should be considered as the first imaging modality in a pregnant patient before using MRI or ionizing radiation.

Table 56-1. Fetal Radiation Exposure With Common Imaging Modalities

PROCEDURE	FETAL EXPOSURE (CGY OR RAD)
Chest radiograph (2 views)	$2\text{-}7 \times 10^{-5}$
Mammogram (4 views)	$7\text{-}20 \times 10^{-3}$
Abdominal radiograph (1 view)	$1\text{-}2 \times 10^{-3}$
Ventilation-perfusion scan	0.01-0.04
Helical CT scan chest	0.1-0.3
CT scan abdomen	1.7-3.5
CT scan pelvis	1-4.6

CT, Computed tomography.

KEY POINTS: SURGERY DURING PREGNANCY

1. The second trimester is the preferred time for nonurgent surgical procedures.
2. Laparoscopy is considered safe for most procedures in the first and second trimester.
3. The rate of appendiceal rupture in pregnancy is two to three times more common because of delays in both diagnosis and making the decision to operate.
4. Surgical treatment of an adnexal mass is advised if concern exists for rupture, torsion, or malignancy.
5. The most common malignant diseases diagnosed during pregnancy are cervical cancer and breast cancer.

BIBLIOGRAPHY

1. American College of Obstetricians and Gynecologists. Nonobstetric surgery during pregnancy. ACOG committee opinion no. 474. *Obstet Gynecol.* 2011;117:420–421.
2. Cheek TG, Baird E. Anesthesia for nonobstetric surgery: maternal and fetal considerations. *Clin Obstet Gynecol.* 2009;52:535–545.
3. Erekson EA, Brousseau EC, Dick-Biascoechea MA, Ciarleglio MM, Lockwood CJ, Pettker CM. Maternal postoperative complications after nonobstetric antenatal surgery. *J Matern Fetal Neonatal Med.* 2012;25:2639–2644.
4. Koren G, Carey N, Gagnon R, Maxwell C, Nulman I, Senikas V. Cancer chemotherapy and pregnancy. *J Obstet Gynaecol Can.* 2013;35:263–280.
5. Kuczkowski KM. Nonobstetric surgery during pregnancy: what are the risks of anesthesia? *Obstet Gynecol Surv.* 2004;59:52–56.
6. Longo SA, Moore RC, Canzoneri BJ, Robichaux A. Gastrointestinal conditions during pregnancy. *Clin Colon Rectal Surg.* 2010;23:80–89.
7. McGrath SE, Ring A. Chemotherapy for breast cancer in pregnancy: evidence and guidance for oncologists. *Ther Adv Med Oncol.* 2011;3:73–83.
8. Niemann T, Nicolas G, Roser HW, Müller-Brand J, Bongartz G. Imaging for suspected pulmonary embolism in pregnancy: what about the fetal dose? A comprehensive review of the literature. *Insights Imaging.* 2010;1:361–372.
9. Schmeler KM, Mayo-Smith WW, Peipert JF, Weitzen S, Manuel MD, Gordinier ME. Adnexal masses in pregnancy: surgery compared with observation. *Obstet Gynecol.* 2005;105:1098–1103.
10. Walsh CA, Tang T, Walsh SR. Laparoscopic versus open appendectomy in pregnancy: a systematic review. *Int J Surg.* 2008;6:339–344.

TRAUMA IN PREGNANCY

Stacy M. Yadava, MD

CHAPTER 57

1. **What is the frequency of trauma in pregnancy, and why is it significant?**
   Trauma, either accidental or intentional (e.g., suicide, homicide, or domestic violence), is a leading cause of death in women of reproductive age. It complicates approximately 1 in every 12 pregnancies and is the leading cause of nonobstetric maternal death.

2. **What are the three most common forms of trauma in pregnancy in industrialized nations?**
   1. Motor vehicle accidents
   2. Interpersonal or domestic violence
   3. Falls

3. **What are risk factors for trauma in pregnancy?**
   - Drug and alcohol use
   - Younger maternal age
   - History of domestic violence

4. **What is the risk of fetal loss with maternal trauma?**
   Life-threatening trauma (e.g., shock, head injury with coma, emergency laparotomy for maternal indications) is associated with a 40% to 50% fetal loss rate. For less severe injuries, the rate ranges from 1% to 5%. Because minor trauma is much more common, it is associated with a higher number of pregnancy losses overall.

5. **How is the risk to the fetus different with blunt trauma compared with penetrating trauma?**
   - **Blunt trauma:** Shearing forces place the fetus at risk for placental abruption, direct fetal injury, uterine rupture, and maternal shock or death.
   - **Penetrating trauma** can cause direct fetal injury or damage to the umbilical cord or placenta. Overall, maternal loss of life is the most frequent cause of fetal death.

6. **How does gestational age affect fetal risk?**
   In pregnancies of less than 13 weeks of gestation, fetal or uterine injury is rare because of the protection afforded by the bony pelvis. As the uterus enlarges, the risk of fetal injury increases. At gestational ages compatible with extrauterine survival, immediate delivery may be warranted if evidence of fetal compromise is present.

7. **Can pregnancy affect maternal outcomes in penetrating abdominal trauma?**
   In some situations, yes. Maternal outcome is overall improved by the shielding effect of the uterus, which absorbs most of the projectile energy in gunshot wounds and can prevent penetrating wounds from reaching vital organs. However, abdominal stab wounds may result in more complex bowel injury than in nonpregnant woman because of the cephalad displacement of bowel by the uterus. It is important to be aware that penetrating injury to the uterus can cause severe maternal hemorrhage.

8. **Does pregnancy alter the initial evaluation of a trauma patient?**
   No. The standard protocol for assessment and stabilization should be followed (airway, breathing, circulation [ABCs]), and the initial focus should be on maternal stabilization. If possible, joint evaluation by trauma and obstetric teams should be performed to expedite management decisions.

9. **Does pregnancy alter radiologic imaging in a trauma patient?**
   No. Any imaging necessary for optimal treatment of the mother should be performed, with shielding of the fetus whenever possible. Ultrasound imaging is preferred in pregnant patients because it is safe for the fetus.

10. **What are the methods used to diagnose intraperitoneal hemorrhage in pregnant patients?**

    The FAST scan (Focused Assessment with Sonography for Trauma) can be performed in pregnancy and is 80% sensitive and 100% specific for detecting intraperitoneal hemorrhage. If a FAST scan result is nondiagnostic, diagnostic peritoneal lavage (DPL) can be considered. Although controversial, DPL has a 98% sensitivity and should be performed using an open, periumbilical technique to avoid uterine injury. If a patient is relatively stable, computed tomography (CT) scan is another option. It is less invasive, can provide injury-specific data, and is superior for the evaluation of retroperitoneal injuries. However, it involves radiation and has a lower sensitivity than DPL.

11. **What physiologic changes associated with pregnancy can complicate the diagnosis of serious injury or affect the pathophysiologic response of the mother?**

    Table 57-1 provides an overview of the effect of physiologic changes of pregnancy on trauma patients.

Table 57-1. Effect of Physiologic Changes of Pregnancy on Trauma Patients

PARAMETER	ADAPTATION	IMPACT ON TRAUMA PATIENT
Plasma volume	50% increase	Relative resistance to limited blood loss
RBC mass	30% increase	Dilutional anemia (plasma volume increase >RBC mass increase)
Cardiac output	30%-50% increase	Relative resistance to limited blood loss
Heart rate	10-15 beat increase	May be interpreted as hypovolemia
Blood pressure	Fall in second trimester	May be interpreted as hypovolemia
Coagulation factors	Increased	Increased risk of deep vein thrombosis
Uteroplacental blood flow	20%-30% shunt	Uterine injury may predispose to increased blood loss
Uterine size	Dramatic increase	Compression of vena cava or aorta (supine hypotension); shifting of abdominal contents
Minute ventilation	25% increase	Decreased $Paco_2$; decreased buffering capacity
Functional residual capacity	Decreased	Increased propensity for atelectasis and hypoxemia
Gastric emptying	Slowed	Increased risk of aspiration
Bladder	Displaced cephalad in second and third trimesters	Increased risk of bladder injury in abdominal trauma

$Paco_2$, Arterial partial pressure of carbon dioxide; *RBC*, red blood cell.

12. **In addition to the standard evaluation, what additional facts must be established for a pregnant trauma patient?**
    - Estimated gestational age
    - Fetal status (heart rate) by ultrasound or external fetal monitoring
    - Assessment for labor, rupture of membranes, placental abruption

13. **What additional laboratory studies should be obtained from a pregnant trauma patient?**

    Blood type and Kleihauer-Betke (KB) test. The KB test screens for fetal cells in the maternal circulation, which indicates fetal-maternal hemorrhage from the placental bed. Coagulation studies (international normalized ratio [INR], fibrinogen) should also be obtained if placental abruption is suspected.

    No evidence indicates that testing can predict immediate adverse sequelae (severe fetal anemia, cardiac arrhythmias, and death) of hemorrhage. However, knowledge of a pregnant patient's Rh status is required because Rh immune globulin (RhoGAM) should be given to prevent alloimmunization in Rh-negative women. In cases of fetal-maternal hemorrhage, the mean estimated blood volume of injected fetal whole blood is less than 15 mL, and more than 90% of cases involve less than 30 mL.

A single dose (300 μg or one ampule) of Rh immune globulin is sufficient for these volumes. If the KB test indicates more than 30 mL of fetal blood, additional Rh immune globulin is required.

Rh immune globulin appears to prevent alloimmunization effectively when it is administered within 72 hours.

14. **How long does a pregnant patient need to be monitored to rule out placental abruption?**
After major trauma, the recommended minimum time of posttrauma monitoring is 4 to 6 hours. Monitoring should be continued and further evaluation performed in patients with uterine contractions, nonreassuring fetal test results, vaginal bleeding, uterine tenderness, serious maternal injury, or signs of amniotic rupture. Because abruption usually becomes apparent shortly after injury, monitoring should be initiated as soon as the woman is stabilized.

In the case of minor trauma with maternal injury limited to cuts and bruises, limited fetal assessment can be performed.

15. **What is the most sensitive predictor of placental abruption?**
Regular contractions on tocometry.

16. **How does hypovolemic shock affect uterine blood flow?**
The fetus is treated as an expendable peripheral organ; blood is preferentially shunted to the maternal brain and heart.

17. **What steps can be taken to increase uterine perfusion?**
- **Left uterine displacement** can relieve compression of the inferior vena cava (IVC) by the uterus and alleviate maternal hypotension, and it is achieved by tilting the patient or manual displacement (if the patient must remain supine).
- **Oxygen** is administered to the mother.
- **Intravenous hydration:** Expansion of intravascular volume increases uteroplacental perfusion.

18. **What must be considered with pelvic fracture during pregnancy?**
Pelvic fracture is associated with a high rate of fetal injury and mortality, especially at later gestational ages, when the fetal head is engaged in the pelvis. Vaginal delivery is not contraindicated in women with a history of pelvic fracture, but these patients should be evaluated on an individual basis.

19. **How does pregnancy affect the outcome of burn victims?**
Pregnancy does not appear to have an impact on maternal outcome. Fetal prognosis is related to the extent of the burns and the development of maternal complications such as hypoxia, hypotension, and sepsis. At later gestational ages, delivery should be considered before the development of complications.

20. **What is the fetal risk following maternal electrical injuries?**
The potential injury to the fetus increases directly with the severity of the electrical injury, with severe electrical injury carrying up to a 70% fetal mortality rate. Other potential effects other than fetal death include placental abruption, fetal cardiac arrhythmias, burns, and fetal end-organ damage such as nervous system injury can also occur. The more common minor electrical injuries (e.g., sustained from batteries or from non-industrial power sources) typically do not pose a major risk to the fetus.

21. **Does pregnancy change the indications for laparotomy after blunt trauma?**
Yes, by adding additional indications: uterine rupture, massive placental abruption, and fetal distress (in cases with a viable fetus).

Standard indications remain: overt peritonitis, massive hemoperitoneum, and significant injury to a hollow viscus or major solid organ noted on imaging.

22. **Does pregnancy change the management of stab wounds?**
This is controversial. The standard management protocol limits laparotomy to patients with violation of the peritoneum or positive results of FAST or DPL. In pregnant trauma patients, some experts advocate further restriction if the injury overlies the uterus because all other organs except the bladder are protected. Observation may be appropriate if fetal test results are reassuring and cystoscopic findings are normal.

23. **In what circumstances is cesarean delivery indicated during laparotomy?**
- Mechanical obstruction by the gravid uterus preventing surgical exposure
- Unstable thoracolumbar spinal injury

- A risk of potential injury to the fetus by continuing the pregnancy that is believed to exceed the risks of prematurity
- Persistent maternal shock or imminent maternal death

Although cesarean delivery adds approximately 500 mL to total blood loss, evacuation of the uterus can increase cardiac output by 60% to 80% and optimize maternal outcome.

24. **Is intrauterine fetal demise an indication for cesarean delivery?**
No. Cesarean delivery for this indication alone incurs increased risk to the mother and may lead to complications that could otherwise have been avoided (e.g., coagulopathy, infection, surgical complications).

25. **In what circumstances is hysterectomy indicated?**
- Severe penetrating injury to the uterus that cannot be repaired
- Damage to uterine vessels or lacerations or rupture of the uterus that cannot be repaired
- Severe coagulopathy causing massive uterine hemorrhage (can occur in placental abruption)

26. **What are the indications for perimortem cesarean delivery?**
Although no clear guidelines are available, cesarean delivery should be considered after 4 minutes of maternal cardiopulmonary arrest for the highest likelihood of fetal and maternal survival. (Delivery of the fetus can improve maternal status by returning blood to the central circulation.) Neurologically intact fetal survival is highly unlikely if more than 15 to 20 minutes have elapsed since the loss of maternal vital signs.
Left uterine displacement should be maintained during cardiopulmonary resuscitation (CPR).

27. **How does trauma affect pregnancy outcome in women who are successfully stabilized?**
These women are at increased risk of premature birth because of labor or premature rupture of membranes.

28. **When and how should pregnant women wear seat belts?**
Pregnant women should position the lap belt low under the abdomen and over both anterior superior iliac spines and the pubic symphysis. The shoulder harness should be positioned diagonally between the breasts. This configuration has been shown to reduce amount of pressure transferred to the uterus in a collision.

KEY POINTS: TRAUMA IN PREGNANCY

1. Trauma is the leading cause of death in women of reproductive age.
2. Initial evaluation of a pregnant trauma patient is the same as in nonpregnant women; stabilize mother with ABCs before evaluating the fetus.
3. Women who are Rh-negative need RhoGAM when abdominal trauma has occurred.
4. The recommended minimum time of fetal monitoring is 4 to 6 hours.
5. Perimortem cesarean delivery should be considered after 4 minutes of CPR in a woman with a pregnancy that is believed to be viable.
6. Blunt trauma may cause placental abruption, whereas penetrating trauma may directly injure the fetus, placenta, or umbilical cord.

BIBLIOGRAPHY

1. Barraco RD, Chiu WC, Clancy TV, et al. Practice management guidelines for the diagnosis and management of injury in the pregnant patient: the EAST Practice Management Guidelines Work Group. *J Trauma.* 2010;69:211–214.
2. Brown HL. Trauma in pregnancy. *Obstet Gynecol.* 2009;114:147–160.
3. Chames MC, Pearlman MD. Trauma during pregnancy: outcomes and clinical management. *Clin Obstet Gynecol.* 2008;51:398–408.
4. Hill CC, Pickinpaugh J. Trauma and surgical emergencies in the obstetric patient. *Surg Clin North Am.* 2008;88: 421–440.
5. Mendez-Figueroa H, Dahlke JD, Vrees RA, Rouse DJ. Trauma in pregnancy: an updated systematic review. *Am J Obstet Gynecol.* 2013;209:1–10.
6. Plante LA, Lerner B. Trauma. In: Berghella V, ed. *Maternal-Fetal Evidence Based Guidelines.* 2nd ed. New York: Informa Healthcare; 2012.

CHAPTER 58

ALCOHOL AND DRUG ABUSE DURING PREGNANCY

Tina A. Nguyen, MD

1. **How are the types of use, abuse, and dependence defined?**
   - Use: sporadic consumption of alcohol or drugs with no adverse consequences
   - Abuse: frequency of consumption varies, some adverse consequences
   - Physical dependence: a state of adaption that is manifested by a substance class-specific withdrawal syndrome
   - Psychological dependence: a subjective sense of a need for a specific psychoactive substance
   - Addiction: a primary, chronic disease of brain reward, motivation, memory, and related circuitry. It involves the pathologic pursuit of reward and relief through substance abuse and is characterized by an inability to abstain from use consistently and to control behavior and cravings, as well as dysfunctional emotional responses and diminished recognition of problems with behaviors and interpersonal relationships.

2. **Why is alcohol use during pregnancy of clinical importance?**
   Maternal alcohol consumption during pregnancy is one of the most common preventable causes of birth defects and childhood disabilities. Varying levels of fetal abnormalities can occur from fetal alcohol exposure. These appear in a spectrum of alcohol-related disabling conditions called fetal alcohol spectrum disorders (FASDs).
   Alcohol is the most commonly abused substance during pregnancy.

3. **What are some common statistics related to alcohol use in pregnancy?**
   One in 13 (7.6%) of known pregnant women report alcohol consumption within the past 30 days. One in 71 (1.4%) of known pregnant women report binge drinking within the past 30 days. Among pregnant women, the highest estimates of reported alcohol use are among those who are:
   - Between 35 and 44 years of age (14.3%)
   - White (8.3%)
   - College graduates (10.0%)
   - Employed (9.6%)

4. **What is a safe amount of alcohol to consume during pregnancy?**
   No safe level of alcohol consumption in pregnancy has been identified. The safest thing to do is not to drink alcohol at all.

5. **Does a dose-response relationship exist between alcohol consumption and pregnancy outcome?**
   Not a direct one; no threshold exists below which FASDs do not occur. Among children of women who consume 5 ounces of alcohol daily, approximately one third of the infants have the most severe form of the FASDs, fetal alcohol syndrome (FAS). Another one third shows some prenatal toxic effects, and the remaining one third appears to be normal. When 1 to 2 ounces of alcohol are consumed daily, approximately 10% of children may exhibit characteristics of FAS. Even smaller amounts of alcohol have been associated with FASDs. Alcohol consumption within the social drinking range has been associated with persistent effects on intelligence quotient (IQ) and learning problems in young children who have no apparent anatomic abnormalities.

6. **What is a standard "drink"?**
   One standard drink is equal to 15 mL of pure ethanol.
   - Beer or wine cooler: 12 ounces
   - Table wine: 5 ounces (25-ounce bottle = five drinks)
   - Malt liquor: 8 to 9 ounces (12-ounce can = 1.5 drink)
   - 80-proof spirits: 1.5 ounce (a mixed drink may contain one to three or more drinks)

7. What are some tools to screen for alcohol abuse in pregnancy?
   - Four Ps
     - Did any of your **parents** have problems with drug or alcohol use?
     - Did any of your **peers (friends)** have problems with drug or alcohol use?
     - Does your **partner** have problems with drug or alcohol use?
     - Before you were pregnant did you have **past** problems with drug or alcohol use?
   - CRAFFT
     - Have you ridden in a **car** driven by someone (including yourself) who was intoxicated?
     - Do you use drugs or alcohol to **relax**, feel better about yourself, or fit in?
     - Do you ever **forget** things you did while using alcohol or drugs?
     - Do your **family or friends** tell you that you should cut down?
     - Have you ever gotten into **trouble** while using alcohol or drugs?
   - TACE (2+ points = positive screen for high-risk drinking)
     - **T**olerance: How many drinks does it take to make you feel high? (>2 drinks = 2 points)
     - **A**nnoyed: Have people annoyed you by criticizing your drinking? (yes = 1 point)
     - **C**ut down: Have you felt that you need to cut down on your drinking? (yes = 1 point)
     - **E**ye opener: Have you ever had a drink first thing in the morning? (yes = 1 point)

8. What are the features of FASDs?
   - Abnormal facial features, such as a smooth ridge between the nose and upper lip (this ridge is called the philtrum)
   - Small head size
   - Shorter than average height
   - Low body weight
   - Poor coordination
   - Hyperactive behavior
   - Difficulty with attention
   - Poor memory
   - Difficulty in school (especially with math)
   - Learning disabilities
   - Speech and language delays
   - Intellectual disability or low IQ
   - Poor reasoning and judgment skills
   - Sleep and sucking problems as a baby
   - Vision or hearing problems
   - Problems with the heart, kidney, or bones

9. How are the FASDs further classified?
   Different terms are used to describe the FASDs, depending on the type of symptoms:
   - **FAS:** This represents the most severe end of the FASD spectrum. People with FAS may have abnormal facial features, growth problems, and central nervous system (CNS) problems. People with FAS can have problems with learning, memory, attention span, communication, vision, or hearing. They may have a mix of these problems. People with FAS often have a difficult time in school and trouble getting along with others. Fetal death is the most extreme outcome.
   - **Alcohol-related neurodevelopmental disorder (ARND):** People with ARND may have intellectual disabilities and problems with behavior and learning. They may do poorly in school and have difficulties with math, memory, attention, and judgment, as well as poor impulse control.
   - **Alcohol-related birth defects (ARBDs):** People with ARBDs may have problems with the heart, kidneys, or bones or with hearing. They may have a mix of these problems.

10. Does alcohol cross the placenta?
    Yes. Fetal blood alcohol levels approximate those of the mother.

11. Should an alcoholic pregnant woman stop drinking on her own?
    No. A pregnant woman who is physically dependent on alcohol requires medically supervised detoxification. The risk of preterm labor is significantly increased with alcohol withdrawal.

12. **What is the timing for the signs and symptoms of alcohol withdrawal to appear in a pregnant woman?**
Withdrawal symptoms begin when blood alcohol concentrations decline sharply after cessation or reduction, usually within 4 to 12 hours. However, it is possible for symptoms to develop even a few days after abstinence. Untreated withdrawal symptoms reach their peak intensity at 48 hours and can persist for up to 3 to 6 months at low levels. Signs and symptoms depend on the severity of previous alcohol dependence and the general condition of the patient and include tremulousness, anxiety, increased heart rate, increased blood pressure, sweating, nausea, hyperreflexia, and insomnia.

13. **Once a pregnancy is recognized, does decreasing alcohol intake affect the rate of fetal abnormalities?**
Alcohol crosses the placenta and the fetal blood-brain barrier freely. It is thought that the effects are caused by the direct toxicity of both alcohol and its metabolites. Stopping or slowing down consumption of alcohol once pregnancy is diagnosed may lead to a decrease in anomaly rates, although clinical studies are needed to evaluate this accurately.

14. **True or false: Cocaine use in pregnancy is increasing.**
True. The rise in the use of cocaine in the pregnant population corresponds to the rise in the general population. The availability of inexpensive crack cocaine is a major reason for this increase.

15. **How does cocaine affect a pregnant patient?**
Cocaine prevents reuptake of norepinephrine and dopamine. The increase in norepinephrine causes vasoconstriction, tachycardia, and rapid rise in maternal and fetal arterial pressure. Uterine and placental blood flow decreases, with resultant fetal tachycardia and increased fetal oxygen consumption. Uterine contractility also increases. *Cocaine readily crosses the placenta and the fetal blood-brain barrier.*

16. **What risks are associated with cocaine use during pregnancy?**
Obstetric risks associated with cocaine use include irregularities in placental blood flow, placental abruption, and premature labor and delivery. Use of cocaine in the third trimester increases the risk of abruption. Abruption and stillbirth have been documented in 8% of cocaine abusers. Cocaine use in the first trimester is associated with a spontaneous abortion rate of 40%.

   In terms of fetal development, reported risks include low birth weight, mild neurodysfunction, transient electroencephalographic abnormalities, intrauterine growth restriction, increased risk of intrauterine fetal demise, cerebral infarction, and seizures. Hypertonicity, spasticity and convulsions, hyperreflexia, and irritability (withdrawal symptoms) have been observed in children exposed to cocaine in utero. These neonates are also at higher risk for other exposure to sexually transmitted infections in utero (e.g., human immunodeficiency virus [HIV] infection, hepatitis, syphilis).

17. **How long do cocaine metabolites remain in the urine?**
Cocaine use can be detected in a urine sample for up to 3 days after last use. Depending on the amount of use (long-term, large amounts) the metabolites can be detected up to 20 days after last use.

18. **What is the prevalence of opiate abuse or dependence during pregnancy?**
The true extent of opiate abuse and dependence by women is unknown. Overall, women account for approximately 25% of all opiate-dependent persons, and most of these estimated 300,000 women are untreated for their addiction.

19. **What risks are incurred by opiate dependence during pregnancy?**
Heroin does not seem to cause an increase in congenital anomaly rates. However, fetal issues include prematurity, intrauterine growth restriction, PPROM, intraamniotic infections, stillbirth, perinatal death, and multiple neonatal problems.

   Maternal risks depend on the route of administration. The common routes are oral, intranasal, and intravenous (IV). All are associated with maternal somnolence, altered mental status and cardiorespiratory depression, and possible overdose. Intranasal and IV administration is associated with hepatitis, HIV infection, endocarditis, and other issues related to what the drug is "cut" with and how it is procured.

20. **What is the standard treatment for opiate dependence during pregnancy?**
    Methadone maintenance confers several treatment benefits for the pregnant opiate-dependent woman. It eliminates the need for illicit behavior to support a drug habit, prevents fluctuations in maternal heroin levels, and removes the patient from a drug-seeking environment.

21. **Is methadone harmful?**
    Methadone is not known to cause an increase in congenital anomalies. However, it has been reported to be associated with low birth weights.

22. **Should a woman receiving methadone be weaned from it during pregnancy?**
    No. Although it is desirable to use the lowest possible dose, reduction to less than 20 mg/day may precipitate in utero withdrawal. Whatever dose is required to prevent symptoms in the mother is also best for the fetus, and no attempt should be made to taper and discontinue methadone until after delivery.

23. **Does methadone prevent withdrawal in the newborn period?**
    No. Approximately 80% of infants exposed to methadone require treatment for neonatal withdrawal (in contrast to 100% of infants exposed to heroin). The incidence of withdrawal is lower in infants of mothers receiving the lowest methadone doses.

24. **What is neonatal abstinence syndrome (NAS)?**
    NAS is a constellation of withdrawal symptoms that is seen with both heroin and methadone use. Classic NAS includes CNS hyperirritability, gastrointestinal dysfunction, respiratory distress, tremors, high-pitched cry, poor feeding, possible seizures, and electrolyte imbalance. Treatment is symptomatic and supportive.

25. **How common is NAS?**
    Reported rates range from 42% to 94%. The timing of maternal withdrawal is important; if more than a week has passed since the last opioid use, the risk is lower. All at-risk infants should be observed in the hospital for 4 to 5 days in case of any late-onset issues.

26. **What is the prevalence of marijuana use in pregnancy?**
    Self-reported prevalence of marijuana use during pregnancy ranges from 2% to 5% in most studies but it increases to 15% to 28% among young, urban, socioeconomically disadvantaged women. Higher rates of use are found when women are asked at the time of delivery rather than at prenatal visits because some users may not seek prenatal care. Notably, 48% to 60% of marijuana users continue use during pregnancy, with many women believing that it is relatively safe to use during pregnancy and less expensive than tobacco.

27. **What are the specific effects of marijuana use during pregnancy?**
    It is difficult to be certain about the specific effects of marijuana on pregnancy and the developing fetus, because women who use it often use other substances as well (e.g., tobacco, alcohol, or illicit drugs). Animal and longitudinal studies have shown impaired cognition and increased sensitivity to drugs of abuse. Given the potential for impaired neurodevelopment, all pregnant women should be encouraged to abstain from marijuana use.

28. **What obstetric complications have been associated with tobacco use?**
    Pregnant mothers who smoke are at increased risk for intrauterine growth restriction, placenta previa, placental abruption, decreased maternal thyroid function, preterm premature rupture of membranes (PPROM), low birth weight, perinatal mortality, and ectopic pregnancy. The risks of smoking during pregnancy extend beyond pregnancy-related complications; children born to mothers who smoke during pregnancy are at an increased risk of asthma, infantile colic, and childhood obesity. Research has shown that infants born to women who use smokeless tobacco during pregnancy have levels of nicotine similar to those born to mothers who smoke. Rates of low birth weight and shortened gestational age are also similar. Prenatal exposure to secondhand tobacco smoke increases the risk of having an infant with low birth weight by as much as 20%.

29. **What are effective and safe smoking cessation techniques for pregnant women?**
    Effective techniques in controlling tobacco addiction include counseling, continued reassurance, periodic and frequent contact with a health provider, and medication.
    Evidence on whether nicotine replacement therapy increases abstinence rates in pregnant smokers is conflicting; it does not appear to increase the likelihood of permanent smoking cessation during postpartum follow-up. If nicotine replacement is used, it should be with clear resolve to quit smoking on the part of the patient.

Alternative smoking cessation agents used in the nonpregnant population include varenicline and bupropion. Varenicline is a drug that acts on brain nicotine receptors, but its safety in pregnancy is unknown. Bupropion is an antidepressant with limited safety data, but at this time it has no known risk of fetal anomalies or adverse pregnancy effects. Both bupropion and varenicline are transmitted to breast milk. Both these medications have also added product warnings mandated by the U.S. Food and Drug Administration about the risk of psychiatric symptoms and suicide associated with their use. In patients at risk for depression, these drugs should be used with caution and in consultation with experienced prescribers.

30. **Should patients who abuse drugs breastfeed?**
No. Alcohol, cocaine, cannabinoid metabolites, and opiates all cross into breast milk to some extent. Cocaine from breast milk may cause significant cardiovascular changes in neonates, and opiates transferred in this manner have been shown to cause somnolence. Data are insufficient to evaluate the effects of marijuana; breastfeeding women should be informed that the potential neonatal risks of exposure to marijuana metabolites are unknown and should be encouraged to discontinue marijuana use.

31. **What are the common signs of substance abuse?**
   - Agitation
   - Sedation
   - Disorientation
   - Tachycardia
   - Hallucinations
   - Hypertension
   - Unusual skin infections

32. **How is substance abuse managed during pregnancy?**
Hospitalization may be necessary for detoxification purposes. Referral to treatment centers, social services, and any other needed form of counseling is important. These women should also be screened for domestic abuse (see Chapter 20).

KEY POINTS: ALCOHOL AND DRUG ABUSE DURING PREGNANCY

1. No safe level of alcohol consumption exists in pregnancy; the best advice is not to drink alcohol at all.
2. Fetal effects of alcohol use in pregnancy include lower IQ scores, learning problems, and the fetal alcohol disorder spectrum.
3. Placental abruption and stillbirth occur in approximately 8% of pregnant cocaine users.
4. Pregnant women addicted to heroin or opiates should be referred to methadone maintenance programs.
5. Tobacco use increases the risk of miscarriage, abruption, preterm birth, PPROM, and small for gestational age infants.
6. The rate of substance abuse varies by region and type of drug; it is important to ask *every* patient about past and present use.

BIBLIOGRAPHY

1. American College of Obstetricians and Gynecologists. Substance abuse reporting in pregnancy: The role of the obstetrician-gynecologist. ACOG committee opinion no. 473. *Obstet Gynecol.* 2011;117(1):200–201. Reaffirmed 2014.
2. American College of Obstetricians and Gynecologists. Marijuana use during pregnancy and lactation. ACOG committee opinion no. 637. *Obstet Gynecol.* 2015;126:234–238.
3. Centers for Disease Control and Prevention. Update: trends in fetal alcohol syndrome—United States, 1979-1993. *MMWR Morb Mortal Wkly Rep.* 1995;44:249–253. Updated 2012.
4. Chasnoff IJ, Griffith DR, Freier C, Murray J. Cocaine/polydrug use in pregnancy: two-year follow-up. *Pediatrics.* 1992;89:284–289.
5. Creasy RK, Resnik R, Iams JD, Lockwood CJ, Moore TR, eds. *Creasy and Resnik's Maternal-Fetal Medicine: Principles and Practice.* 6th ed. Philadelphia: Saunders; 2009:145–164.
6. Cyr MG, Moulton AW. Substance abuse in women. *Obstet Gynecol Clin North Am.* 1990;17:905–925.

7. Dombrowski M, Wolfe H, Welch R, Evans M. Cocaine abuse is associated with abruptio placentae and decreased birth weight, but not shorter labor. *Obstet Gynecol*. 1991;77:139.

8. Finnegan LP, Kandall SR. Maternal and neonatal effects of alcohol and drugs. In: Lowinsin JH, Ruiz P, Millman RB, Langrod JG, eds. *Substance Abuse: A Comprehensive Textbook*. 2nd ed. Baltimore: Williams & Wilkins; 1992: 628–656.

9. Mastrogiannis D, Decavalas G, Verma U, Tejani N. Perinatal outcome after recent cocaine usage. *Obstet Gynecol*. 1990;76:8.

10. Wiemann CM, Berenson AB. San Miguel VV. Tobacco, alcohol, and illicit drug use among pregnant women. *J Reprod Med*. 1994;39:769–776.

OBESITY IN PREGNANCY

Jared Roeckner, MD

CHAPTER 59

1. **What is the definition of obesity?**
   A body mass index (BMI) of 30 or more is considered obese. Different classes of obesity include class I (BMI of 30 to 34.9), class II (35 to 39.9), and class III (>40), although they do not change management during pregnancy.

2. **What is the incidence of obesity among women?**
   Approximately one third of women are obese.

3. **Does obesity affect the recommended amount of weight to gain during a pregnancy?**
   Yes. Women who are obese should only gain 11 to 20 pounds total. The recommended weight gain for overweight women (BMI of 25 to 25.9) is 15 to 25 pounds. This is in contrast to the 25 to 35 pounds considered appropriate for women of normal weight (BMI of 18.5 to 24.9) and the 28 to 40 pounds that underweight women (BMI <18.5) are recommended to gain.

4. **What key points should be included in the preconception counseling of an obese patient?**
   - Assessment of height and weight to determine BMI
   - Recommendations for weight gain
   - Nutritional counseling
   - Encouragement of an exercise program

5. **How does prenatal care for an obese patient differ from prenatal care in a woman of normal weight?**
   Ideally, these women should be screened for preexisting diabetes early in pregnancy. This can be done with an early 1-hour glucose tolerance test. This testing does not eliminate the need to screen for gestational diabetes at 24 to 28 weeks.

   Because of the difficulty in measuring fundal height (used to screen for abnormal fetal growth), obese women are often followed with monthly growth ultrasound examinations. Although evidence does not show a clear improvment in pregnancy outcome, antenatal testing is often performed in the late 3rd trimester.

   Obese pregnant women are at an increased risk of obstructive sleep apnea (OSA) and should be referred to a sleep medicine specialist if OSA is suspected.

6. **What fetal complications are associated with obesity?**
   Obesity is associated with higher rates of early pregnancy loss and stillbirth. Neural tube defects are about twice as common compared with women of normal weight. The rate of fetal macrosomia (defined as >4000 g) is increased as well.

7. **What maternal complications are associated with obesity?**
   Obese women have increased rates of gestational diabetes, gestational hypertension, OSA, and preeclampsia. Outside of pregnancy, obesity is linked to increased rates of diabetes, heart disease, and uterine cancer.

8. **What intrapartum complications are associated with obesity?**
   Obesity makes estimation of fetal weight, neuraxial anesthesia placement, and emergency cesarean delivery more technically challenging. Obese women have been shown to have a longer first stage of labor and should be allowed to labor longer before performing cesarean for arrest of labor.

9. **How does the rate of cesarean delivery change with BMI?**
   Obesity is an independent risk factor for cesarean delivery. One study found the rate of cesarean delivery to be increased twofold in patients with morbid obesity compared with normal-weight controls. The success of vaginal birth after cesarean (VBAC) declines with increasing BMI.

10. **What postpartum complications are more common in obese patients?**
    Wound separation, wound infection, and venous thromboembolism. These risks can be addressed by suturing the subcutaneous tissue and skin (as opposed to the use of surgical staples), and by administering unfractionated or low-molecular-weight heparin post partum.

11. **What considerations need to be made for pregnant women with a history of bariatric surgery?**
    The types of bariatric surgery are malabsorptive and restrictive. Nutritional deficiencies are common after malabsorptive procedures (e.g., Roux-en-Y), and these women should be followed each trimester with folate, vitamin B_{12}, and vitamin D levels as well as a complete blood count. Supplementation with extended-release preparations should be avoided. Nutritional deficiencies can also occur after restrictive procedures (e.g., gastric banding) because of decreased food intake and intolerance to certain foods. The degree of restriction may need to be adjusted during pregnancy, and these women

KEY POINTS: OBESITY IN PREGNANCY

1. One third of women are obese (BMI ≥30); this increases the risk of many fetal and maternal complications.
2. For obese women, recommended weight gain during the entire pregnancy is only 11 to 20 pounds.
3. Nutritional deficiencies are more common after malabsorptive bariatric procedures, but they can also occur after restrictive procedures.
4. Women who have had a malabsorptive bariatric procedure should not be given an oral glucose challenge test because of the risk of dumping syndrome.

should continue to be followed by a bariatric surgeon. For more information on nutrition after bariatric surgery, see Chapter 37.

Women who have had a malabsorptive procedure should not be given an oral glucose challenge test due to the risk of dumping syndrome. They can be screened for diabetes by recording blood glucose levels at home (fasting and 2-hour postprandial) for 1 week.

BIBLIOGRAPHY

1. American College of Obstetricians and Gynecologists. Bariatric surgery and pregnancy. ACOG practice bulletin no. 105. *Obstet Gynecol.* 2009;113:1405–1413.
2. American College of Obstetricians and Gynecologists. Weight gain during pregnancy. ACOG committee opinion no. 548. *Obstet Gynecol.* 2013;121:210–212.
3. American College of Obstetricians and Gynecologists. Obesity in pregnancy. ACOG committee opinion no. 156. *Obstet Gynecol.* 2015;126:112–126.
4. Baeten JM, Bukusi EA, Lambe M. Pregnancy complications and outcomes among overweight and obese nulliparous women. *Am J Public Health.* 2001;91:436–440.
5. Kabiru W, Raynor BD. Obstetric outcomes associated with increase in BMI category during pregnancy. *Am J Obstet Gynecol.* 2004;191:928–932.
6. Stothard KJ, Tennant PW, Bell R, Rankin J. Maternal overweight and obesity and the risk of congenital anomalies: a systematic review and meta-analysis. *JAMA.* 2009;301:636–650.
7. Weiss JL, Malone FD, Emig D, et al. Obesity, obstetric complications and cesarean delivery rate: a population-based screening study. *Am J Obstet Gynecol.* 2004;190:1091–1097.

CHAPTER 60

MULTIPLE GESTATION

Erin Burnett, MD

1. **How often do twins occur?**
   Over the past several decades, the rate of twin birth has increased annually to a current rate of 3.3%. This is a 76% relative increase from 1980.

2. **What is causing the increased rate of multiple gestations?**
   Assisted reproductive technology (ART) and increasing maternal age at childbirth have caused the rate of multiple gestations to increase.

3. **What is superfecundation?**
   Superfecundation is the fertilization of two different eggs during the same menstrual cycle, and it results in dizygotic or "fraternal" twinning (Fig. 60-1). Approximately two thirds of all twin pregnancies are dizygotic. This phenomenon appears to have a genetic component, with certain areas in Africa reporting twin rates nearly twice as high as in the United States.

4. **What are monozygotic twins?**
   Monozygotic twins (also known as "paternal" or "identical") result from a single fertilized ovum splitting into two separate embryos. The timing of this split determines what type of chorionicity (number of placentas) and amnionicity (number of amniotic sacs) will result (see Fig. 60-1). Approximately one third of all twin pregnancies are monozygotic.
   - Division at 3 days or less results in **dichorionic, diamniotic** (di/di) twins and represents 30% of monozygotic twins. This split occurs before the inner and outer layers of the blastocyst have formed.
   - Division at days 4 to 8 results in **monochorionic, diamniotic** (mono/di) twins and represents the majority (68%) of monozygotic pregnancies.
   - Division at days 8 to 13 results in **monochorionic, monoamniotic** (mono/mono) twins and represents only 1% of twin pregnancies. This was historically associated with an extremely high mortality rate (>50%), which has now decreased to approximately 13%.
   - Attempted division of the embryonic disk at 14 days and beyond leads to **conjoined** twins. The estimated frequency is 1.5 per 100,000 births.

5. **How is chorionicity diagnosed?**
   Ultrasound examination is used to establish chorionicity, and it is most accurate in the first trimester (96% to 100%). Before 8 weeks, separate gestational sacs can be seen; if a thick echogenic ring surrounds each sac, the pregnancy is likely dichorionic. If separate chorionic rings are not visible, monochorionicity is likely. The number of yolk sacs can be used to assess amnionicity—visualization of two indicates the presence of two amniotic sacs.

   Later in pregnancy, fetal sex, intertwin membrane thickness, placental location, and the appearance of where fetal membranes insert into the placenta or placentas can be used to help determine chorionicity. Two different fetal sexes or two distinctly separate placentas indicate dichorionicity, as well as a thick intertwin membrane (≥2 mm). The presence or absence of the "lambda" or "twin peak" sign can also be used; if present, a dichorionic pregnancy is suggested. Images of the lambda sign can be seen in Chapter 38 (see Fig. 38-3, *A*).

6. **What are higher-order multiples, and how do they form?**
   Higher-order multiples are gestations with more than two embryos (e.g., triplets, quadruplets). They can occur from any number of combinations of division, ranging from multiple divisions of the same conceptus to fertilization of multiple ova.

7. **Are twins at an increased risk for aneuploidy?**
   Twin pregnancies have a higher overall rate of aneuploidy compared with singletons, mainly because of advanced maternal age. Zygosity determines the degree of risk and whether two fetuses may be concordant for a specific chromosomal anomaly.

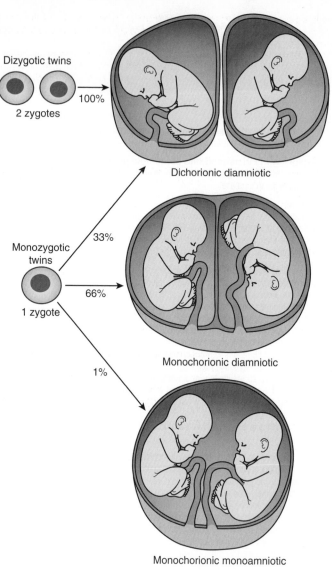

Figure 60-1. Dizygotic and monozygotic twins. *(Modified from* Diagnostic Ultrasound, *4th ed. Philadelphia: Mosby; 2011.)*

8. What are the options for aneuploidy screening in a twin pregnancy?
   For more information on aneuploidy screening and diagnosis, see Chapter 39.
   - **Nuchal translucency** is not significantly different from singletons and has similar detection rates.
   - **First trimester serum markers combined with nuchal translucency:** Levels of pregnancy-associated plasma protein-A (PAPP-A) and β-human chorionic gonadotropin (hCG) are approximately twice as high in twins compared with singletons, and corrective adjustments are made for each biochemical.

- **Integrated screening** (first and second trimester serum markers combined with nuchal translucency) can be offered in twin pregnancies, although no prospective validation studies have been reported.
- **Second trimester serum markers:** Levels of hCG, estriol, inhibin-A, and α-fetoprotein (AFP) are approximately twice as high in twins compared with singletons, and corrective adjustments are made for each biochemical. Second trimester serum screening has been associated with higher false-positive rates compared with singleton pregnancies, but it is still considered an acceptable option for women who miss first trimester screening.
- **Noninvasive prenatal testing (NIPT)** can be offered in twin pregnancy, although no large validation studies have been reported.

9. **Do twin pregnancies have a higher rate of congenital anomalies?**
   Yes. Both monochorionic twins and twins conceived using in vitro fertilization (IVF) or intracytoplasmic sperm injection (ICSI) have increased rates of congenital anomalies, particularly cardiac defects. Compared with less than 1% of singleton pregnancies, the incidence of cardiac defects in at least one twin has been reported to be approximately 7% to 9% for mono/di twins and as high as 57.1% for mono/mono twins. The risk of cardiac defects associated with IVF and ICSI is four times greater than the baseline rate.

10. **What is twin-twin transfusion syndrome (TTTS)?**
    TTTS is overperfusion of one twin and underperfusion of the other. It complicates approximately 10% of monochorionic twin pregnancies and occurs when an imbalance exists between placental anastomoses, especially arteriovenous ones. Death of one or both twins can result, and neurologic morbidity in the surviving twin is as high as 20% to 26%.

11. **How is TTTS diagnosed and staged?**
    TTTS is diagnosed and staged using ultrasound examination. The most commonly used system is Quintero staging, which describes the progression of this condition (Table 60-1).

Table 60-1. Quintero Staging System for Twin-Twin Transfusion Syndrome

STAGE	CRITERION
I	Oligohydramnios (deepest vertical pocket <2 cm) in one twin and polyhydramnios (deepest vertical pocket >8 cm) in the other
II	Donor twin bladder no longer visible
III	Donor twin bladder no longer visible and fetal Doppler values abnormal
IV	Fetal hydrops present in one or both twins
V	Death of one or both twins

From Creasy RK, Resnick R, Iams JD, et. al. Multiple gestations. In *Creasy and Resnik's Maternal-Fetal Medicine: Principles and Practice*. 7th ed. Philadelphia: Saunders; 2014:578-596.e4.

12. **How is TTTS treated?**
    Treatment is based on staging and gestational age.
    - **Expectant management:** Among pregnancies diagnosed with stage I TTTS, 85% will remain stable or regress, and the overall survival rate is 86%.
    - **Serial amnioreduction:** Amniocentesis is performed to remove fluid from the sac of the twin with polyhydramnios. This reduces intrauterine and placental intravascular pressure, which may improve placental blood flow and reduce the risk of preterm labor associated with polyhydramnios. Overall survival is 60% to 65%.
    - **Selective fetoscopic laser coagulation:** Anastomotic placental vessels are identified and coagulated. This treatment is generally reserved for cases at 15 to 26 weeks of gestation with stage II or higher TTTS. Compared with serial amniocentesis, laser ablation has been shown to increase survival rates of at least one twin (51% vs. 76%) at 6 months of age and decrease the incidence of major neurologic damage (10% vs. 5%).
    - If at less than 24 weeks of gestation, **termination** of the entire pregnancy or **selective reduction** (see question 13) can be performed.

Amniotic septostomy (deliberately perforating the intertwin membrane) offers no therapeutic advantage and is no longer performed.

13. **What is multifetal reduction, and what is selective reduction?**
In *multifetal reduction*, a higher-order multiple gestation is usually reduced to a twin or singleton pregnancy. This increases the chance of live birth, decreases the risk of losing the entire pregnancy, decreases the risks associated with preterm delivery, and decreases maternal risks such as preeclampsia and diabetes. To minimize the difficulty of the procedure and risk to the pregnancy, the decision of which fetus or fetuses to reduce is usually based on location. In *selective reduction*, fetuses are chosen for a medical indication such as aneuploidy, the presence of an anomaly, or abnormal health status (e.g., growth restriction).

   If a fetus does not share a placenta, reduction is performed using ultrasound-guided, intracardiac injection of potassium chloride. If a fetus is part of a monochorionic pair, radiofrequency ablation of the umbilical cord is used. The overall the pregnancy loss rate associated with a reduction is approximately 4%, although data for later gestations are limited.

14. **What are the major obstetric risks associated with multiple gestation?**
    - Fetal risks
      - Spontaneous abortion
      - Stillbirth (1.61% for twins, 2.15% for triplets)
      - Congenital anomalies
      - Intrauterine growth restriction (66%)
      - Placenta previa
      - Preterm birth (twins: 50%; triplets: 75%)
      - Fetal malpresentation
      - Perinatal mortality (0.5%, 2%, 4.7%, and 9.4% for twins, triplets, quadruplets, and quintuplets, respectively)
    - Maternal risks
      - Hypertension, preeclampsia (26%), and HELLP (hemolysis, elevated liver enzymes, low platelets) syndrome (9%)
      - Anemia (24%)
      - Gestational diabetes (14%)
      - Preterm premature rupture of membranes (24%)
      - Acute fatty liver of pregnancy (4%)

15. **How are pregnancies complicated by the intrauterine demise of one twin managed?**
The main risk to the surviving twin is prematurity. However, neurologic injury can also occur. In monochorionic twins, this rate is 20% to 26% of surviving twins. This rate is thought to be caused by a shared placenta, and it can result in hemodynamic changes and hypotension immediately after the demise of one twin. For dichorionic twins, the rate of neurologic injury in the survivor is 2%. Magnetic resonance imaging (MRI) can be performed after 2 weeks have passed to determine the presence and extent of injury in the surviving twin. These pregnancies are followed closely with ultrasound growth assessments and antepartum surveillance and generally undergo delivery in the late preterm period (i.e., between 34 and 37 weeks).

16. **What additional considerations should be made during prenatal care for patients with a multiple gestation?**
    - **Supplementation:** Each day, women should take extra folic acid (1 mg/day), extra iron (60 to 100 mg/day), and consume an additional 300 calories per fetus.
    - **Weight gain:** Patients with twins should gain 37 to 54 pounds if their prepregnancy weight was normal, 31 to 50 pounds if they are overweight, and 25 to 42 pounds if they are obese. No set guidelines have been issued for higher-order multiples, but ideal weight gain is generally thought to be greater than what is recommended for twins. (For more information on nutrition in pregnancy, see Chapter 37.)
    - **Ultrasound examinations:** In addition to ruling out congenital anomalies with a second trimester anatomy assessment, multiple gestations should also receive a fetal echocardiogram. Growth should be monitored using serial ultrasound examinations for the remainder of the pregnancy, with the timing determined by chorionicity and amnionicity. Monochorionic twins are monitored more

frequently because of the risk of TTTS (see questions 10 to 12), starting at 16 weeks of gestation and repeated every 2 weeks.
- **Number of visits:** Because of their higher risk of both fetal and maternal complications, women with multiple gestations should be seen more frequently than women with singleton gestations.

17. **What is the mean gestational age for delivery of multiples gestations?**
On average, twins undergo delivery at 35.3 weeks, triplets at 31.9 weeks, and quadruplets at 29.4 weeks. These numbers include deliveries resulting from preterm labor, as well as fetal or maternal indications.

18. **What is the incidence of delivery at less than 32 weeks of gestation in multiple gestations?**
Eleven percent of twins and 37% of triplets undergo delivery at gestations of less than 32 weeks, compared with only 1.6% of singletons.

19. **What are the mean birth weights for twins and triplets?**
The mean birth weight for twins is 2333 g (5 pounds 2 ounces). The mean birth weight for triplets is 1700 g (3 pounds 12 ounces). These weights are both significantly lower than those of singletons, which average 3316 g (7 pounds 5 ounces).

20. **How are twin pregnancies managed during labor?**
Both fetuses should be monitored (see Chapter 62). If a vaginal delivery is planned, epidural anesthesia and delivery in an operating room are recommended because of an increased risk of cesarean delivery. No contraindications to induction, augmentation, or trial of labor after cesarean exist solely because of the presence of twins. Women should be thoroughly counseled on the possibility of needing a cesarean section after delivery of the first twin, and equipment for both vaginal and cesarean delivery should be readily available.

21. **How common are the different combinations of twin presentation at the time of delivery?**
- Vertex/vertex: 40%
- Vertex/breech: 26%
- Breech/vertex: 20%
- Breech/breech: 10%
- Vertex/transverse: 8%
- Miscellaneous: 6%
For more information on malpresentation, see Chapter 67.

22. **How are vertex/vertex twins delivered?**
It is reasonable to plan for a vaginal delivery at all estimated fetal weights. As is the case with singleton pregnancies, women may still elect to have a cesarean delivery.

23. **How are breech/breech and breech/vertex twins delivered?**
Cesarean delivery is recommended at all fetal weights.

24. **How are vertex/breech and vertex/transverse twins delivered?**
The recommended route of delivery depends on the estimated fetal weights, the amount of difference or **discordance** between the fetal weights, and the experience of the delivering physician. Cesarean delivery is recommended if the second twin is more than 20% larger or if the estimated fetal weights are less than 1500 g.
   If vaginal delivery is attempted, the presenting infant is allowed to deliver. Then either an external cephalic version or breech extraction of the second twin is performed. Breech extraction is successful in approximately 95% of attempts, and it should be done quickly after delivery of the first twin while the cervix is still at full dilation. The major associated risks are fetal injury and head entrapment. External cephalic version of the second twin is successful in up to 70% of cases; associated risks are umbilical cord prolapse and placental abruption.

25. **How are higher-order multiples delivered?**
Cesarean delivery is recommended.

26. **What is a major postpartum risk associated with multiple gestations regardless of the route of delivery?**
Uterine atony, which can lead to postpartum hemorrhage. Uterotonic agents should be readily available, and patients should be typed and crossmatched for blood products.

KEY POINTS: MULTIPLE GESTATION

1. The later the division of an embryo occurs after fertilization, the more structures are shared (amnion, chorion, fetal parts).
2. Ultrasound examination is used to establish chorionicity, and it is most accurate in the first trimester (96% to 100%).
3. Both monochorionic twins and twins conceived using IVF or ICSI have increased rates of congenital anomalies, particularly cardiac defects.
4. TTTS complicates approximately 10% of monochorionic twin pregnancies. It occurs when an imbalance exists between placental anastomoses, and it can result in death of one or both twins.
5. Preterm labor and delivery are much more common in multiple gestations; the mean gestational age at delivery is 35.3 weeks for twins, 31.9 weeks for triplets, and 29.4 weeks for quadruplets.
6. The most common presentation for twins at the time of delivery is vertex/vertex.

BIBLIOGRAPHY

Abuhamad A, Chaoui R. *A Practical Guide to Fetal Echocardiography: Normal and Abnormal Hearts.* 2nd ed. Philadelphia: Lippincott Williams & Wilkins; 2010:3–6.

American College of Obstetricians and Gynecologists. Multifetal pregnancy reduction. ACOG committee opinion no. 553. *Obstet Gynecol.* 2013;121:405–410.

Audibert F, Gagnon A. Genetics Committee of the Society of Obstetricians and Gynaecologists of Canada, Prenatal Diagnosis Committee of the Canadian College of Medical Geneticists. Prenatal screening for and diagnosis of aneuploidy in twin pregnancies. *J Obstet Gynaecol Can.* 2011;33:754–767.

D'Alton M, Fuchs K. *Twins, Triplets and Beyond: Protocols for High Risk Pregnancies.* 5th ed. Malden, Mass: Blackwell; 2010:535–544.

Hansen M, Bower C, Milne E, et al. Assisted reproductive technologies and the risks of birth defects: a systematic review. *Hum Reprod.* 2005;20:328–338.

Malone FD, D'Alton ME. Multiple gestation: clinical characteristics and management. In: Creasy R, Resnik R, Iams JD, Lockwood CJ, Moore TR, eds. *Creasy and Resnik's Maternal-Fetal Medicine: Principles and Practice.* 7th ed. Philadelphia: Saunders; 2014:578–596.

Manning N, Archer N. A study to determine the incidence of structural congenital heart disease in monochorionic twins. *Prenat Diagn.* 2006;26:1062–1064.

Pettit KE, Merchant M, Machin GA, Tacy TA, Norton ME. Congenital heart defects in a large, unselected cohort of monochorionic twins. *J Perinatol.* 2013;33:457–461.

Society for Maternal-Fetal Medicine, Simpson LL. Twin-twin transfusion syndrome. *Am J Obstet Gynecol.* 2013;208:3–18. [Erratum in: Am J Obstet Gynecol. 2013;208:392.]

Vink J, Wapner R, D'Alton M. Prenatal diagnosis in twin gestations. *Semin Perinatol.* 2012;36:169–174.

LABOR AND VAGINAL DELIVERY

Kelly A. Best, MD

CHAPTER 61

1. **What is the definition of labor?**
   Labor begins when uterine contractions of sufficient frequency, intensity, and duration are attained to bring about effacement and progressive dilation of the cervix.

2. **What two steps are theorized to be crucial to the initiation of labor in human pregnancy?**
   1. Retreat from pregnancy maintenance
   2. Uterotonic induction
   Despite extensive investigation into the associated physiologic and biochemical changes, the physiologic processes in human pregnancy that result in the onset of labor are still not defined.

3. **In which patients is induction of labor considered?**
   Awaiting the onset of normal labor may not be an option in certain circumstances. At preterm gestations, indications for labor induction include severe preeclampsia, fetal growth restriction with abnormal antepartum surveillance or other evidence of fetal compromise, and deterioration of maternal disease to the point that continuation of pregnancy is believed to be detrimental. In cases of rupture of membranes without labor (i.e., premature rupture of membranes) at term (37 to 42 weeks) or postterm (≥42 weeks), induction of labor is often performed.

4. **What is a Bishop score, and how is it used?**
   A Bishop score is a quantifiable method to assess the likelihood of a successful induction. Elements include dilation, effacement, station, consistency, and position of the cervix (Table 61-1). A score of 6 or less translates into a need to ripen the cervix and is associated with less successful inductions. A score 8 or greater generally means the cervix does not need ripening and induction is more likely to be successful.

Table 61-1. Bishop Scoring System for Assessment of Inducibility

SCORE	DILATION (cm)	EFFACEMENT (%)	STATION (-3 TO +3 SCALE)	CERVICAL CONSISTENCY	CERVICAL POSITION
0	Closed	0-30	−3	Firm	Posterior
1	1-2	40-50	−2	Medium	Midposition
2	3-4	60-70	−1, 0	Soft	Anterior
3	≥5	≥80	+1, +2	—	—

5. **What methods are available for cervical ripening?**
   Mechanical methods provide local pressure and stimulate endogenous release of prostaglandins, which results in cervical ripening. Options include a transcervical Foley catheter (filled with 30 to 60 mL after insertion) or hydroscopic dilators (laminaria or a similar synthetic product).
   Pharmacologic methods include low-dose oxytocin, prostaglandin E_2 (dinoprostone), and prostaglandin E_1 (misoprostol). Prostaglandin E_1 can be administered intravaginally or orally, and prostaglandin E_2 can be applied within the vagina in either gel or suppository form.

6. **When is cervical ripening contraindicated?**
   Contraindications to labor induction are the same as those for spontaneous labor and vaginal delivery. They include—but are not limited to—vasa previa, placenta previa, fetal malpresentation (e.g., breech

or transverse lie), umbilical cord prolapse, and previous transfundal uterine surgical procedures. Because of an increased risk of uterine rupture during induction of labor with prostaglandins among women with previous low-transverse cesarean sections, the American College of Obstetricians and Gynecologists (ACOG) advises against the use of prostaglandins in these cases. For more information on a trial of labor after cesarean section (TOLAC), see Chapter 63.

7. **How is the pelvis assessed clinically?**
   Historically, clinical assessment of the pelvis (known as **pelvimetry**) was used to predict whether vaginal birth was possible and provide information about a patient's overall pelvic dimensions and configuration. However, this has been shown not to be reliable; the best way to assess whether a pelvis is adequate is to allow for a trial of labor.
   - The **pelvic inlet** is bounded in the anteroposterior dimension (obstetric conjugate) by the sacral promontory and the pubic symphysis. Laterally, it is bound by the linea terminalis. The size of the pelvic inlet can be estimated by palpating the sacral promontory, which provides the measurement for the *diagonal conjugate*, which is approximately 1.5 to 2 cm greater than the *obstetric conjugate*.
   - The **pelvic midplane** is bounded laterally by the inferior margins of the ischial spines, anteriorly by the lower margin of the symphysis pubis, and posteriorly by the sacrum (usually S4 or S5).
   - The **pelvic outlet** consists of two triangular areas that are not in the same plane but share a common base, which is the distance between the two ischial tuberosities. The apex of the posterior triangle is at the tip of the sacrum, and the anterior triangle is formed by the area under the pubic arch (Fig. 61-1).
   Most patients have an intermediate form of the four classically described pelvic types (Fig. 61-2).

8. **What are the three stages of labor?**
   The first stage begins with the onset of labor and ends when the cervix is fully dilated (10 cm). The second stage begins when dilation of the cervix is complete and ends with delivery of the infant. The third stage begins immediately after delivery of the infant and ends with delivery of the placenta.

9. **How are uterine contractions monitored?**
   Uterine monitoring can be either external or internal.
   - **External monitoring:** performed by securing a displacement transducer to the maternal abdomen. When the uterus contracts, the transducer moves; this movement is translated into an electronic signal and is transcribed as a vertical displacement from the resting uterine tone. This form of monitoring provides information only about the *frequency* of contractions.

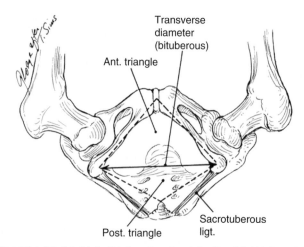

Figure 61-1. The pelvic outlet. Ant., Anterior; ligt., ligament; post., posterior. *(From Hobel CJ, Chang AB. Normal labor, delivery, and postpartum care. In: Hacker NF, Moore JG, Gambone JC, eds. Essentials of Obstetrics and Gynecology. 4th ed. Philadelphia: Saunders; 2004:108.)*

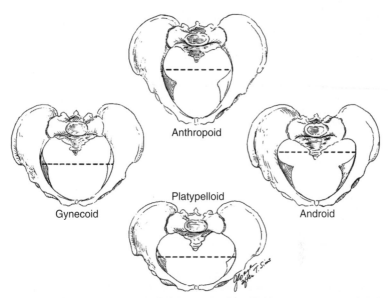

Figure 61-2. The four basic pelvic types (Caldwell-Moloy classification). The *dotted line* indicates the transverse diameter of the inlet. *(From Hobel CJ, Chang AB. Normal labor, delivery, and postpartum care. In: Hacker NF, Moore JG, Gambone JC, eds.* Essentials of Obstetrics and Gynecology. *4th ed. Philadelphia: Saunders; 2004:109.)*

- **Internal monitoring:** performed by threading a pressure catheter through the cervix, around the presenting part of the fetus, and into the uterine cavity. This method provides information on both the *strength and frequency* of contractions.

10. What is a normal contraction pattern?
    A normal contraction pattern during labor consists of three to five contractions in 10 minutes, averaged over a 30-minute period.

11. What is an "adequate" contraction pattern?
    An adequate contraction pattern refers to contractions of sufficient frequency and strength to cause cervical change.
    Uterine contractions can be measured in **Montevideo units.** To calculate Montevideo units, total vertical displacement above resting uterine tone is multiplied by contraction frequency over a 10-minute period (Fig. 61-3). An intrauterine pressure catheter must be used. Contractions are considered adequate when they reach 200 Montevideo units or greater.

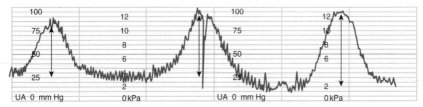

Figure 61-3. Calculation of Montevideo units. *UA,* Uterine activity. *(From Bashore RA, Koos BJ. Fetal surveillance during labor. In: Hacker NF, Gambone JG, Hobel CJ, eds.* Hacker and Moore's Essentials of Obstetrics and Gynecology. *5th ed. Philadelphia: Saunders; 2010.)*

12. **What are the two phases of the first stage of labor?**
    The first stage is divided into a latent phase and an active phase. The duration of the latent phase is variable and has little bearing on the subsequent course of labor, whereas the characteristics of the active phase are usually predictive of the outcome of a particular labor.

13. **What is the Friedman curve?**
    In the 1950s, Emanuel A. Friedman popularized the use of an objective measure of labor progression. He constructed a graphic representation of expected cervical dilation against time, with varying expectations for nulliparous and multiparous patients. Used in conjunction with fetal descent, these curves were used to provide clinical feedback about the normalcy of a patient's labor progress.
    "Labor curves" have since been updated in light of changing demographics, improved statistical and experimental methods, and more robust study designs.

14. **What cervical changes generally take place during the latent phase of labor?**
    Although little cervical dilation occurs during this time, considerable changes take place in the extracellular matrix (collagen and other connective tissue components) of the cervix. Cervical ripening generally includes palpable softening, effacement, and anterior rotation of the cervix in the pelvic axis.

15. **When does conversion from the latent to active phase occur?**
    During labor, the transition is characterized by increased regularity and intensity of contractions, accompanied by progressive and predictable cervical change. The active phase of labor begins at 6 cm dilation and accelerates at different rates based on parity.

16. **What is the duration of the first stage of labor?**
    - **Latent phase:** The median duration and 95th percentile duration of the latent phase depend on baseline cervical dilation and are similar between nulliparous and parous women. If a patient is admitted to the hospital at 2 cm dilation, the median duration of the latent phase is approximately 6 hours, and the 95th percentile is 15.7 hours. If a patient is admitted at 3 cm, the median duration is approximately 4 hours, and the 95th percentile is 12.5 hours. The term *prolonged latent phase* is used to indicate that a patient has been in the latent phase of labor for longer than the 95th percentile.
    - **Active phase:** The median duration and 95th percentile duration of the active phase in nulliparous women are 2.1 and 8.6 hours, respectively. In parous women, these times are 1.5 and 7.5 hours. The term *prolonged active phase* is used to indicate that cervical dilation is occurring at a rate of less than the 5th percentile.

17. **What is the management of a prolonged latent phase?**
    Options include maternal sedation (also known as "therapeutic rest"), augmentation with oxytocin, or discharge home if the patient and fetus are stable.

18. **What is the management of a prolonged active phase?**
    Treatment is either observation or augmentation with oxytocin.

19. **How is arrest of the active phase defined, and how is it managed?**
    Arrest of the active phase is defined as cessation of dilation when an adequate contraction pattern (≥200 Montevideo units in a 10-minute period) has been present for 2 hours. Cesarean section is generally indicated in these cases.

20. **At how many centimeters is a cervix considered to be fully dilated?**
    At 10 cm, it is considered fully dilated because this is the approximate diameter of the fetal vertex at term. For preterm infants, however, full dilation may be less than 10 cm; the cervix will not dilate past the maximal point of the presenting part.

21. **What are the two possible abnormalities of the second stage of labor?**
    Prolonged descent and arrest of descent. Although prolonged descent has traditionally been defined as descent occurring at less than 1 cm/hour in nulliparas and more than 2 cm/hour in multiparas, it does not usually affect clinical management. Arrest of descent is defined as generally considered to occur when there has been no progress (descent or rotation) for a specified amount of time based on parity and whether regional anesthesia is being used:
    - 4 hours or longer in nulliparous women with an epidural
    - 3 hours or longer in nulliparous women without an epidural
    - 3 hours or longer in multiparous women with an epidural
    - 2 hours or longer in multiparous women without an epidural

If the patient is a candidate for operative vaginal delivery, this may be an acceptable option as long as fetal macrosomia and cephalopelvic disproportion are not suspected; otherwise, cesarean delivery is indicated.

22. **What should be assessed during a vaginal examination?**
    - Cervical dilation
    - Degree of effacement (thinning of the cervix, usually expressed as a percentage)
    - Fetal station (presenting part described in centimeters in relation to the maternal ischial spines)
    - Presenting part (e.g., vertex, breech, shoulder) and orientation

23. **What are the cardinal movements of labor?**
    Engagement
    Descent
    Flexion
    Internal rotation
    External rotation
    Extension
    Restitution
    Expulsion
    Figure 61-4 illustrates the cardinal movements of labor.

24. **What is the Ritgen maneuver?**
    Moderate upward pressure is applied to the fetal chin by the operator's posterior hand, which is covered with a sterile towel, while the vertex is held against the symphysis (Fig. 61-5). This maneuver allows control of the delivery of the head and favors extension, so that the head is delivered with its smallest diameter passing through the introitus and over the perineum.

25. **What is shoulder dystocia and how is it managed?**
    Shoulder dystocia is impaction of the fetal shoulders within the maternal pelvis after delivery of the fetal head, thus preventing further expulsion of the infant. Special maneuvers are required to free the anterior shoulder:
    - McRobert maneuver (acute flexion of the maternal legs)
    - Suprapubic pressure
    - Woods corkscrew maneuver (rotating the posterior shoulder of the fetus 180 degrees in a corkscrew fashion)
    - Delivery of the posterior shoulder (by sweeping the posterior arm of the fetus across the chest)
    - Rubin maneuver (displacing the anterior shoulder toward the chest of the fetus within the pelvis)
    - Deliberate fracture of the clavicles
    - Zavanelli maneuver (involving flexion of the fetal head, replacement of the fetus within the uterine cavity, and emergency cesarean section delivery)

26. **How often does shoulder dystocia occur?**
    Although it has traditionally been associated with fetal macrosomia, up to 50% of cases of shoulder dystocia occur in neonates weighing less than 4000 g. Among infants weighing 4000 to 4499 g, the incidence of shoulder dystocia is 1% to 10% in nondiabetic women and 5% to 23% in diabetic women. These numbers rise to 3% to 23% and 20% to 50%, respectively, for infants weighing more than 4500 g.

27. **What are the potential complications of shoulder dystocia?**
    For the fetus, shoulder dystocia may be associated with transient brachial plexus palsies, clavicular fractures, humeral fractures, and neonatal death. For the mother, severe perineal lacerations and postpartum hemorrhage can occur.

28. **What is an episiotomy, and why is it performed?**
    An episiotomy is incision of the perineum to enlarge the vaginal opening. It was historically thought to prevent excessive stretching of the perineum, but it has now been abandoned for lack of evidence. Episiotomy has been associated, however, with an increased risk of injury to the rectal sphincter. The two types of episiotomy are median (midline) and mediolateral. A median episiotomy is considered easier to repair and to have a less painful recovery, but it also has a higher rate of extension into the rectum. Mediolateral episiotomies are made at a 45-degree angle to the base of the introitus; they have a lower extension rate and may be considered for large infants, a small perineal body, and in some cases of operative vaginal delivery.

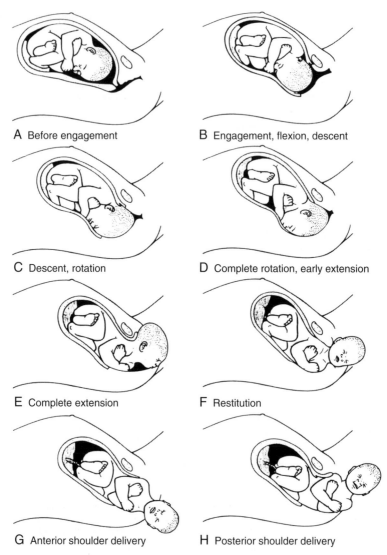

A Before engagement

B Engagement, flexion, descent

C Descent, rotation

D Complete rotation, early extension

E Complete extension

F Restitution

G Anterior shoulder delivery

H Posterior shoulder delivery

Figure 61-4. The cardinal movements of labor. Although labor is a continuous process, eight discrete cardinal movements of labor occur. **A,** Before engagement. **B,** Engagement, flexion, and descent. **C,** Descent and rotation. **D,** Complete rotation and early extension. **E,** Complete extension. **F,** Restitution. **G,** Anterior shoulder delivery. **H,** Posterior shoulder delivery. *(From Norwitz ER, Robinson JN, Repke JT. Labor and delivery. In: Gabbe SG, Niebyl JR, Simpson JL, eds.* Obstetrics: Normal and Problem Pregnancies. *4th ed. Philadelphia: Churchill Livingstone; 2002:365.)*

29. What tissue layers are involved in each of the four types of obstetric laceration?
    - **First-degree:** the fourchette, perineal skin, and vaginal mucosa, but not the underlying fascia and muscle
    - **Second-degree:** as in first-degree lacerations, with the addition of the fascia and muscles of the perineal body
    - **Third-degree:** as in second-degree lacerations, with the addition of the anal sphincter
    - **Fourth-degree:** as in third-degree lacerations, with the addition of the rectal mucosa (exposing the lumen of the rectum)

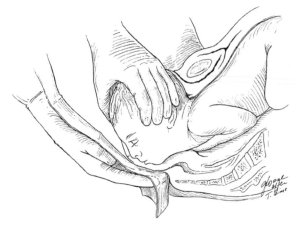

Figure 61-5. Ritgen maneuver. The fingers of the right hand, pressing posterior to the rectum, are used to extend the head while counterpressure is applied to the occiput by the left hand to allow controlled delivery of the fetal head. *(From Hobel CJ, Chang AB. Normal labor delivery and postpartum care. In: Hacker NF, Moore JG, Gambone JC, eds. Essentials of Obstetrics and Gynecology. 4th ed. Philadelphia: Saunders; 2004:118.)*

30. **What are the indications for operative vaginal delivery?**
    The indications for operative vaginal delivery include any condition threatening the mother or fetus during the second stage of labor that is likely to be relieved by delivery. Examples of *maternal* indications are heart disease, pulmonary injury or compromise, certain neurologic conditions, and maternal exhaustion. An common *fetal* indication is a nonreassuring fetal heart rate pattern.

31. **What are general prerequisites for performing an operative vaginal delivery (ABCs)?**
    - There must be adequate **a**nesthesia.
    - The maternal **b**ladder should be emptied.
    - The **c**ervix must be completely **d**ilated.
    - The fetal head must be **e**ngaged.
    - The **f**ontanels and direction of the occiput must be precisely known.
    - Membranes must be ruptured ("**g**ush of amniotic fluid").
    - The maternal pelvis must be assessed to be adequate ("**hips**").
    - An **i**ndication should be present.

32. **What is asynclitism?**
    Asynclitism is failure of the vertex to descend with the sagittal suture in the middle plane between the front and back of the pelvis. It is detected clinically on examination when either the anterior or posterior parietal bones precede the sagittal suture. When accompanied by molding, asynclitism can lead to erroneous assessments of the true fetal position.

33. **How are the different levels of operative delivery described?**
    - In a *high* operative delivery, the fetal head is not engaged; this type of operative delivery is no longer performed.
    - A *mid* operative delivery is when the fetal station is greater than +2 cm but the head is engaged.
    - A *low* operative delivery is when the leading point of the fetal skull is at station +2 cm or greater and not on the pelvic floor.
    - An *outlet* operative delivery is when the fetal skull has reached the pelvic floor; scalp should be visible at the introitus without separating the labia, the sagittal suture is in an anteroposterior orientation, and rotation of the fetal head does not exceed 45 degrees (i.e., in right or left occiput anterior or posterior position).

34. **What are the two general types of operative delivery?**
    Vacuum-assisted delivery and forceps-assisted delivery.

35. What are following forceps: Simpson, Elliot, Tucker-McLane, Kielland, and Piper?
- **Simpson:** fenestrated blades with divergent handles. The greater cephalic curve of the blade is suited for the molded head and when traction is desired. The Luikart modification employs a pseudofenestrated or semifenestrated blade.
- **Elliot:** fenestrated blades with convergent handles. The lesser cephalic curve is suited for the unmolded head and when traction is desired.
- **Tucker-McLane:** solid blades with convergent handles. The lesser cephalic curve is suited for the unmolded head in situations requiring minimal traction; the Luikart modification employs a pseudofenestrated or semifenestrated blade.
- **Kielland:** minimal pelvic curve. It is ideal for rotation of the vertex from the occiput posterior or transverse position to the occiput anterior position.
- **Piper:** used for delivering the aftercoming head of the breech fetus. The pelvic curve is opposite that of other forceps so that the handles are below the level of the blades

Figure 61-6 illustrates the classification of forceps.

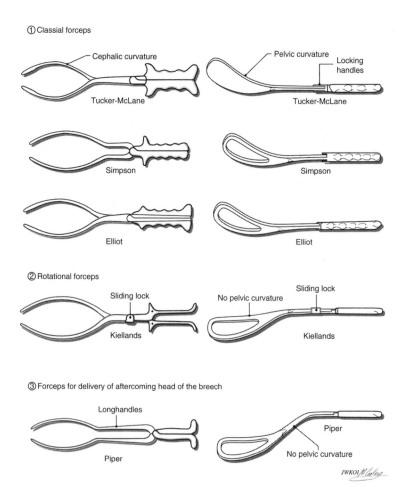

① Classial forceps

Cephalic curvature

Tucker-McLane

Pelvic curvature
Locking handles

Tucker-McLane

Simpson

Simpson

Elliot

Elliot

② Rotational forceps

Sliding lock

Kiellands

No pelvic curvature

Sliding lock

Kiellands

③ Forceps for delivery of aftercoming head of the breech

Longhandles

Piper

Piper

No pelvic curvature

Figure 61-6. Classification of forceps. *(From Norwitz ER, Robinson JN, Repke JT. Labor and delivery. In: Gabbe SG. Niebyl JR, Simpson JL, eds, Obstetrics: Normal and Problem Pregnancies. 4th ed. Philadelphia: Churchill Livingstone; 2002:381.)*

KEY POINTS: LABOR AND VAGINAL DELIVERY

1. Labor begins when uterine contractions of sufficient frequency, intensity, and duration are attained to bring about effacement and progressive dilation of the cervix.

2. A Bishop score is a quantifiable method to assess the likelihood of a successful induction. If unfavorable, cervical ripening can be done by mechanical (e.g., large Foley catheter) or pharmacologic (e.g., prostaglandins, oxytocin) means.

3. Labor has three stages. The first stage (from the onset of contractions to complete dilation) is divided into latent and active phases. Stage 2 is from complete dilation to delivery of fetus, and stage 3 is from delivery of the fetus to delivery of the placenta.

4. The cardinal movements of labor are engagement, descent, flexion, internal rotation, extension, external rotation, and expulsion.

5. Indications for operative vaginal delivery include any condition threatening the mother or fetus during the second stage of labor that is likely to be relieved by delivery.

BIBLIOGRAPHY

1. American College of Obstetricians and Gynecologists. Induction of labor. ACOG practice bulletin no. 107. *Obstet Gynecol.* 2009;114:386–397.
2. American College of Obstetrics and Gynecologists. Vaginal birth after previous cesarean delivery. ACOG practice bulletin no. 115. *Obstet Gynecol.* 2010:1143–1156.
3. Ananth CV, et al. Electronic fetal monitoring in the US: temporal trends and adverse perinatal outcomes. *Obstet Gynecol.* 2013;121:927–933.
4. Baskett TF, Allen AC. Perinatal implications of shoulder dystocia. *Obstet Gynecol.* 1995;86:15.
5. Bishop EH. Pelvic scoring for elective induction. *Obstet Gynecol.* 1964;24:266–268.
6. Buser D, Mora G, Arias F. A randomized comparison between misoprostol and dinoprostone for cervical ripening and labor induction in patients with unfavorable cervices. *Obstet Gynecol.* 1997;89:581–585.
7. Creasy RK, Resnik RI, Iams JD, Lockwood CJ, Moore TR, eds. *Creasy and Resnik's Maternal-Fetal Medicine: Principles and Practice.* 6th ed. Philadelphia: Saunders; 2009.
8. Cunningham F, Leveno KJ, Bloom SL, et al., eds. *Williams Obstetrics.* 24th ed. New York: McGraw-Hill; 2013.
9. Frigoletto FD, Lieberman E, Lang J, et al. A clinical trial of active management of labor. *N Engl J Med.* 1995;333:745–750.
10. Gherman RB, Ouzounian JG, Goodwin TM. Obstetric maneuvers for shoulder dystocia and associated fetal morbidity. *Am J Obstet Gynecol.* 1998;178:1126.
11. Gilson GJ, Russell DJ, Izquiedero LA. A prospective randomized evaluation of a hygroscopic cervical dilator, Dilapan, in the preinduction ripening of patients undergoing induction of labor. *Obstet Gynecol.* 1996;175:145.
12. Kazzi FM, Bottoms SF, Rosen MG. Efficacy and safety of laminaria digitata for preinduction ripening of the cervix. *Obstet Gynecol.* 1982;60:440–443.
13. Lydon-Rochelle M, Holt VL, Easterling TR, Martin DP. Risk of uterine rupture during labor among women with a prior cesarean delivery. *N Engl J Med.* 2001;345:3–8.
14. Osterman MJ, Martin JA. Recent declines in induction of labor by gestational age. *NCHS Data Brief.* 2014;155:1–8.
15. Spong CY, Berghella V, Wenstrom KD, Mercer BM, Saade GR. Preventing the first cesarean delivery: summary of a joint Eunice Kennedy Shriver National Institute of Child Health and Human Development, Society for Maternal-Fetal Medicine, and American College of Obstetricians and Gynecologists Workshop. *Obstet Gynecol.* 2012;120:1181–1193.
16. Ventura SJ, Martin JA, Curtin SC, Mathews TJ. Births: final data for 1997. *Natl Vital Stat Rep.* 1999;47:1–96.
17. Zhang J, Landy HJ, Branch DW, et al. Contemporary patterns of spontaneous labor with normal neonatal outcomes. *Obstet Gynecol.* 2010;116:1281–1287.

CHAPTER 62

INTRAPARTUM FETAL SURVEILLANCE

Laurin Cristiano, MD

1. **What is intrapartum fetal surveillance, and why is it done?**
   Intrapartum fetal surveillance is how obstetricians monitor the fetal response to labor, and the goals are to identify fetal hypoxia or acidemia and intervene early enough to prevent neurologic injury or death. It most frequently refers to fetal heart rate monitoring. Additional, less common techniques include fetal pulse oximetry, fetal scalp blood sampling, vibroacoustic stimulation, and fetal electrocardiography.

2. **How is fetal heart rate monitoring performed?**
   Fetal heart rate monitoring can be divided into intermittent and continuous monitoring. Continuous monitoring can then be further classified as external or internal (Fig. 62-1).
   - **Intermittent auscultation:** Intermittent auscultation is performed using a handheld Doppler device to assess the fetal heart rate periodically. The optimal frequency has not been established, but the most commonly cited protocol involves auscultation every 30 minutes during the first stage of labor and every 15 minutes during the second stage.
   - **Electronic fetal monitoring, external:** An ultrasound transducer and detector device are secured to the maternal abdomen over an area where the fetal heart rate is best detected. The transducer sends out ultrasound waves that are reflected from the motion of the fetal heart back to the transducer. A microprocessor analyses these reflections and transcribes them onto a moving paper reel or through a computer program that displays the fetal heart tracing on a computer screen. The provider can then evaluate the fetal heart pattern.
   - **Electronic fetal monitoring, internal:** A bipolar electrode is attached directly to the fetal scalp, inserted just under the skin. The electrical fetal cardiac signal is then amplified, and the heart rate is calculated. Because the fetal heart rate is measured directly, as opposed to being measured through the maternal abdomen, internal monitoring is a more precise measure of fetal status.

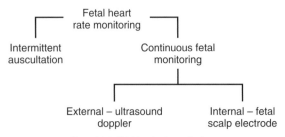

Figure 62-1. Fetal heart rate monitoring.

3. **Is electronic fetal monitoring superior to intermittent auscultation?**
   Multiple clinical trials comparing electronic monitoring with intermittent auscultation showed no clear benefit. However, these studies were limited to normal, uncomplicated pregnancies. Data also suggest that the protocol for intermittent auscultation is successfully followed only a small percentage of the time. For these reasons, electronic monitoring is most frequently the method of intrapartum surveillance in labor and delivery units.

4. What parameters should be documented when electronic fetal monitoring is used?
   When reading a fetal heart tracing, it is important to make note of the following:
   • Baseline
   • Variability
   • Presence or absence of accelerations
   • Presence or absence of decelerations

5. What is meant by the term "baseline"?
   The baseline is the mean fetal heart rate rounded to increments of 5 beats per minute (bpm) during a 10-minute segment. The baseline must be present for at least 2 minutes during this period; a change lasting more than 2 minutes represents the establishment of a new baseline (not necessarily an acceleration or a deceleration).

6. What is a normal baseline, and what are some causes of baseline abnormalities?
   A normal baseline is 110 to 160 bpm. Tachycardia is a baseline greater than 160 bpm, and it can be caused by maternal infection (e.g., viral illness, pyelonephritis, or chorioamnionitis), a fetal arrhythmia, or administration of drugs such as terbutaline. It can also be an early indication of fetal compromise. Bradycardia is a baseline lower than 110 bpm, and it can be caused by maternal hypovolemia, fetal heart block, and late or severe fetal compromise.

7. What is meant by the term "variability"?
   Beat-to-beat variability is the small-scale oscillation of the baseline heart rate; it results from the interplay between sympathetic and parasympathetic activity on the sinoatrial node. Variability is characterized by the amplitude of the difference in peaks and troughs in beats per minute:
   • Absent variability: No change in the amplitude occurs from beat to beat.
   • Minimal variability: Change in amplitude is detectable, but less than 5 bpm.
   • Moderate variability: Change in amplitude is 6 to 25 bpm; this is considered normal.
   • Marked variability: Change in amplitude is greater than 25 bpm.

8. What can cause changes in variability?
   Increased variability can be caused by fetal breathing or fetal movement. Decreased variability can result from fetal acidemia, maternal administration of analgesic drugs, or maternal administration of magnesium sulfate. Decreased variability is considered to be the most reliable warning sign of fetal compromise, and it should always prompt heightened awareness and close surveillance.

9. What is meant by the term "acceleration"?
   Accelerations are visually apparent increases in the fetal heart rate, and they are often associated with fetal movement or stimulation. Before 32 weeks of gestation, the acceleration must be at least 10 bpm from the baseline and last 10 seconds or more. After 32 weeks of gestation, this increase must be at least 15 bpm higher than the baseline and last 15 seconds or more.

10. What is meant by the term "deceleration"?
    A deceleration is a visually apparent decrease in the fetal heart rate from an established baseline. The four types of decelerations are early, late, variable, and prolonged.

11. What is an early deceleration?
    Early decelerations are usually caused by fetal head compression during active labor. They are characterized by a gradual decrease in the fetal heart rate, and they last 30 seconds or more from onset to nadir, which coincides with the peak of a uterine contraction (Fig. 62-2). These decelerations are *not* associated with tachycardia, loss of variability, fetal hypoxia, academia, or low Apgar scores.

12. What is a late deceleration?
    Late decelerations indicate decreased oxygen delivery to the fetus secondary to uteroplacental insufficiency, maternal hypotension, excessive uterine activity, or placental abruption. Similar to early decelerations, they are characterized by a gradual decrease in fetal heart rate lasting 30 seconds or more from onset to nadir (Fig. 62-3). Unlike early decelerations, the nadir occurs *after* the peak of a contraction.

13. What is a variable deceleration?
    Variable decelerations are caused by umbilical cord compression. They are characterized by an abrupt decrease in the fetal heart rate, and they reach a nadir in less than 30 seconds. The decrease is 15 bpm or more and lasts between 15 seconds and 2 minutes (Fig. 62-4).

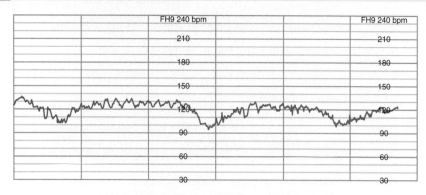

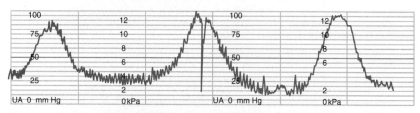

Figure 62-2. Early decelerations. *bpm,* Beats per minute; *FH,* fetal heart rate; *UA,* uterine activity. *(From Bashore RA, Koos BJ. Fetal surveillance during labor. In: Hacker NF, Gambone JG, Hobel CJ, eds.* Hacker and Moore's Essentials of Obstetrics and Gynecology. *5th ed. Philadelphia: Elsevier; 2010.)*

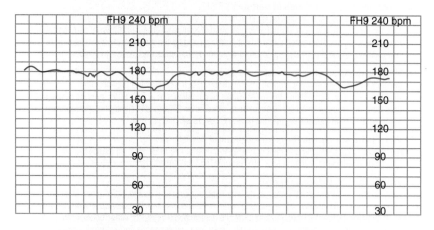

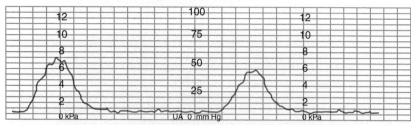

Figure 62-3. Late decelerations. *bpm,* Beats per minute; *FH,* fetal heart rate; *UA,* uterine activity. *(From Bashore RA, Koos BJ: Fetal surveillance during labor. In: Hacker NF, Gambone JG, Hobel CJ, eds.* Hacker and Moore's Essentials of Obstetrics and Gynecology. *5th ed. Philadelphia: Elsevier; 2010.)*

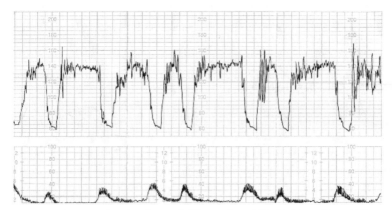

Figure 62-4. Variable deceleration. *(From Westgate JA, Wibbens B, Bennet L, Wassink G, Parer JT, Gunn AJ. The intrapartum deceleration in center stage: a physiologic approach to the interpretation of fetal heart rate changes in labor. Am J Obstet Gynecol. 2007;197:236.e1-236.e11.)*

14. What is a prolonged deceleration?

Prolonged decelerations are caused by sustained interruption of oxygen delivery to the fetus. They can result from uterine tachysystole, placental abruption, tightening of umbilical cord knots, umbilical cord prolapse, maternal shock, maternal hypoxia, or maternal hypotension. (Fig. 62-5). They are characterized by a decrease in the fetal heart rate of 15 bpm or more and last between 2 and 10 minutes; any deceleration lasting longer than 10 minutes is considered a baseline change.

Prolonged decelerations are associated with fetal death if they are not managed appropriately.

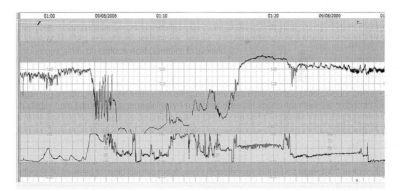

Figure 62-5. Prolonged deceleration. *(From Ugwumadu A. Understanding cardiotocographic patterns associated with intrapartum fetal hypoxia and neurologic injury. Best Pract Res Clin Obstet Gynaecol. 2013;27:509-536.)*

15. What is a sinusoidal fetal heart rate pattern?

A sinusoidal pattern is a smooth, sine wave–like undulation of the fetal heart rate. It has regular oscillations with an amplitude between 5 and 15 bpm around a fixed baseline anywhere between 120 and 160 bpm. The cycle frequency is two to five cycles/minute, and both variability and accelerations are absent. This pattern can occasionally be seen following maternal use of intravenous opioids for pain control (e.g., meperidine, butorphanol, and nalbuphine).

A true sinusoidal pattern not associated with maternal medication is an ominous finding and can be associated with severe fetal hypoxia and acidemia. It has also been reported in cases of severe fetal anemia secondary to causes such as intracranial hemorrhage, Rh alloimmunization, or bleeding vasa previa.

16. **What is the three-tiered fetal heart rate interpretation system?**
To help guide management, fetal heart tracings are placed into three categories based on their characteristics (Table 62-1). Category I is considered normal, category II is indeterminate, and category III is abnormal. The presence of one criterion from a higher category necessarily places the fetus into that category. For example, if the fetal heart rate baseline is 110 to 160 bpm with moderate variability, accelerations, and a prolonged deceleration, the tracing is considered to be category II because of the prolonged deceleration.

Table 62-1. Category Classification Based on Fetal Heart Tracing

CATEGORY	BASELINE	VARIABILITY	ACCELERATIONS	LATE OR VARIABLE DECELERATIONS	EARLY DECELERATIONS
Category I	110-160 bpm	Moderate	Present or absent	Absent	Present or absent
Category II	Bradycardia with variability Tachycardia	Minimal Absent, with no recurrent decelerations Marked	Absent, even after fetal stimulation	Recurrent late or variable decelerations with some variability Prolonged decelerations	Absent
Category III	Bradycardia without variability Sinusoidal pattern	Absent with recurrent decelerations	Absent	Present without variability	Absent

bpm, Beats per minute.

17. **How are category I fetal heart tracings managed?**
Patients can be managed with either continuous electronic monitoring or intermittent auscultation.

18. **How are category II fetal heart tracings managed?**
Because category II includes a wide spectrum of patterns, several different interventions may be helpful in reverting category II to category I tracings (Table 62-2).

Table 62-2. Interventions for Common Category II Findings

FINDING	ETIOLOGY	INTERVENTIONS	RATIONALE
Variable decelerations	Umbilical cord compression	1. Change maternal position 2. Amnioinfusion	1. Move fetus off cord 2. Increase fluid around fetus to relieve compression
Late decelerations	Uteroplacental insufficiency	1. Change maternal position 2. Fluid bolus 3. Supplemental oxygen 4. Decrease/turn off Pitocin 5. Tocolytic (terbutaline)	1. Decrease pressure on inferior vena cava 2. Relieve maternal hypotension 3. Increase maternal oxygenation 4. Resolve tachysystole 5. Stop contractions; relieve tetanic contractions
Tachycardia	Maternal infection	1. Antibiotics 2. Heightened surveillance	1. Treat infection 2. Evaluate for signs of fetal compromise, such as placental abruption or fetal bleeding

Table 62-2. Interventions for Common Category II Findings *(Continued)*

FINDING	ETIOLOGY	INTERVENTIONS	RATIONALE
Prolonged decelerations, fetal bradycardia	Cord prolapse, rapid fetal descent, tachysystole	1. Examine for umbilical cord 2. Noninvasive resuscitation 3. Terbutaline 4. If no resolution, immediate delivery	1. Rule out cord prolapse 2. Increase uteroplacental perfusion as above 3. Stop contractions 4. Prolonged fetal bradycardia, especially with minimal variability or absent variability, is a sign of impending fetal compromise
Minimal variability	Fetal sleep cycle, uteroplacental insufficiency	1. Expectant management 2. VAS, scalp stimulation 3. Noninvasive resuscitation	1. Sleep cycles last 20-60 minutes 2. Wake fetus if in a sleep cycle 3. Increase uteroplacental perfusion

VAS, Vibroacoustic stimulation.

19. **What is amnioinfusion?**

    Amnioinfusion is the introduction of fluid into the uterus to relieve umbilical cord compression after fetal membranes have been ruptured. Although protocols can vary, they all involve placement of an intrauterine catheter, an initial bolus of fluid, and subsequent infusion at a steady rate (frequently 2 to 3 mL/minute). Either normal saline or lactated Ringer solution is acceptable.

20. **How are category III fetal heart tracings managed?**

    Because of their association with acidemia and poor neonatal outcomes, category III tracings require immediate attention. If resuscitative interventions are successful and the tracing reverts to category I or II, labor may proceed with heightened surveillance. If resuscitative interventions fail, delivery should be expedited (often by cesarean section).

21. **What are the other methods of intrapartum fetal surveillance?**

    Table 62-3 is an overview of ancillary methods of intrapartum fetal surveillance.

Table 62-3. Ancillary Methods of Intrapartum Fetal Surveillance

METHOD	DESCRIPTION	EVIDENCE	COMMENTS
Fetal pulse oximetry	Evaluates fetal oxyhemoglobin saturation	No change in cesarean rates No difference in outcomes	Not used outside of research
Fetal scalp sampling	Assesses blood pH to identify or confirm fetal acidemia	Slight decrease in cesarean rates	Rarely used because of difficulty obtaining and analyzing an adequate sample
Fetal electrocardiography	Known ST-segment and T-wave changes occur with fetal hypoxia	No change in cesarean rates No reduction in cases of fetal acidemia	Not used outside of research
Vibroacoustic stimulation (VAS)	In nonacidotic fetuses, fetal heart rate accelerates in response to VAS	Can predict fetal acidosis in the setting of variable decelerations, but not late decelerations	Currently used in clinical practice

22. **What is the role of uterine monitoring in intrapartum fetal surveillance?**
    Placental perfusion is temporarily decreased during a contraction, which challenges fetal oxygen reserves and may result in late decelerations. Monitoring uterine contractions can help identify the type of decelerations present and determine the cause of an abnormal fetal heart tracing. For more information on uterine monitoring, see Chapter 61.

KEY POINTS: INTRAPARTUM FETAL SURVEILLANCE

1. The goals of intrapartum fetal surveillance are to identify fetal hypoxia or acidemia and intervene early enough to prevent neurologic injury or death.
2. Accelerations are visually apparent increases in the fetal heart rate. After 32 weeks of gestation, the minimum requirements are an increase of 15 bpm or more above baseline and a duration of 15 seconds or more.
3. Accelerations and moderate beat-to-beat variability on a fetal heart tracing are considered reassuring.
4. A three-tiered system is used to categorize fetal heart rate and help guide management; Category I is considered normal.
5. Repeat variable, late, and prolonged decelerations are abnormal. They should prompt noninvasive interventions and heightened surveillance.
6. Monitoring uterine contractions can help identify the type of decelerations present and determine the cause of an abnormal fetal heart tracing.

BIBLIOGRAPHY

1. American College of Obstetricians and Gynecologists. Intrapartum fetal heart rate monitoring: nomenclature, interpretation, and general management principles. ACOG practice bulletin no. 106. *Obstet Gynecol*. 2009;114:192–202.
2. American College of Obstetricians and Gynecologists. Management of intrapartum fetal heart rate tracings. ACOG practice bulletin no. 116. *Obstet Gynecol*. 2010;116:1232–1240.
3. Bashore R, Koos B. Fetal surveillance during labor. In: Hacker N, Gambone J, Hobel C, eds. *Hacker and Moore's Essentials of Obstetrics and Gynecology*. 5th ed. Philadelphia: Saunders; 2010:119–127.
4. Beckmann C, Ling F, Barzandsky B, et al. *Obstetrics and Gynecology*. 6th ed. Baltimore: Lippincott Williams & Wilkins; 2010.
5. Creasy R, Resnik R, Iams J, Lockwood CJ, Moore TR, eds. *Creasy and Resnik's Maternal-Fetal Medicine: Principles and Practice*. 6th ed. Philadelphia: Saunders; 2009.
6. Cunningham F, Leveno K, Bloom S, Spong C, Dash J. *Williams Obstetrics*. 24th ed. New York: McGraw-Hill; 2014.
7. Modanlou HD, Murata Y. Sinusoidal heart rate pattern: reappraisal of its definition and clinical significance. *J Obstet Gynaecol Res*. 2004;30:169–180.
8. Ugwumadu A. Understanding cardiotocographic patterns associated with intrapartum fetal hypoxia and neurologic injury. *Best Pract Res Clin Obstet Gynaecol*. 2013;27:509–536.
9. Westgate JA, Wibbens B, Bennet L, Wassink G, Parer JT, Gunn AJ. The intrapartum deceleration in center stage: a physiologic approach to the interpretation of fetal heart rate changes in labor. *Am J Obstet Gynecol*. 2007;197:236. e1–236.e11.

CHAPTER 63

CESAREAN DELIVERY AND VAGINAL BIRTH AFTER CESAREAN DELIVERY

Erin C. Chong, MD

1. **What is a cesarean delivery (CD)?**
   A CD is an abdominal (as opposed to vaginal) delivery. The rate of CDs has dramatically increased over recent decades, from 5% in 1970 to more than 30% in 2007; it is one of the most common surgical procedures performed worldwide.

2. **What are the indications for a CD?**
   The three most common indications are (1) labor dystocia, (2) nonreassuring fetal heart tracing, and (3) fetal malpresentation. Other indications include the following:
   - Fetal or placental indications
     - Fetal anomaly that precludes vaginal delivery (e.g., large omphalocele, macrocephaly)
     - Malpresentation (e.g., breech presentation, transverse lie)
     - Fetal macrosomia (>4500 g in a diabetic woman or >5000 g in a nondiabetic woman)
     - Placenta previa
     - Vasa previa
     - Placental abruption with nonreassuring fetal heart tracing
     - Umbilical cord prolapse
   - Maternal indications
     - History of a classical CD or CD with a T-shaped incision
     - History of more than two previous CDs
     - History of myomectomy or significant uterine surgical intervention
     - Inability to labor (e.g., severe cardiac disease in which the Valsalva maneuver should be avoided)
     - Mechanical obstruction (e.g., uterine fibroids or pelvic mass obstructing the internal os)
     - Infection (active or prodromal herpes, human immunodeficiency virus [HIV] infection with a viral load >1000 copies/mL)
     - Maternal request (elective)
     - Worsening maternal illness requiring urgent or emergency delivery (e.g., HELLP [hemolysis, elevated liver enzymes, low platelets] syndrome, preeclampsia with severe features)

3. **How is a CD performed?**
   A CD begins with a low transverse skin incision; vertical incisions are used in a minority of cases. The underlying layers of fat and fascia are incised and extended to accommodate the size of the infant. In general, the rectus muscles are dissected off the fascia before entering the peritoneum.

   Once the uterus is exposed, it is inspected to determine which type of uterine incision to use. The most common choice is a transverse incision made across the lower uterine segment, referred to as a "low transverse incision." If the lower uterine segment is poorly developed (which can occur in preterm deliveries) or the fetus is in a position that may render delivery difficult, a vertical incision may be chosen.

   Once the uterine incision is made, an amniotomy is performed if necessary, and the infant is delivered. The umbilical cord is clamped and cut, and the infant is handed to a waiting pediatric or nursing team. The placenta is delivered, and the uterine incision is closed with suture. After hemostasis is confirmed, the abdominal incision is closed and the skin is reapproximated with suture or surgical staples.

4. **What other types of uterine incisions may be used during a CD, and why?**
   - **Classical** incision: a vertical incision through the contractile portion of the uterus. The lower margin may begin as low as the lower uterine segment, and the upper margin may cross the

fundus. This incision is used in cases of preterm deliveries when the lower segment is poorly developed, in the presence of an anterior placenta previa (to avoid disrupting the placental bed before delivery of the infant), and with fetal malpresentation (i.e., transverse lie with the back oriented toward the cervix).

- **Low vertical** incision: This begins within the lower uterine segment and ends at a point below the insertion of the round ligaments. This incision is chosen for similar reasons as a classical incision, but it attempts to preserve the potential for vaginal delivery in subsequent pregnancies. Extending the incision upward and converting it into a classic incision may be necessary.
- **T-shaped** incision: This occurs after a low transverse incision is made and found to be inadequate for delivery of the infant; the myometrium is incised upward as high into the uterus as needed to allow for delivery.

5. **What are the potential complications of a CD?**
The most common complications are the same as those for most major surgical procedures. They include pain, infection, bleeding, and injury to adjacent organs. An estimated blood loss up to 1000 mL is considered normal, and transfusions (with their own associated risks) are not uncommon. A risk of intraoperative fetal injury also exists. Less common complications include venous thromboembolism, pulmonary embolism, adverse reaction to anesthesia, ileus, and small bowel obstruction. Rarely, a hysterectomy must be performed because of uncontrollable bleeding or placenta accreta (known or unexpected). Other uncommon complications include maternal or fetal death, which can also occur in vaginal deliveries.

A long-term risk associated with CD is a higher rate of complications in future pregnancies. A history of a previous CD increases blood loss and operative time in subsequent CDs, conveys the risk of uterine rupture during an attempted vaginal delivery, and increases the risk of abnormal placentation (placenta previa, accreta, or increta; for more information on this topic, see Chapter 66).

6. **What are the risks and benefits of CD versus vaginal delivery?**
Both CDs and vaginal deliveries have risks. Overall, CDs have a higher rate of maternal morbidity (9.2% for CD versus 8.6% for vaginal delivery). These morbidities include wound infection, hematoma, hemorrhage requiring transfusion, hysterectomy, venous thromboembolism, and longer hospital stay. However, women who had vaginal deliveries are more likely to develop pelvic organ prolapse and urinary incontinence compared with those who had CDs.

With respect to fetal risks, shoulder dystocia complicates approximately 1% to 3% of vaginal deliveries and 0% of CDs. Brachial plexus injuries, however, can still occur before or during CD. Infants delivered by CD without preceding labor are more likely to experience respiratory distress.

Maternal mortality is higher for CDs compared with vaginal delivery (13.3 in 100,000 vs. 3.6 in 100,000, respectively); vaginal delivery is recommended over CD, particularly in women who plan to have multiple pregnancies.

7. **Can CDs be performed by maternal request in the absence of maternal or fetal indications?**
Yes. CDs on maternal request comprise an estimated 2% of all CDs in the United States. To avoid neonatal risks associated with early term delivery, these CDs are performed at or after 39 weeks of gestation. Reasons given by patients who request a CD include fear of pain during childbirth, convenience, negative past experiences in labor, concerns for long-term changes in pelvic floor function (e.g., pelvic organ prolapse, incontinence), and concern for fetal well-being. Providers must be sure that these women have been adequately counseled on the risks and benefits of both modes of delivery.

8. **Does having one CD commit a woman to having CDs for all subsequent pregnancies?**
No. As long as the previous uterine incision did not extend into the contractile portion of the uterus, a trial of labor after cesarean (referred to as TOLAC) may be considered.

9. **What is the difference between a TOLAC and vaginal birth after cesarean (VBAC)?**
A TOLAC refers to the attempt at a vaginal delivery. It may result in either a vaginal birth (VBAC) or a repeat CD (i.e., failed TOLAC).

10. **What are the benefits of VBAC compared with repeat CD?**
- Faster recovery time
- Avoidance of a major surgical procedure
- Improved infant outcomes

- Lower blood loss
- Lower chance of abnormal placentation in future pregnancies

11. **What are the risks of TOLAC compared with repeat CD?**
Both TOLAC and repeat CD are associated with risks of hemorrhage, infection, thromboembolic disease, uterine rupture, and even maternal and fetal death. However, most of the morbidity surrounding a TOLAC is associated with the need for an eventual CD; compared with an elective repeat CD, a failed TOLAC has a higher complication rate.

12. **What is uterine rupture, and how is it managed?**
Uterine rupture is the separation of the layers of the uterine wall that results in a direct communication between the uterine and abdominal cavities. Potential sequelae include placental abruption, hemorrhage requiring transfusion, hysterectomy, fetal neurologic injury from hypoxia, and fetal death.
Uterine rupture is an obstetric emergency; once it is suspected, an emergency CD should be performed as quickly and safely as possible. Obstetric, anesthesia, pediatric, and nursing teams should all be made aware of the situation. Blood products should be ordered and readily available.

13. **What are the signs and symptoms of uterine rupture?**
- Nonreassuring fetal heart tracing
- Loss of fetal station
- Sudden severe abdominal or supraclavicular pain
- Heavy vaginal bleeding
- Maternal hemodynamic instability

14. **What are risk factors for uterine rupture, and what are the rates associated with each?**
Table 63-1 provides an overview of risk factors for uterine rupture.

Table 63-1. Risk Factors for Uterine Rupture and Their Associated Rates

RISK FACTOR	RATE OF RUPTURE
One prior low transverse uterine incision	<1%
One prior low vertical uterine incision	<1%
Two prior low transverse uterine incisions	<2%
Labor induction or augmentation	~1%
Short interpregnancy interval (<18 months)	4.8%
Prior classic or T-shaped uterine incision	4%-9%

15. **What characteristics make a patient more likely to have a successful TOLAC?**
Factors that increase the likelihood of success include a history of a previous vaginal delivery or VBAC and the onset of spontaneous labor (as opposed to labor induction).

16. **What characteristics make a patient less likely to have a successful TOLAC?**
TOLAC success rates are lower for women who are obese, are older than 35 years of age, have preeclampsia, have a macrosomic fetus, are not of white ethnicity, and are at more than 40 weeks of gestational age. Success is also less likely for women with a history of CD for labor dystocia.

17. **What are contraindications to TOLAC?**
Any features that preclude vaginal delivery also preclude TOLAC. Other contraindications reflect an unacceptably high risk of uterine rupture: more than two earlier CDs, history of a classical or T-shaped uterine incision, history of uterine rupture in a previous TOLAC, or history of significant uterine surgical intervention (e.g., transfundal uterine surgical procedure, repair of developmental anomaly). With the exception of having more than two previous CDs, patients with these contraindications should be delivered by repeat CD before the onset of labor (usually 37 to 38 weeks of gestation).

18. **Can women attempting TOLAC undergo induction of labor?**
Yes. Although rates of uterine rupture associated with induction of labor (without use of prostaglandins) are greater than rates in women who present in spontaneous labor, this risk is still approximately 1%. Augmentation with oxytocin also increases the risk of rupture, but this risk is also approximately 1%.
Prostaglandins are not recommended for induction of labor in women with a previous CD because of the increased risk of uterine rupture (>2%).

19. **Can TOLAC be attempted in twin pregnancies?**
Yes. For more information about vaginal delivery of twins, see Chapter 60.

20. **What about patients who desire an elective or elective repeat CD but have a pregnancy with poor dating?**
Two options exist for these patients: (1) await an indication for delivery (spontaneous labor, rupture of membranes, abnormal fetal surveillance) or (2) perform amniocentesis to assess for fetal lung maturity. For more information on adequate pregnancy dating, see Chapter 38.

21. **How is fetal lung maturity assessed?**
Amniocentesis is performed using ultrasound guidance, and then the sample of amniotic fluid is tested for signs of lung maturity by using either biochemical or biophysical tests. These tests include the lecithin-to-sphingomyelin ratio, lamellar body count, and testing for the presence of phosphatidylglycerol (Table 63-2).

Table 63-2. Tests Used to Determine Fetal Lung Maturity

TEST	POSITIVE VALUE	COMMENTS
Lecithin-to-sphingomyelin ratio (L/S ratio)	2:1	Affected by blood and meconium
Lamellar body count (LBC)	50,000 lamellar bodies/μL	Affected by blood, meconium, and severe polyhydramnios
Phosphatidylglycerol (PG)	Present	*Not* affected by blood or meconium

KEY POINTS: CESAREAN DELIVERY AND VAGINAL BIRTH AFTER CESAREAN

1. A CD is one of the most common surgical procedures performed worldwide, and it usually involves a transverse incision in the lower segment of the uterus.
2. The three most common indications for a CD are labor dystocia, nonreassuring fetal heart tracing, and malpresentation.
3. Compared with vaginal deliveries, CDs have higher rates of maternal morbidity and mortality. A long-term risk associated with CD is a higher rate of complications in future pregnancies.
4. As long as a patient has not had more than two CDs and any previous uterine incisions did not extend into the contractile portion of the uterus, a TOLAC may be considered.
5. A successful TOLAC is associated with fewer maternal and neonatal complications compared with a scheduled repeat CD. However, a scheduled repeat CD has fewer complications than a failed TOLAC.

BIBLIOGRAPHY

1. American College of Obstetrics and Gynecologists. Vaginal birth after previous cesarean delivery. ACOG practice bulletin no. 115. *Obstet Gynecol.* 2010;116:1143–1156.
2. American College of Obstetricians and Gynecologists. Cesarean delivery on maternal request. ACOG committee opinion no. 559. *Obstet Gynecol.* 2013;121:904–907.
3. American College of Obstetricians and Gynecologists. Society for Maternal-Fetal Medicine, Caughey AB, Cahill AG, Guise JM, Rouse DJ. Safe prevention of the primary cesarean delivery. *Am J Obstet Gynecol.* 2014;210:179–193.
4. Bujold E, Gauthier RJ. Risk of uterine rupture associated with an interdelivery interval between 18 and 24 months. *Obstet Gynecol.* 2010;115:1003–1006.

5. Ecker J. Elective cesarean delivery on maternal request. *JAMA*. 2013;309:1930.

6. Guise J, McDonach M, Osterweil P. Systematic review of the incidence and consequences of uterine rupture in women with previous cesarean section. *BMJ*. 2004;329:1–7.

7. Hofmeyr GJ, Barrett JF, Crowther CA. Planned caesarean section for women with a twin pregnancy. *Cochrane Database Syst Rev*. 2011;12. CD006553.

8. Landon M. Predicting uterine rupture in women undergoing trial of labor after cesarean delivery. *Semin Perinatol*. 2010;34:267–271.

9. Liu S, Liston RM, Joseph KS, Heaman M, Sauve R, Kramer MS. Maternal mortality and severe morbidity associated with low-risk planned cesarean delivery versus planned vaginal delivery at term. Maternal Health Study Group of the Canadian Perinatal Surveillance System. *CMAJ*. 2007;176:455–460.

10. Leung AS, Leung EK, Paul RH. Uterine rupture after previous cesarean delivery: maternal and fetal consequences. *Am J Obstet Gynecol*. 1993;169:945–950.

11. Mercer B. Assessment and induction of fetal pulmonary maturity. In: 7th ed. Creasy R, Resnik R, Iams JD, Lockwood CJ, Moore TR, eds. *Creasy and Resnik's Maternal-Fetal Medicine: Principles and Practice*. Philadelphia: Saunders; 2014. 507.e3–515.e3.

12. Silver RM, Landon MB, Rouse DJ, et al. Maternal morbidity associated with multiple repeat cesarean deliveries. *Obstet Gynecol*. 2006;107:1226–1232.

CHAPTER 64

OBSTETRIC ANESTHESIA

Daniela Karagyozyan, MD, Lee Coleman, MD, and Mark Zakowski, MD

1. **What is an obstetric anesthesiologist?**
   The obstetric anesthesiologist is a physician who is board certified in anesthesiology and has a special interest and focus in obstetric anesthesia. His or her primary objective is to deliver comprehensive perioperative and critical care to the obstetric patient. Although the most common activity is to provide pain control during delivery that is safe for both mother and fetus, the obstetric anesthesiologist serves as a consultant to the obstetrician to assist not only with pain management but also with management of complex medical conditions, surgical emergencies, and complications that arise from pregnancy and delivery.

2. **Why have a physician dedicated to pain management during labor and delivery?**
   Labor and delivery result in severe pain for most women. The pain of childbirth was rated greater than that of a fractured arm and cancer pain; only causalgia and amputation of a digit exceeded the pain of labor and delivery (Fig. 64-1). Patients describe the pain as sharp, cramping, aching, throbbing, stabbing, hot, shooting, and tight. The American College of Obstetricians and Gynecologists (ACOG) and the American Society of Anesthesiologists (ASA) state: "There is no other circumstance where

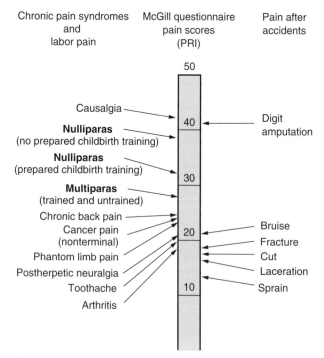

Figure 64-1. Patient ratings of labor pain compared with general patient ratings of other pain. Comparison of pain scores obtained through the McGill pain questionnaire. *(Modified from Melzack R. The myth of painless childbirth [the John J. Bonica lecture]. Pain. 1984;19:321-337. As modified in Pan PH, Eisenach JC. The pain of childbirth and its effect on the mother and the fetus. In: Chestnut DH, Wong CA, Tsen LC, et al, eds. Chestnut's Obstetric Anesthesia: Principles and Practice. 5th ed. Philadelphia: Saunders; 2014:410-426.)*

it is considered acceptable for an individual to experience untreated severe pain, amenable to safe intervention, while under a physician's care. In the absence of a medical contraindication, maternal request is sufficient medical indication for pain relief during labor."

3. **What are the stages of labor?**
   Stage 1: Onset of uterine contractions and cervical dilation. It ends with complete dilation (10 cm) of the cervix.
   Stage 2: It begins with full dilation of the cervix and ends with delivery of the infant.
   Stage 3: It extends from delivery of the infant to delivery of the placenta.

   Anesthesiologists are actively involved in managing pain and the hemodynamic changes and complications during all three stages of labor and into the postpartum period.

4. **What causes pain in the first stage of labor?**
   Pain during the first stage of labor is primarily the result of dilation of the cervix and uterine contractions. Pressure and stretching of the uterine muscles activate high-threshold mechanoreceptors. The pain is visceral, being strong and dull and occurring over the lower abdomen between the umbilicus and the symphysis pubis. It responds only partially to opioids, with epidural analgesia being the "gold standard" for pain relief. Use of oxytocin, which increases the strength and frequency of uterine contractions, increases labor pain (and thus epidural analgesia usage).

5. **What is the perceived location of pain during the first stage of labor?**
   The location can be explained by the concept of referred pain. The sensory nerves of the uterus and cervix leave the cervix and join the sympathetic nerves as they pass through the hypogastric plexus to the sympathetic chain, synapsing within the dorsal horn of the spinal cord at T10, T11, T12, and L1 (Fig. 64-2). This area of the spinal cord receives not only these visceral high-threshold afferents, but also low-threshold cutaneous afferents of the skin. Because of the convergence of somatic and visceral fibers in the same area of the spinal cord, patients interpret uterine pain as originating from the cutaneous afferents of these spinal segments and localize it to the lower abdomen.

6. **What causes pain in the second stage of labor?**
   Pain during the second stage occurs as the fetus descends through the birth canal, a movement that results in the stretching and tearing of fascia, skin, and subcutaneous tissue. This somatic pain is transmitted primarily through the pudendal nerve. Unlike visceral pain, it is best treated with local anesthetics. The pudendal nerve is derived from the anterior primary divisions of sacral nerves S2, S3, and S4 (see Fig. 64-2).
   Fetal descent begins during the first stage of labor; patients therefore experience both visceral (uterine) and somatic (birth canal) pain during this time.

7. **How do psychological factors influence labor pain, and how does pain affect the progress of labor?**
   Different psychological factors affect pain perception. Anxiety, depression, and neuroticism have all been implicated as contributing to pain during labor. All these factors are influenced by a patient's age, parity, marital status, and the presence of emotional support and labor coaching, among other factors. Effective childbirth training may help reduce anxiety and the perceived intensity of pain.
   Normal physiologic responses to labor pain such as the release of stress hormones (e.g., cortisol and endorphins) can influence maternal and fetal well-being as well as the progress of labor. The sympathetic nervous system responds to pain by increasing the amount of circulating catecholamines, and this action in turn can (1) decrease uterine activity by β-adrenergic agonism and (2) decrease placental blood flow by α-adrenergic agonism and vasoconstriction. Effective pain relief by epidural analgesia reduces these responses and improve uterines blood flow.

8. **What physiologic changes of pregnancy must an obstetric anesthesiologist consider when designing a plan for analgesia?**
   Major changes occur in maternal physiology throughout pregnancy; those changes occurring early in pregnancy are a result of hormonal factors, whereas those occurring later in pregnancy are a combination of hormonal factors and mechanical effects from the enlarging uterus (Table 64-1).

9. **What is aortocaval compression, and why is it important?**
   Approximately 15% of pregnant women will develop hypotension when lying supine. In this position the gravid uterus obstructs the inferior vena cava, thus decreasing venous return to the heart. This in turn decreases cardiac output. The gravid uterus also compresses the aorta, which decreases

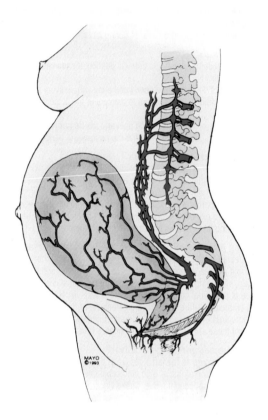

Figure 64-2. Pain pathways during labor and delivery. The afferent pain pathways from the cervix and uterus involve nerves that accompany sympathetic fibers and enter the neuraxis at T10 to L1. The pain pathways for the pelvic floor and perineum include the pudendal nerve fibers, which enter the neuraxis at S2 to S4. *(From Nathan N, Wong CA. Spinal, epidural, and caudal anesthesia: anatomy, physiology, and technique. In: Chestnut DH, Wong CA, Tsen LC, et al, eds. Chestnut's Obstetric Anesthesia: Principles and Practice. 5th ed. Philadelphia: Saunders; 2014:229-260.)*

uterine blood flow. Collateral venous return (through the epidural and azygos veins) and activation of the sympathetic nervous system (resulting in peripheral vasoconstriction and increased heart rate) compensate for this effect in most patients. However, both general anesthesia and regional anesthesia cause sympathetic blockade.

For these reasons, all patients receiving anesthesia or analgesia should maintain left uterine displacement to prevent decreased venous return to the heart, decreased blood pressure and cardiac output, and decreased uterine perfusion. This can be achieved by placing a wedge under the right hip (which tilts the uterus to the left) or tilting the entire operating room table to the left.

10. **How do medications administered to the mother gain access to the fetus?**
The transfer of drugs across the placenta is based primarily on simple diffusion, although other mechanisms such as active transport and facilitated diffusion play a role. Placental transfer is directly proportional to the area available for transfer and to the difference in free drug serum concentrations between the mother and fetus. It is also indirectly proportional to the distance across the intervillous space. Molecular size, lipophilicity, protein binding, degree of ionization, and pH differences can all influence the process of placental transfer. Nearly all anesthetic drugs—opioids, inhaled agents, and local anesthetics—can cross the placenta. Neuromuscular paralyzing agents, however, are large charged molecules and do not cross the placenta in clinically significant amounts.

Table 64-1. Physiologic Changes in Pregnancy and Their Relevance to Obstetric Anesthesia

SYSTEM	PHYSIOLOGIC CHANGES	ANESTHETIC IMPLICATIONS
Cardiovascular	Increased cardiac output Aortocaval compression Decreased systemic vascular resistance	Supine hypotension syndrome Decrease in systolic and diastolic BP
Airway	Capillary engorgement and edema of respiratory mucosa Obesity, breast enlargement	Difficult intubation, smaller endotracheal tube Difficult airway manipulations
Respiratory	Decreased FRC Increased oxygen consumption	Rapid development of hypoxia and acidosis Vulnerable to hypoxia
Gastrointestinal	Delayed gastric emptying Decreased tone of esophageal sphincter	Full stomach consideration Aspiration risk
Neurologic	Increased progesterone	Increased sensitivity to volatile anesthetics Increased sensitivity to local anesthetics
Hematologic	Increased plasma volume > increase in RBC volume Hypercoagulable state: Increased level of fibrinogen and coagulation factors	Physiologic anemia Thromboembolism risk

BP, Blood pressure; *FRC,* functional residual capacity; *RBC,* red blood cell.

11. **What systemic analgesic options are available for labor?**
    Although neuraxial (epidural or spinal) techniques are the preferred form of pain relief, certain comorbidities and conditions such as coagulopathies preclude their use and leave systemic analgesia as the only option.
    - Parenteral: **Meperidine** is used for labor analgesia worldwide, but concerns about its analgesic efficacy and potential neonatal depression (from the active metabolite normeperidine) have limited its use. **Remifentanil** has become a popular alternative because of its very short half-life (6 minutes) and its minimal effect on neonatal outcomes. Patient-controlled analgesia (PCA) with remifentanil provides good analgesia, but it requires close monitoring of the patient because of the risk of sedation and desaturation.
    - Inhalational: **Nitrous oxide (N_2O)** combines analgesic and antianxiety properties. A combination of equal parts N_2O and oxygen is popular in England, especially where access to epidural analgesia is reduced. It is self-administered by a facemask or mouthpiece on an intermittent basis, usually 30 to 60 seconds before a contraction. N_2O is not as effective as epidural analgesia, and major reviews have found insufficient evidence with regard to its efficacy. Side effects include nausea, vomiting, dizziness, and desaturation. Concerns also exist about occupational exposure and fetal effects, although no significant difference in Apgar scores is noted. At present, few locations in the United States offer N_2O for labor analgesia.

12. **What are the differences among the various regional anesthesia techniques?**
    - Neuraxial: epidural block, spinal block, and combined spinal and epidural analgesia
        - **Lumbar epidural analgesia:** the most popular and effective analgesia for both the first and second stages of labor. In 2008, 61% of laboring women in the United States received an epidural block. Analgesia is achieved by injecting local anesthetic, with or without an added opioid, through an epidural catheter. The epidural space is located peripherally to the dura mater and extends from foramen magnum to the sacral hiatus. The ligamentum flavum forms the posterior boundary. The contents of the epidural space include nerve roots, fat, lymphatic tissue, and blood vessels. The epidural space is entered with a needle through the ligamentum flavum and identification relies on the anesthesiologist's sense of feel (loss of resistance technique) (Fig. 64-3). Analgesia is tailored to the patient's labor, medical condition, and individual preferences (e.g., ambulation may be possible with dilute solutions of local anesthetic). Different administration regimens are available: intermittent boluses, continuous infusion, or continuous

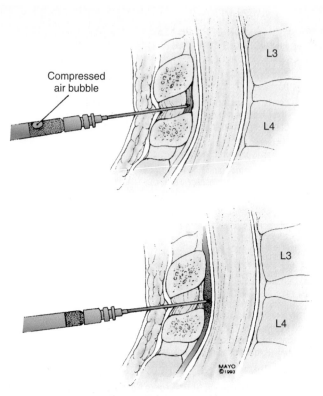

Figure 64-3. Loss-of-resistance technique for identifying the epidural space. The needle is first inserted into the interspinous ligament or ligamentum flavum, and a syringe containing an air bubble in saline is attached to the hub. After compression of the air bubble by pressure on the syringe-plunger, the needle is carefully advanced until a loss of resistance to syringe-plunger pressure is noted as the needle enters the epidural space. *(From Nathan N, Wong CA. Spinal, epidural, and caudal anesthesia: anatomy, physiology, and technique. In: Chestnut DH, Wong CA, Tsen LC, et al, eds. Chestnut's Obstetric Anesthesia: Principles and Practice. 5th ed. Philadelphia: Saunders; 2014:229-260.)*

infusion with boluses administered by the patient. The latter is known patient-controlled epidural analgesia (PCEA). The epidural catheter can also be used to provide surgical anesthesia for a cesarean delivery.

- **Spinal analgesia:** a highly effective, single-shot technique with rapid onset. The total time of analgesia, however, is limited. Medication (local anesthetic or opioid) is injected into the subarachnoid space using a specially designed needle that makes a small hole that tends to self-seal (Fig. 64-4). Because of the lipophilic nature of the drugs that are used, redistribution out of the intrathecal compartment limits the duration of analgesia.
- **Combined spinal-epidural analgesia** involves locating the epidural space with an epidural needle, advancing a spinal needle through the epidural needle until cerebrospinal fluid (CSF) is obtained, injecting local anesthetic or opioid into the CSF, removing the spinal needle, and then threading a catheter into the epidural space. This technique allows for rapid onset of analgesia (because of the spinal portion) and for continuous analgesia (because of the presence of the epidural catheter). Intrathecal use of opioid alone or with a small amount of local anesthetic may not produce a motor blockade, thus allowing for ambulation if desired. Many people refer to this type of block as a "walking epidural," although other epidural analgesic techniques can also allow ambulation.

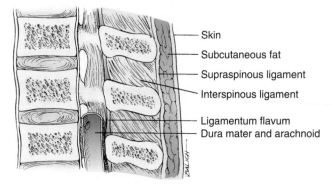

Figure 64-4. Midline sagittal anatomy of the vertebral column. When a needle is placed into the cerebrospinal fluid, it must pass through skin, subcutaneous fat, the supraspinous ligament, the interspinous ligament, the ligamentum flavum, the epidural space, and finally the dura mater and arachnoid. *(From Wong CA, Nathan N, Brown DL. Spinal, epidural, and caudal anesthesia: anatomy, physiology, and technique. In: Chestnut DH, Polley LS, Tsen LC, et al, eds.* Chestnut's Obstetric Anesthesia: Principles and Practice. *4th ed. Philadelphia: Mosby; 2009:223-245.)*

- Alternative regional anesthetic techniques: paracervical block, pudendal block
  - **Paracervical nerve block** involves submucosal injection of local anesthetic into the fornix of the vagina lateral to the cervix (generally at the 4 o'clock and 8 o'clock positions). Somatic sensory fibers of the perineum are not affected, and this technique is effective only for the first stage of labor. It is associated with a relatively high (15%) incidence of fetal bradycardia because of a high rate of uptake of the anesthetic by the fetus. At present, its main analgesic role is in dilation and curettage in the office setting.
  - **Pudendal nerve block** involves transvaginal injection of local anesthetic below the ischial spines (the approximate location of the pudendal nerve). This technique is used during the second stage of labor and may be a good option for operative vaginal delivery if epidural analgesia is not being used.

13. **What are local anesthetics, and which ones are most frequently used for regional blocks in obstetrics?**
    Local anesthetics interfere with the rapid sodium channels in neurons and produce reversible blockade of neural conduction. Their molecular structure consists of an aromatic ring, a linking chain, and a carbon chain bearing an amino group. The two groups of local anesthetics are esters and amides. To remember which class an anesthetic belong to, esters have one "i" in the name (e.g., tetracaine), whereas amides have two "i"s in the name (e.g., lidocaine, bupivacaine). Patients with an allergy to an ester do not necessarily have allergies to amides and vice versa.

    The most frequently used ester local anesthetics in obstetric anesthesia are tetracaine for spinal anesthesia and 2-chloroprocaine for epidural analgesia or anesthesia. Plasma pseudocholinesterase metabolizes ester local anesthetics in the bloodstream and produces the metabolite para-aminobenzoic acid. This metabolite can be a significant allergen.

    The most frequently used amide local anesthetics in obstetric anesthesia are bupivacaine, ropivacaine, and lidocaine. Hypersensitivity reactions to amides are rare, and systemic toxicity involves both the central nervous and cardiovascular systems. At high concentration and dosages, bupivacaine has caused maternal cardiac arrest. However, careful, fractional dosing (i.e., use of a "test dose") almost entirely eliminates these cases. Treatment of local anesthetic toxicity from bupivacaine or ropivacaine includes administration of intravenous (IV) intralipid, which serves as a lipophilic drug sink.

14. **What are the complications of epidural analgesia use in labor and delivery?**
    - **Pain** at the needle insertion site is probably the most common complaint, typically because of a small bruise and lasting for approximately 48 hours. Although retrospective studies suggested that epidural analgesia may be associated with postpartum backache, high-quality prospective studies have found the frequency of postpartum backache similar between patients who do and do not receive epidural analgesia (up to 44%).

- **Hypotension** may result from sympathetic nervous system blockade caused by an epidural. This effect can be attenuated by IV hydration before placement; in the case of significant or persistent hypotension, medical management is required. The most commonly used medications are ephedrine (a mixed α- and β-adrenergic agonist) and phenylephrine (a pure α-adrenergic agonist).
- **Maternal fever:** Women in labor who receive epidural analgesia are more likely to experience fever compared with patients electing other forms of analgesia. The mechanism is unclear, and factors such as altered thermoregulation, the antipyretic effect of systemic opioids, or inflammation are thought to play a role. On average, temperature elevation is 0.5° C over a few hours.
- **Neurologic injury** is almost always related to the birthing process rather than neuraxial anesthetic placement; the incidence of nerve injuries are related epidural analgesia is less than 0.01%. They include trauma to the nerve root, epidural hematoma, and epidural abscess. The lumbosacral trunk, lateral femoral cutaneous nerve, femoral nerve, and the common peroneal nerve are among the more commonly injured nerves.
- **Postdural puncture (also known as "spinal") headache** results from accidental or intended dural puncture. Its incidence is 0.6% to 2.6 % of all epidural procedures and varies based on both the experience level of the practitioner and certain patient characteristics such as maternal age and obesity.

15. What is a "spinal headache," and how is it treated?

Postdural puncture headache (PDPH), formerly called spinal headache, may follow intentional or unintentional puncture of the dura mater. PDPH results from leakage of CSF into the epidural space resulting in loss of the cushion effect when sitting or standing. Pain results from traction on pain-sensitive structures within the cranial cavity and includes severe headache, neck pain, and possible cranial nerve involvement (vision or hearing changes). The headache is frontal and occipital in location, and symptoms are worse with upright positioning. In obstetric patients, the incidence of PDPH is 45% to 80% after accidental dural puncture with an epidural needle and 5% to 8% after puncture with a cutting-edge spinal needle. The lowest rate is for the rounded, "pencil point" spinal needle at 1% to 1.6%.

PDPH generally occurs within 48 hours of dural puncture, but it can occur later than 3 days in up to 25% of cases. It usually resolves within 7 to 10 days (75% of patients). Symptomatic treatment consists of bed rest, IV caffeine, theophylline, sumatriptan, and hydration. The gold standard for treatment is an epidural blood patch, in which 15 to 20 mL of aseptic autologous blood is placed into the epidural space. The blood acts as a plug against further CSF leakage, and 65% to 95% are effective after the first 24 hours. Prophylactic placement before development of PDPH in patients with a known incidental dural puncture has not been shown to be effective.

16. What are contraindications to epidural analgesia in obstetrics?

- Patients' refusal or inability to cooperate
- Increased intracranial pressure
- Frank coagulopathy
- Infection at the site of needle insertion
- Maternal fever or sepsis
- Thrombocytopenia
- Hypovolemia
- Mild isolated coagulation abnormalities are relative contraindications; the decision to proceed with placement depends on the severity of the abnormality and judgment of the anesthesiologist.

17. Does epidural analgesia affect the course of labor?

No. High-quality prospective studies have found that use of epidural analgesia during labor does **not** have a significant effect on cesarean delivery rates. In addition, early initiation of epidural analgesia (usually defined as placement at cervical dilation <4 cm) does **not** increase the risk of cesarean delivery. A Cochrane review of 27 trials involving 8417 patients estimated the relative risk of cesarean delivery associated with epidural analgesia to be 1.1 (95% confidence interval: 0.97 to 1.25). Epidural analgesia was associated with a slightly longer second stage of labor (by an average of 13.66 minutes), as well as increased risks of instrument-assisted vaginal delivery and oxytocin use. However, patients who received epidural analgesia were more satisfied compared with those who received parenteral analgesia and experienced no increased rate of adverse neonatal effects. Studies have also shown no benefit to discontinuing an epidural infusion during the second stage of labor.

18. **What anesthetic options are available for cesarean delivery?**
    Neuraxial anesthesia (spinal, epidural, or combined spinal and epidural) is the preferred method for cesarean deliveries, used for 95% of cesarean deliveries in the United States. Compared with general anesthesia, regional anesthesia provides better hemodynamic control, blunts the neuroendocrine stress response, avoids potentially difficult airway management, and allows a patient to remain awake and able to interact with her newborn.
    - **Spinal anesthesia** is a single-shot technique that has rapid onset and produces a dense surgical block. It requires approximately 5 to 10 minutes before the patient is ready for surgical incision.
    - **Epidural anesthesia** is beneficial when extending the duration of the surgical anesthetic may be needed or when using an existing epidural catheter that was placed for pain management during labor. With a catheter in place, surgical anesthesia can be obtained within 3 to 5 minutes with chloroprocaine.
    - **Combined spinal and epidural anesthesia** offers the benefits of both spinal and epidural techniques.

    General anesthesia is used for emergency cesarean deliveries when no epidural anesthetic has already been placed and no time exists to place a neuraxial block. It is also used in the presence of comorbidities that preclude neuraxial anesthesia.

19. **What is the anesthetic-related mortality rate in obstetric cases?**
    Anesthesia-related maternal mortality accounts for 1.6% of all pregnancy-related deaths. For general anesthesia, mortality has decreased from 16.8 per million live births during 1991 to 1996 to 6.5 per million during 1997 to 2002. During these same time intervals, regional anesthesia rates were 2.5 and 3.8 per million, respectively. In 1997 to 2002, the relative risk ratio for maternal death from general anesthesia compared with regional anesthesia was 1.7.

20. **Why is general anesthesia riskier?**
    Failed intubation and subsequent hypoxia are the primary reasons. Several pregnancy-associated factors increase these risks: (1) capillary engorgement of the mucosa causes swelling of the nasal and oral pharynx, larynx, and trachea; (2) gastric emptying is delayed, increasing the risk for aspiration; and (3) the gravid uterus elevates the diaphragm, thus decreasing the functional residual capacity by 20% in the setting of increased oxygen consumption (by 20% to 35%) because of a higher metabolic rate. Not only are pregnant patients more difficult to intubate, but also intubation must be accomplished quickly. The gravid uterus or abdominal obesity can make mask ventilation difficult, and hypoxemia can develop rapidly.
    Proper airway evaluation and management are the most effective ways of preventing airway problems during induction of general anesthesia. Patients with suspected difficult airways should be identified and treated with alternative techniques such as video laryngoscopy, nonsedated fiberoptic intubation, or regional anesthesia. These patients should also receive consideration for early placement of an epidural catheter during labor.

21. **What is aspiration?**
    Aspiration is when the contents of the stomach gain access to the lungs. Patients who aspirate are at risk for development of aspiration pneumonitis (Mendelson syndrome), which may be fatal. Risk factors for the development of aspiration pneumonitis include the aspiration of a large volume, the aspiration of food, and the aspiration of highly acidic material.

22. **What can be done to prevent aspiration?**
    Aspiration has decreased tremendously in the last 3 decades because of NPO (nothing by mouth) policies for patients in labor, decrease in the use of general anesthesia, and use of nonparticulate antacids, histamine (H_2)-receptor antagonists, and metoclopramide. Although a nonparticulate antacid such as sodium bicitrate instantly neutralizes the acidity of the stomach, H_2-receptor antagonists require more than 40 minutes to become effective. Metoclopramide immediately increases gastroesophageal sphincter tone, but it requires more than 30 minutes to have an effect on gastric emptying.
    General anesthesia abolishes the protective reflexes of the larynx and trachea. When it is used for obstetric patients, rapid-sequence induction with cricoid pressure is standard practice. The cricoid cartilage is the only complete cartilaginous ring of the trachea; application of gentle pressure can occlude the esophagus and prevent passive regurgitation.

23. **Are neonatal outcomes any different between regional and general anesthesia?**

    In general, well-performed general anesthesia with rapid delivery of the infant results in a vigorous infant. A 2012 Cochrane review found no significant difference between regional and general anesthesia in terms of neonatal Apgar scores and the need for neonatal resuscitation with oxygen. Neurobehavioral testing has shown some subtle early differences between infants delivered with general anesthesia and regional anesthesia (better scores in the regional group) but essentially no differences at 24 hours.

    Infants born to mothers who receive general anesthesia have slightly lower Apgar scores at 1 minute but little difference at 5 minutes. The longer a fetus is exposed to a general anesthetic, the greater is the tendency toward a lower Apgar score. Longer intervals between uterine incision and delivery also increase the risk of fetal hypoxia and acidosis from fetal hypoperfusion.

24. **What are the anesthetic risks associated with preeclampsia?**

    Preeclampsia is characterized by a variety of pathophysiologic derangements:
    - Contracted plasma volume: Judicious administration of IV fluids is recommended because these patients are at risk for development of pulmonary edema.
    - Hypersensitivity to catecholamines, both endogenous and exogenous, accompanied by an exaggerated hypertensive response: Epidural analgesia blunts the hypertensive response to pain, dilates arteries, and improves cardiac output and uterine blood flow.
    - Thrombocytopenia or disseminated intravascular coagulation: Platelet count (and sometimes clotting studies) should be obtained *before* placing neuraxial anesthesia, to minimize the risk of spinal or epidural hematoma.
    - Seizures: Magnesium sulfate is the preferred prophylactic treatment for seizures in these patients; however, magnesium can exacerbate the hypotension caused by a neuraxial block and can potentiate neuromuscular blocking agents.

    It is important for the anesthesiologist to be involved early as part of a multidisciplinary team in the management of the blood pressure, fluid status, and delivery method.

25. **What are the causes of obstetric hemorrhage?**

    Obstetric hemorrhage is a major cause of maternal morbidity and mortality worldwide. In the United States, it complicates 3% of deliveries and accounts for 20% of hospital deaths after delivery. Defined as blood loss greater than 500 mL for vaginal delivery and greater than 1000 mL for cesarean delivery, it can be massive and associated with rapid consumption of coagulation factors.

    Uterine blood flow increases from 50 mL/minute during the nonpregnant state to 500 to 700 mL/minute at term. Risk factors for antepartum hemorrhage include placental abruption, placenta previa, uterine rupture, and trauma. After birth and following separation of the placenta, cessation of bleeding in the uterus depends primarily on the ability of the uterus to contract. Uterine atony can cause life-threatening hemorrhage and is present in 80% of cases with postpartum hemorrhage (PPH). Atony is associated with chorioamnionitis, multiparity, polyhydramnios, macrosomia, multiple gestation, prolonged labor, prolonged oxytocin use, medications with tocolytic effects (e.g., magnesium and volatile anesthetic agents), retained placenta, and coagulation abnormalities.

26. **How is an anesthesiologist involved in cases of PPH?**

    An anesthesiologist plays a leading role in resuscitating and monitoring patients with PPH by placing IV access and arterial lines, transfusing blood products, treating coagulopathies, and maintaining maternal homeostasis. (For more information on the management of PPH, see Chapter 68.) For massive transfusions, current recommendations are to transfuse packed red blood cells, fresh frozen plasma, and platelets at a 6:4:1 ratio.

27. **What are the anesthetic implications of tocolytic drugs?**

    - Magnesium sulfate: Side effects include nausea, weakness, and increased sensitivity to muscle relaxants.
    - β-Adrenergic agents: Side effects include hypokalemia, hyperglycemia, and tachycardia, and these drugs increase the risk of pulmonary edema.
    - Calcium channel blockers can cause hypotension.

    For more information on tocolytics, see Chapter 65.

28. **What options are available for postoperative pain control after cesarean delivery?**
    This depends on the anesthetic technique used for the surgical procedure.
    - If **spinal anesthesia** was used, preservative-free morphine is typically included with the local anesthetic. Intrathecal morphine (0.15 to 0.25 mg) provides analgesia for 16 to 24 hours. Side effects include pruritus, nausea and vomiting, and rarely respiratory depression. Respiratory depression has a higher risk of occurring if the patient receives supplemental IV opioids or sedatives.
    - If **epidural anesthesia** was used, 2.5 to 5 mg of morphine administered into the epidural space provides 16 to 24 hours of analgesia. Risks are the same as for intrathecal morphine. Occasionally, epidural infusion of low concentrations of local anesthetic and an opioid can be extended into the postoperative period and the patient given a controller device to augment a basal infusion rate (PCEA).
    - If **general anesthesia** was used, the patient can be offered postoperative IV PCA. With PCA, a pump allows for the continuous infusion of an opioid and for the patient to self-administer boluses when desired. Although programmed limits prevent overdosing, continuous monitoring of ventilation and sedation level is required.
    - **Ultrasound-guided transverse abdominal plane (TAP) block** is an alternative method for postoperative pain control. With this method, local anesthetic is deposited bilaterally between the internal oblique and transverse abdominis muscles. This can help control pain in the abdominal wall, but not the uterus. TAP is usually supplemented with IV pain medications such as ketorolac (a nonsteroidal antiinflammatory drug [NSAID]). Overall, the analgesic effect is inferior to that of intrathecal morphine, but TAP is associated with fewer opioid-related side effects. A TAP block may be a reasonable alternative when opioids are contraindicated or not appropriate.

29. **What are the basic steps in the resuscitation (Advanced Cardiac Life Support [ACLS]) of an obstetric patient?**
    Cardiac arrest during pregnancy occurs in less than 1 in 20,000 women. Leading causes are amniotic fluid embolism (AFE), hemorrhage, preexisting heart disease, trauma, sepsis, and iatrogenic causes (e.g., local anesthetic toxicity, high spinal, allergic reactions). ACLS protocols are applicable to the pregnant patient, but with additional considerations. In 2014 the Society of Obstetric Anesthesia and Perinatology issued a consensus statement that addressed resuscitation efforts in the pregnant patient to optimize maternal and neonatal outcomes:
    - High-quality chest compressions should be performed with hands placed higher on the sternum. This is secondary to elevation of the diaphragm associated with pregnancy.
    - Manual uterine displacement to the left is vital to help achieve adequate venous return to the heart. Tilting the patient may compromise the adequacy of chest compressions.
    - Treat reversible causes (e.g., local anesthetic toxicity, transfuse).
    - If no return of spontaneous circulation occurs within 4 minutes and the fetus is viable, a perimortem cesarean delivery should be performed. The best chance for fetal survival is if delivery is achieved within 5 minutes of the onset of cardiac arrest.

KEY POINTS: OBSTETRIC ANESTHESIA

1. Pain during the first stage of labor is primarily visceral; it results from cervical dilation and uterine contractions and is transmitted by afferents originating in the T10 to L1 segments of the spinal cord.
2. Pain during the second stage of labor is both visceral and somatic; it is transmitted by the same afferents as in the first stage, in addition to afferents from S2 to S4.
3. Lumbar epidural analgesia is the most popular method for pain relief during labor. It is effective for both the first and second stages.
4. Although epidural analgesia is associated with slight prolongation of the second stage and an increased rate of operative vaginal delivery, it does not increase the risk of cesarean delivery or neonatal depression.
5. Spinal anesthesia is the most common method of anesthesia for cesarean delivery; general anesthesia has a higher rate of maternal morbidity.

BIBLIOGRAPHY

1. Afolabi BB, Lesi FE. Regional versus general anesthesia for cesarean section. *Cochrane Database Syst Rev.* 2012;10. CD004350.
2. American College of Obstetricians and Gynecologists. Pain relief during labor. ACOG committee opinion no. 295. *Obstet Gynecol.* 2004;104:213.
3. Bateman BT, Berman MF, Riley LE, Leffert LR. The epidemiology of postpartum hemorrhage in a large, nationwide sample of deliveries. *Anesth Analg.* 2010;110:1368–1373.
4. Baysinger C. Nitrous Oxide for Labor Analgesia. Available at: www.asahq.org/resources/resources-from-ASA-committee/nitrous-oxide
5. Bucklin BA, Hawkins JL, Anderson JR, Ullrich FA. Obstetric anesthesia workforce survey: twenty-year update. *Anesthesiology.* 2005;103:645–653.
6. California Maternal Quality Care Collaborative. OB Hemorrhage Toolkit V 2.0. Available at: https://www.cmqcc.org/ob_hemorrhage. Accessed November 10, 2015.
7. Cambic C, Wong C. Labour analgesia and obstetric outcomes. *Br J Anaesth.* 2010;105:i50–i60.
8. D'Angelo R, Smiley RM, Riley ET, Segal S. Serious complications related to obstetric anesthesia: the serious complication repository project of the Society for Obstetric Anesthesia and Perinatology. *Anesthesiology.* 2014;120:1505–1512.
9. Dutton RP, Lee LA, Stephens LS, Posner KL, Davies JM, Domino KB. Massive hemorrhage: a report from the Anesthesia Closed Claims Project. *Anesthesiology.* 2014;121:450–468.
10. Hawkins JL, Chang J, Palmer SK, Gibbs CP, Callaghan W. Anesthesia-related maternal mortality in the United States:1979-2002. *Obstet Gynecol.* 2011;117:69–74.
11. Kinsella SM, Lohmann G. Supine hypotensive syndrome. *Obstet Gynecol.* 1994;83:774–788.
12. Lang AJ, Sorrell JT, Rogers CS, Lebeck MM. Anxiety sensitivity as a predictor of labor pain. *Eur J Pain.* 2006;10: 263–270.
13. Likis FE, Andrews JC, Collins MR, et al. Nitrous oxide for the management of labor pain: a systematic review. *Anesth Analg.* 2014;118:153–167.
14. Lipman S, Cohen S, Einav S, et al. The Society for Obstetric Anesthesia and Perinatology consensus statement on the management of cardiac arrest in pregnancy. *Anesth Analg.* 2014;118:1003–1016.
15. Loane H, Preston R, Douglas MJ, Massey S. A randomized controlled trial comparing intrathecal morphine with transversus abdominis plane block for post cesarean delivery analgesia. *Int J Obstet Anesth.* 2012;21:112–118.
16. Melzack R. The myth of painless childbirth (the John J. Bonica lecture). *Pain.* 1984;19:321–337.
17. Sachs A, Smiley R. Post-dural puncture headache: the worst common complication in obstetric anesthesia. *Semin Perinatol.* 2014;38:386–394.
18. Segal S. Labor epidural analgesia and maternal fever. *Anesth Analg.* 2010;111:1467–1475.
19. Somuah M, Smyth RMD, Howell CJ. Epidural versus non-epidural or no analgesia in labour. *Cochrane Database Syst Rev.* 2011;12. CD000331.
20. Stocki D, Matot I, Einav S, et al. A Randomized Controlled Trial of the Efficacy and Respiratory Effects of Patient-Controlled Intravenous Remifentanil Analgesia and Patient-Controlled Epidural Analgesia in Laboring Women. *Anesth & Analg.* 2014;118:589–597.
21. Ullman R, Smith LA, Burns E, Mori R, Dowswell T. Parenteral opioids for maternal pain relief in labor. *Cochrane Database Syst Rev.* 2010;9. CD007396.
22. Wali A, Suresh M. Maternal morbidity, mortality, and risk assessment. *Anesthesiol Clin.* 2008;26:197–230.
23. Zakowski MI. Complications associated with regional anesthesia in the obstetric patient. *Semin Perinatol.* 2002;26:154–168.
24. Zakowski MI, Geller A. The placenta: anatomy, physiology, and transfer of drugs. In: Chestnut DH, Wong CA, Tsen LC, et al., eds. *Chestnut's Obstetric Anesthesia: Principles and Practice.* 5th ed. Philadelphia: Saunders; 2014.

PRETERM LABOR AND PRETERM PREMATURE RUPTURE OF MEMBRANES

Enid T. Kuo, MD

CHAPTER 65

1. **How is preterm labor defined?**

   Preterm labor is defined as regular uterine contractions, with or without pain, accompanied by progressive cervical dilation or effacement and occurring between 20 0/7 weeks and 36 6/7 weeks of gestation.

2. **What causes preterm labor?**

   In the majority of cases, the cause of preterm labor is unknown. Most experts agree that infection (urogenital or systemic) may be largest contributor.

3. **What are the risk factors associated with preterm labor?**

   The strongest risk factor is a previous preterm birth, and a history of a previous preterm delivery increases the risk of subsequent preterm birth by up to twofold. Other risk factors are listed in Box 65-1.

Box 65-1. Risk Factors for Preterm Labor

- Previous preterm delivery
- Multiple gestation
- Preterm premature rupture of membranes
- Polyhydramnios
- Placental abruption
- Placenta previa
- Uterine anomalies
- Previous cervical surgical procedures
- Diethylstilbestrol (DES) exposure
- Congenital anomalies or aneuploidy
- Fetal demise
- Extremes of maternal age (<18 or >35 years)
- Low socioeconomic status
- Smoking
- Substance abuse
- Short interpregnancy interval
- Poor nutritional status or low body mass index
- Poor pregnancy weight gain
- Infections (e.g., chorioamnionitis, pyelonephritis, other serious systemic infection)

---

4. **What is the incidence of preterm birth?**

   Although incidence varies with the population studied, preterm birth complicates approximately 12% of all live births in the United States; it is the leading cause of neonatal mortality.

5. **What are the consequences of preterm birth?**

   Prematurity results in increased risk of neonatal morbidity and death, with the majority of neonatal deaths occurring in infants born before 28 weeks of gestation (Fig. 65-1). Major neonatal complications include the following:
   - Neonatal respiratory distress syndrome (RDS)
   - Persistent pulmonary hypertension

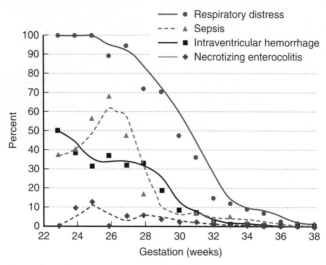

Figure 65-1. Neonatal morbidity by gestational age at birth. Results of a community-based evaluation of 8523 deliveries, 1997 to 1998, Shelby County, Tennessee. Curves are smoothed by a two-point average. *(From Mercer BM. Preterm premature rupture of membranes.* Obstet Gynecol. *2003;101:178.)*

- Bronchopulmonary dysplasia (BPS)
- Intraventricular hemorrhage (IVH)
- Periventricular leukomalacia (PVL)
- Necrotizing enterocolitis (NEC)

6. **What are the rates of survival for preterm infants?**
   Survival estimates by gestational age are as follows:
   - More than 50% at 24 weeks
   - 68% at 25 weeks
   - More than 75% at 26 to 28 weeks
   - More than 90% at 28 weeks and beyond

   These estimates are for mortality alone; although most infants born after 28 weeks survive, only approximately 80% will be free of long-term morbidity. Survival is also affected by accessibility to tertiary neonatal support, as well as the level of provider expertise in neonatal resuscitation and subsequent care. Data suggest that birth weight may correlate better with morbidity and mortality (Table 65-1). An even more accurate estimate can be obtained using the National Institute of Child Health and Human Development (NICHD) website, which takes into account gestational age, birth weight (estimated), sex, and whether antenatal steroids were given: www.nichd.nih.gov/about/org/der/branches/ppb/programs/epbo/Pages/epbo_case.aspx.

Table 65-1. Survival Estimates Based on Birth Weight

WEIGHT (g)	SURVIVED	SURVIVED WITHOUT MORBIDITY
501-750	55%	35%
751-1000	88%	57%
1001-1250	94%	78%
1251-1500	96%	89%

7. **What are common symptoms of preterm labor?**
   - Regular uterine contractions (with or without pain)
   - Pelvic pressure
   - Lower back pain, typically described as dull and constant
   - Abdominal cramping
   - Vaginal spotting or bleeding

8. **How should a patient with possible preterm labor be evaluated?**
   A careful history should be taken and potential risk factors identified. Physical examination should include a pelvic examination to collect cultures for group B streptococcus (GBS), gonorrhea, and *Chlamydia;* if concern exists for ruptured fetal membranes, this should be ruled out first (see question 24). Cervical dilation and effacement should be assessed, and laboratory studies ordered (see question 9). Continuous fetal monitoring with tocometry should be performed in pregnancies of more than 24 weeks of gestation.

9. **What laboratory studies should be ordered?**
   - Complete blood count
   - Urine analysis and culture
   - Cultures for GBS, gonorrhea, and *Chlamydia*
   - Urine toxicology screen if indicated
   - Fetal fibronectin (fFN), which can also help to stratify risk (see question 12)

10. **What imaging studies should be performed?**
    - Transabdominal ultrasound for fetal weight and presentation
    - Transvaginal ultrasound for cervical length

11. **How is cervical length measured, and what is considered normal?**
    After a patient has emptied her bladder, a transvaginal probe is placed in the anterior fornix of the vagina, and the distance of the closed portion of the cervix is measured (Fig. 65-2). In symptomatic women, cervical length is used to assess a patient's risk of preterm delivery within the next 7 days and help direct management.
    - A length less than 20 mm indicates an increased risk of preterm delivery; these patients are generally admitted for closer monitoring and administration of antenatal steroids.
    - A length of 30 mm or greater indicates a low risk of preterm delivery.
    - A length of 20 to 29 mm is an indeterminate range. fFN can be used to provide additional risk assessment (see question 12).

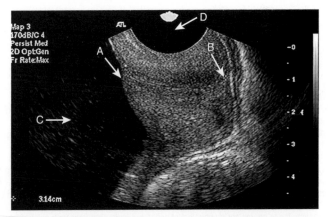

Figure 65-2. Transvaginal ultrasound and sagittal long-axis view of the endocervical canal. The cervical length is measured from the internal os to the external os along the endocervical canal. *A,* Internal os. *B,* External os. *C,* Amniotic fluid. *D,* Ultrasound probe. *(From Bahtiyar MO, Nayeri UA, Shaffer WK. Atlas of selected normal images. In: Copel JA, D'Alton ME, Gratacos E, et al, eds. Obstetric Imaging. Philadelphia: Saunders; 2012:1-12.)*

12. **What is fFN, and how is it used in patients with symptoms of preterm labor?**
fFN is a large glycoprotein found at the interface between the chorion and uterine decidua. It promotes cellular adhesion and is released into the extracellular matrix when the interface between the chorion and decidua is disrupted. A negative test result is fairly reassuring that delivery will not occur in the next 7 to 14 days, with a negative predictive value near 99%. The positive predictive value, however, is only 30%. fFN is valid between 22 and 34 weeks of gestation and is typically used in combination with transvaginal cervical length measurement. However, it must be collected before any other swabs, cultures, or examination because results are affected by cervical manipulation, semen, blood, and lubricant. It has not been shown to be helpful as a screening tool in asymptomatic women.

13. **How is preterm labor treated?**
At present, *no medication has been proven effective in treating preterm labor*; medical interventions are directed at decreasing morbidity and mortality for the infant.
   - **Antenatal corticosteroids** are the most beneficial in improving neonatal outcome and should be given for all cases between 24 and 34 weeks of gestation. These drugs have been demonstrated to decrease the risk of RDS, IVH, NEC, and neonatal death. Two different regimens are using, both given intramuscularly: two 12-mg doses of betamethasone 24 hours apart, or four 6-mg doses of dexamethasone every 12 hours. Even a single dose has been shown to reduce morbidity and mortality, so treatment should be initiated even if delivery is likely to occur in less than 24 hours. Additional benefit may be derived from a repeat course (referred to as a "rescue" course) if more than 2 weeks have passed and delivery is anticipated before 34 weeks; however, additional benefit has not been demonstrated for accelerated rescue dosing or three or more courses. Weekly administration of corticosteroids has been associated with a reduction in head circumference and birth weight and is not recommended.
   - **Magnesium sulfate** has been shown to reduce the severity and overall risk of cerebral palsy in surviving infants and is administered for neuroprotection when delivery is anticipated before 32 weeks of gestation. Several different regimens exist, and all are believed to be efficacious; treatment for this purpose typically does not extend past 24 hours.
   - **Tocolytic therapy** has not been shown to prolong pregnancy more than 48 hours and is generally reserved for cases in which a brief delay in delivery would be beneficial, such as to allow for a full course of antenatal corticosteroids. No evidence exists to support any direct favorable effects on neonatal outcome from tocolysis alone.
   - **GBS prophylaxis** is administered in the majority of cases of preterm labor; the only exception is if the patient has had a negative GBS culture result within the past 5 weeks.

   Strict bed rest has not been shown be beneficial and increases the risk of venous thromboembolism (VTE). It is no longer recommended for the management of preterm labor.

14. **What are common tocolytic agents, their mechanisms of action, and side effects?**
Terbutaline, a β-adrenergic agonist. Generally reserved for short-term tocolysis, it is given as 0.25 mg subcutaneously every 4 hours as needed. Total dosage is not to exceed 5 mg in 24 hours, and treatment should not extend beyond 48 hours.
   - Mechanism: It activates β-adrenergic receptors to increase adenyl cyclase and increases intracellular cyclic adenosine monophosphate (cAMP). cAMP reduces intracellular calcium levels and decreases sensitivity of the myosin-actin contractile unit to calcium.
   - Side effects: hypotension, pulmonary edema, cardiac arrhythmias, chest pain, tachycardia, myocardial ischemia, hyperglycemia, hypokalemia, and glucose intolerance

Nifedipine, a calcium channel blocker. It is given orally as a 30-mg load, then 10 to 30 mg orally every 3 to 6 hours.
   - Mechanism: It interferes with influx of calcium through voltage-gated calcium channels.
   - Side effects: flushing, headache, maternal hypotension; increased risk of respiratory depression with concomitant use of magnesium sulfate

Magnesium sulfate. It is given as a 4- to 6-g intravenous bolus over 20 minutes and then continued at 2 to 4 g/hour.
   - Mechanism: It has an unclear mechanism of action but likely competes with calcium at voltage-gated calcium channels in smooth muscle.
   - Side effects: hypotension, flushing, lethargy, pulmonary edema, loss of deep tendon reflexes (DTR), and respiratory and cardiac depression or arrest

Indomethacin, a prostaglandin synthetase inhibitor. Given orally 25 to 50 mg every 8 hours, it is reserved for gestations of less than 32 weeks because of potential in utero closure of the ductus arteriosus.
- Mechanism: It competes with arachidonic acid for cyclooxygenase (COX), thus inhibiting prostaglandin synthesis.
- Side effects: oligohydramnios, gastric irritation, and platelet dysfunction

15. **Do any contraindications to tocolysis exist?**
Yes. Tocolysis is contraindicated in any instance when continuing the pregnancy would cause undue risk to the fetus, mother, or both. Examples include chorioamnionitis, intrauterine fetal demise, placental abruption, lethal fetal anomaly, preeclampsia with severe features or eclampsia (see Chapter 49), and known intolerance to tocolytics.

16. **Can preterm labor be prevented?**
Spontaneous preterm birth cannot always be prevented, but interventions to reduce it are available. These interventions are divided into two categories based on whether or not a patient has a history of preterm birth.
- In women with a singleton pregnancy, no history of preterm birth, and short cervical length (defined as ≤20 mm at <24 weeks of gestation), daily vaginal progesterone is recommended until 36 weeks of gestation. It can be given as a 200-mg suppository or 90-mg gel and is usually taken at night.
- In women with a singleton pregnancy and earlier spontaneous preterm birth between 20 and 36 weeks of gestation, intramuscular 17α-hydroxyprogesterone caproate should be administered weekly from 16 weeks to 36 weeks of gestation. Transvaginal ultrasound for cervical length assessment should be performed every 1 to 2 weeks, and cerclage should be offered if a length shorter than 25 mm is observed (Fig. 65-3) before 24 weeks of gestation.

17. **What is premature rupture of membranes (PROM), and what is preterm PROM (PPROM)?**
PROM is defined as rupture of membranes before the onset of labor. PPROM is defined as rupture of membranes before the onset of labor and before 37 weeks of gestation. The exact cause of PPROM is often unknown, but it is thought to be secondary to an underlying process that weakens the amnion.

18. **What is the incidence of PROM and PPROM?**
In the United States, PROM occurs in 8% of term pregnancies, and PPROM occurs in 3% of all pregnancies.

19. **What are risk factors for PPROM?**
- Previous history of PPROM
- Vaginal or cervical infection
- Cigarette smoking
- Substance abuse
- Cervical insufficiency
- Previous cervical surgical procedures
- Vaginal bleeding during pregnancy
- Polyhydramnios
- Long-term steroid use
- Connective tissue disease (e.g., Ehlers-Danlos syndrome)
- Amniocentesis (risk of PROM is 1%; iatrogenic rupture has a high chance of spontaneous "resealing" of membranes and often carries a good prognosis in the absence of infection)

20. **What are the major complications of PPROM?**
In addition to fetal and neonatal infection, PPROM is associated with risks of prematurity (see question 5). Maternal complications include placental abruption (2% to 5%), intraamniotic infection (15% to 25%), and postpartum infection (15% to 20%). Cesarean delivery for nonvertex presentation and cord prolapse also occur more commonly in cases of PPROM.

21. **What organisms have been associated with intraamniotic infection in patients with PPROM?**
Although infections are typically polymicrobial, organisms cultured from amniotic fluid include GBS, *Escherichia coli,* enterococci, *Bacteroides* species, *Ureaplasma* or *Mycoplasma* species, peptostreptococci, fusobacteria, and *Gardnerella vaginalis.*

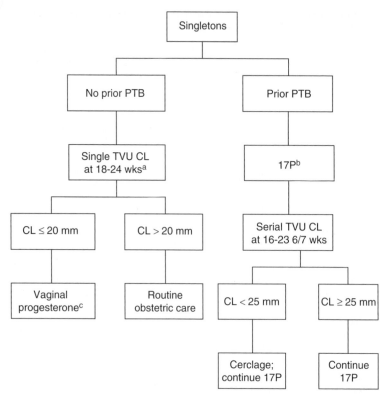

Figure 65-3. Algorithm for the clinical use of progesterone supplementation. [a]If transvaginal ultrasound (TVU) cervical length (CL) screening is performed; [b]17α-hydroxyprogesterone caproate (17P) 250 mg intramuscularly every week from 16 to 20 weeks to 36 weeks ([c]e.g., daily 200-mg suppository or 90-mg gel from the time of diagnosis of short CL to 36 weeks). PTB, preterm birth. *(From Society for Maternal-Fetal Medicine Publications Committee, with assistance of Vincenzo Berghella. Progesterone and preterm birth prevention: translating clinical trials data into clinical practice. Am J Obstet Gynecol. 2012;206:376-386.)*

22. **What is the significance of PPROM before pregnancy viability?**
   Rupture of fetal membranes before viability (<24 weeks of gestation) occurs in less than 1% of pregnancies. Lung development relies largely on the presence of a normal amniotic fluid volume, and pulmonary hypoplasia affects 10% to 20% of fetuses with PPROM before viability. Survival is far greater after 22 weeks of gestation compared with rupture before this time (57.7% versus 14.4%, respectively). Prolonged oligohydramnios can also result in **Potter sequence**, which is characterized by abnormal facial characteristics and limb contractures.

23. **What are common symptoms of PROM?**
   Patients typically complain of fluid leakage, either as a sudden, large-volume loss or as a small but continuous flow. Contractions may or may not be present.

24. **How should a patient with possible PPROM be evaluated?**
   Three key components of an evaluation for PPROM:
   1. Visualization of amniotic fluid pooling in the vaginal vault or passing through the cervix
   2. Using nitrazine paper to test the pH of vaginal fluid. The pH of amniotic fluid is generally 7.1 to 7.3, which turns the paper from yellow to blue. Contaminants such as blood, semen, and occasionally bacterial vaginosis may yield a false-positive result.

3. Assessment for ferning. Vaginal fluid is placed on a microscope slide and allowed to dry; amniotic fluid has a classic arborization or "fernlike" pattern when examined under a microscope.

A sterile speculum examination should be used during the evaluation, and cultures should be collected to rule out any infection. Digital examinations are avoided because of the potential increased risk of infection, and lubricants should be minimized or avoided because they are pH neutral and can crystalize.

25. **What other tests can be used to determine whether PPROM has occurred?**
Transabdominal ultrasound to assess amniotic fluid volume may be helpful, although normal volume does not necessarily rule out ruptured membranes. If a definitive diagnosis cannot be made and determination of PPROM is needed for crucial management decisions, indigo carmine dye can be injected into the amniotic cavity by using ultrasound guidance. A pad or tampon is then placed; visualization of blue dye confirms membrane rupture. Methylene blue should be used for this purpose because of the risk of fetal methemoglobinemia.

26. **How is PPROM managed?**
Patients with gestations of less than 34 weeks should receive antenatal corticosteroids, and those with gestations of less than 32 weeks should receive magnesium sulfate for neuroprotection. Latency antibiotics have been shown to prolong pregnancy and reduce maternal and neonatal infections, and they are given in gestations of less than 34 weeks. The recommended regimen is intravenous ampicillin (2 g every 6 hours) and erythromycin (250 mg every 6 hours) for 48 hours, followed by oral amoxicillin (250 mg every 8 hours) and erythromycin base (333 mg every 8 hours) for an additional 5 days. This antibiotic regimen also acts as GBS prophylaxis, although if the patient begins laboring after the 7-day course of latency antibiotics has finished, GBS prophylaxis should still be given.

27. **Should tocolysis be considered for patients with PPROM?**
Tocolytics are not recommended in the setting of PPROM with active preterm labor because of an increased risk of chorioamnionitis.

28. **What is the latency period, and how is it defined?**
Latency refers to the interval between rupture of membranes and the onset of labor. It is inversely correlated with the gestational age at time of membrane rupture. On average, at least half of patients with PPROM will deliver within 1 week.

29. **What are the recommendations for delivery in the setting of PPROM?**
Indications for expeditious delivery are the same as in term patients and include intrauterine infection, nonreassuring fetal status, placental abruption, suspicion of uterine rupture, and cord prolapse. In the absence of an indication, patients can be managed expectantly and delivery planned for 34 0/7 weeks of gestation or later. If PPROM occurs at a gestation of more than 34 weeks, it is actively managed by inducing labor or delivery by cesarean section (if indicated; for more information on this topic, see Chapter 63).

KEY POINTS: PRETERM LABOR AND PRETERM PREMATURE RUPTURE OF MEMBRANES

1. Preterm labor is defined as cervical change with regular contractions between 20 and 36 6/7 weeks of gestation.
2. Antenatal corticosteroids administered before 34 weeks of gestation significantly reduces the risk of neonatal RDS, IVH, and NEC.
3. Magnesium sulfate for the purpose of fetal neuroprotection is administered in gestations of less than 32 weeks when birth appears imminent.
4. PROM is the rupture of fetal membranes before the onset of labor. Rupture before 37 weeks of gestation is PPROM.
5. Broad-spectrum antibiotics administered in cases of PPROM at less than 34 weeks of gestation significantly reduce maternal and neonatal infectious morbidity.

BIBLIOGRAPHY

1. American College of Obstetricians and Gynecologists. Magnesium sulfate before anticipated preterm birth for neuroprotection. ACOG committee opinion no. 455. *Obstet Gynecol.* 2010;115:669–671.
2. American College of Obstetricians and Gynecologists. Management of preterm labor. ACOG practice bulletin no. 127. *Obstet Gynecol.* 2012;119:1308–1317.
3. American College of Obstetricians and Gynecologists. Prediction and prevention of preterm birth. ACOG practice bulletin no. 130. *Obstet Gynecol.* 2012;120:964–973.
4. American College of Obstetricians and Gynecologists. Premature rupture of membranes. ACOG practice bulletin no. 139. *Obstet Gynecol.* 2013;122:918–930.
5. Creasy RK, Resnik R, Iams JD, Lockwood CJ, Moore TR. *Creasy and Resnik's Maternal-Fetal Medicine: Principles and Practice.* 6th ed. Philadelphia: Saunders; 2009.
6. Creasy R, Resnik R, Iams JD, Lockwood CJ, Moore TR. *Creasy and Resnik's Maternal-Fetal Medicine: Principles and Practice.* 7th ed. Philadelphia: Saunders; 2014.
7. Fanaroff AA, Stoll BJ, Wright LL, et al. NICHD Neonatal Research Network: trends in neonatal morbidity and mortality for very low birthweight infants. *Am J Obstet Gynecol.* 2007;196:147.e1–147.e8.
8. Morse SB, Haywood JL, Goldenberg RL, Bronstein J, Nelson KG, Carlo WA. Estimation of neonatal outcome and perinatal therapy use. *Pediatrics.* 2000;105:1046–1050.
9. Kenyon SL, Taylor DJ, Tarnow-Mordi W. ORACLE Collaborative Group. Broad-spectrum antibiotics for preterm, prelabour rupture of fetal membranes: the ORACLE I randomised trial. *Lancet.* 2001;357:979–988.
10. Lau C, Ambalavanan N, Chakraborty H, Wingate MS, Carlo WA. Extremely low birth weight and infant mortality rates in the United States. *Pediatrics.* 2013;131:855–860.
11. Martin JA. Preterm births—United States, 2006 and 2010. *MMWR Morb Mortal Wkly Rep.* 2013;62:136–138.
12. McManemy J, Cooke E, Amon E, Leet T. Recurrence risk for preterm delivery. *Am J Obstet Gynecol.* 2007;196:576. e1–576.e6. discussion 576.e6.
13. Mercer BM, Miodovnik M, Thurnau GR, et al. Antibiotic therapy for reduction of infant morbidity after preterm premature rupture of the membranes: a randomized controlled trial. National Institute of Child Health and Human Development Maternal-Fetal Medicine Units Network. *JAMA.* 1997;278:989–995.
14. National Institute of Child Health and Human Development (NICHD) Neonatal Research Network (NRN). Extremely Preterm Birth Outcome Data. Available at www.nichd.nih.gov/about/org/der/branches/ppb/programs/epbo/Pages/epbo_case.aspx. Accessed August 20, 2015.
15. National Institutes of Health (NIH) Consensus Developmental Panel. The effect of corticosteroids for fetal maturation on perinatal outcomes. *JAMA.* 1995;273:413.

CHAPTER 66

PLACENTA PREVIA AND PLACENTAL ABRUPTION

Christine Djapri, MD

1. **What is a low-lying placenta?**
   When the edge of the placenta is less than 2 cm from the internal cervical os but does not cover it. In general, women can still be delivered vaginally without an increased risk of complication if the placenta is at least 1 cm from the internal os.

2. **What is a placenta previa?**
   Placenta previa is a condition in which placental tissue abuts or overlies the internal cervical os.

3. **To what does the term "placental migration" refer?**
   Placental migration is a term used to explain the common occurrence of placenta previa diagnosed early in pregnancy that resolves by the late third trimester. Two hypotheses have been proposed for this phenomenon. First, the development of the lower uterine segment at later gestations increases the distance between the lower placental edge and the internal os. Second, **trophotropism** results in the preferential growth of trophoblastic tissue in more vascularized areas of the uterus, which is in the direction toward the fundus (i.e., away from the cervix).

4. **Why does placenta previa cause bleeding?**
   Physiologic changes in the cervix and lower uterine segment, as well as contractions, can produce shearing forces at the inelastic placental attachment site. Vaginal examination or coitus can also disrupt the intervillous space and cause bleeding (placental location should always be verified to ensure that there is no placenta previa before a digital cervical check is performed). Bleeding is primarily maternal, but fetal bleeding can occur if a fetal vessel is disrupted.

5. **What is the incidence of placenta previa at term, and in the second trimester?**
   The overall reported incidence of placenta previa at delivery is 4 in 1000. In the second trimester, placenta previa may be found in 4% to 6% of pregnancies.

6. **What are the common risk factors for placenta previa?**
   - Multifetal gestation
   - Increasing parity and maternal age
   - Previous cesarean delivery
   - Previous placenta previa
   - Previous intrauterine surgical procedure (e.g., curettage)
   - Cigarette smoking

7. **What role does cigarette smoking play in the risk of placenta previa?**
   Cigarette smoking increases the risk of placenta previa at least twofold. The reason is thought to be chronic carbon monoxide hypoxemia causing compensatory placental hypertrophy that covers a larger surface area.

8. **What other obstetric complications are associated with placenta previa?**
   - Preterm labor and rupture of membranes
   - Fetal malpresentation
   - Intrauterine growth restriction
   - Congenital anomalies
   - Placenta accreta, increta, or percreta

9. **What are maternal complications of placenta previa?**
   Maternal complications include hemorrhage, uterine atony, and increased risk of blood transfusions. If bleeding cannot be controlled, postpartum hysterectomy or pelvic artery embolization may be required.

10. **What are potential fetal complications of placenta previa?**
Potential fetal complications include poor growth, morbidity related to preterm delivery, hypoxia, and neonatal demise.

11. **How is placenta previa diagnosed?**
Ultrasound examination is the mainstay of diagnosis and should be used to exclude placenta previa in any woman beyond 20 weeks of gestation who presents with vaginal bleeding before any digital pelvic examination is performed. For this purpose, transvaginal ultrasound and translabial ultrasound are both more sensitive than transabdominal ultrasound. Magnetic resonance imaging (MRI) is usually reserved for complicated cases in which placenta accreta is suspected (see later).

12. **How does placenta previa manifest?**
In the majority of cases, no symptoms are present, and the diagnosis is made at the time of a routine ultrasound examination. If women become symptomatic, the characteristic clinical presentation is painless vaginal bleeding. Some women (10% to 20%) present with both bleeding and uterine contractions. The amount of bleeding can vary from light spotting to overt hemorrhage.

13. **How is placenta previa managed?**
Management of placenta previa depends on the clinical situation, although all deliveries of a living fetus are performed by cesarean section.
   - **Asymptomatic women** are followed with ultrasound examinations to assess placental location and fetal growth. To avoid labor and peripartum hemorrhage, delivery is scheduled between 36 and 37 weeks of gestation. Cervical examinations and sexual intercourse should be avoided throughout the pregnancy.
   - **Women with vaginal bleeding:** Maternal hemodynamic stability should be closely monitored, and continuous fetal monitoring with tocometry (assess for contractions) should be performed in all viable pregnancies. Laboratory tests that should be performed immediately include a complete blood count, coagulation studies (fibrinogen level, activated partial thromboplastin time, prothrombin time, and D-dimer), and a Kleihauer-Betke test to check for fetal bleeding. A large-bore intravenous access should be secured and intravenous fluids administered as needed. Patients should be crossmatched for blood and transfused as needed. Nonreassuring fetal status and refractory maternal hemorrhage are indications for delivery.

Other considerations:
   - Tocolysis can be given if vaginal bleeding is accompanied by uterine contractions.
   - For patients who are at 24 to 32 weeks of gestation and delivery is likely to occur within the next 24 hours, magnesium sulfate can be administered for fetal neuroprotection.
   - Antenatal corticosteroids should be administered to patients between 24 and 34 weeks of gestation to enhance fetal pulmonary maturity.
   - Rh(D) immune globulin should be given to all Rh-negative, unsensitized women who experience bleeding.

14. **In which cases of placenta previa is a classic uterine incision preferred over a low transverse incision?**
To avoid cutting through the placenta, an anterior placenta previa is best managed with a low vertical or classical uterine incision. With posterior, central, or lateral placenta previa, a low transverse incision can often be used, provided the lower uterine segment is sufficiently developed (i.e., the fetus is not severely preterm).

15. **What is the risk of recurrence for placenta previa?**
Placenta previa recurs in 4% to 8% of subsequent pregnancies.

16. **What is vasa previa?**
When fetal blood vessels are positioned over the internal os. Vasa previa is usually associated with a velamentous cord insertion or a succenturiate lobe (see Chapter 34). If these vessels rupture, fetal exsanguination and death can occur.

17. **What is placenta accreta?**
Placenta accreta is a condition in which trophoblastic invasion occurs past the Nitabuch layer (a fibrinoid zone where the trophoblasts normally meets the decidua basalis). Placental detachment does not readily occur at the time of delivery, and massive hemorrhage can ensue. This condition is considered life-threatening to the mother and should be followed by experts. When the placenta invades into the myometrium, the term placenta increta is used. Invasion past the uterine serosa into adjoining pelvic structures (bladder, bowel, and/or vessels) is called placenta percreta.

18. **What is the association between placenta previa and placenta accreta?**
Although placenta accreta can occur in the absence of placenta previa, the presence of placenta previa increases the risk of abnormal placental invasion. The risk of having a placenta accreta in the presence of a placenta previa is 1% to 5%; this increases to 25% with a history of one previous cesarean delivery and to 45% with two or more.

19. **What are risk factors for placenta accreta?**
    - Advanced maternal age (≥35 years of age)
    - Multiparity
    - Placenta previa
    - Previous cesarean section (higher risk when combined with placenta previa)

KEY POINTS: PLACENTA PREVIA

1. The overall incidence of placenta previa in the second trimester (4%) is 10-fold more than the incidence of placenta previa at term (0.4%).
2. Placenta previa is diagnosed with ultrasound examination. Digital pelvic examination is contraindicated.
3. Placenta previa classically manifests as painless third trimester vaginal bleeding; management depends on the severity as well as on maternal and fetal status.

20. **What is placental abruption?**
Detachment of the placenta from its implantation site before delivery of the fetus. The three predominant locations are subchorionic (between the placenta and membranes), retroplacental (between the placenta and myometrium), and preplacental (between the placenta and amniotic fluid). Retroplacental hematomas are associated with the worst prognosis for fetal survival.

21. **What is chronic placental abruption?**
Abruption that occurs early in pregnancy but is not severe enough to result in immediate fetal demise. It is often associated with maternal hypertension and ischemic placental disease.

22. **What is the incidence of placental abruption?**
The overall incidence of placental abruption ranges from 0.4% to 1% of pregnancies.

23. **What are common risk factors for placental abruption?**
    - Maternal hypertensive disorders, including preeclampsia
    - Preterm premature rupture of membranes
    - Rapid uterine decompression associated with multiple gestations and polyhydramnios
    - Cigarette smoking
    - Cocaine abuse
    - Previous history of placental abruption
    - Trauma

24. **How does placental abruption manifest?**
Fetal distress and acute abdominal or back pain are common, as well as vaginal bleeding. Uterine tenderness or rigidity can also occur. Ten percent to 20% of all abruptions are concealed and do not cause vaginal bleeding; in these cases, the blood is retained between the detached placenta and the uterus (Fig. 66-1, *A*).

25. **What are other potential causes of bleeding in the third trimester?**
    - Placenta previa
    - Vasa previa
    - Placental abruption
    - Early labor (bloody show)
    - Lesions of the lower genital tract (e.g., herpes, cervical cancer)
    - Vaginal trauma or foreign bodies

26. **Is the bleeding associated with an abruption maternal or fetal in origin?**
Similar to placenta previa, bleeding associated with an abruption is mostly maternal. Significant fetal bleeding is much more likely in cases associated with trauma.

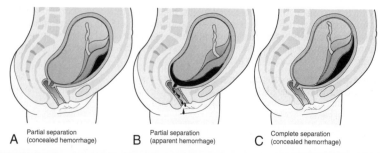

A Partial separation (concealed hemorrhage)   B Partial separation (apparent hemorrhage)   C Complete separation (concealed hemorrhage)

Figure 66-1. Drawings demonstrating different degrees of placental separation. **A,** Partial retroplacental abruption (concealed hemorrhage): blood collects behind the placenta. **B,** Partial abruption: bleeding is observed dissecting along the chorion and manifest (in this case) with vaginal bleeding. **C,** Complete abruption: blood collection anterior to the placenta as the placenta completely separates from the uterine wall. *(From Drife J, Magowan B.* Clinical Obstetrics and Gynaecology. *Edinburgh: Saunders; 2004.)*

27. **How is the diagnosis of placental abruption made?**
    The diagnosis is usually clinical; the classic triad is vaginal bleeding, abdominal or back pain, and nonreassuring fetal status or fetal demise. Some, but not all, abruptions can be seen with ultrasound; it should not be the sole method used to eliminate this disorder from a differential diagnosis.

28. **What are maternal complications of placental abruption?**
    Potential maternal complications include excessive blood loss resulting in hypovolemic shock, end-organ damage (especially renal), need for blood transfusion, and death. Another major complication is disseminated intravascular coagulation (DIC), which is most likely to occur in cases severe enough to cause fetal death or massive hemorrhage. DIC is thought to result from entry of thromboplastins into the circulation from the site of placental injury that results in intravascular activation of the clotting cascade.

29. **What are the potential fetal complications of placental abruption?**
    The most significant fetal complications are morbidity associated with preterm delivery, hypoxemia, and death. A higher incidence of cerebral palsy has been seen in survivors of placental abruption. In cases of chronic abruption, complications include intrauterine growth restriction and oligohydramnios.

30. **How should placental abruption be managed?**
    Management depends on severity, gestational age, and maternal-fetal status.
    - **Severe abruptions** are indicated by fetal distress or maternal hemodynamic instability. Initial efforts should be focused on stabilization of the mother and delivery of the fetus. Hemorrhagic shock requires vigorous blood and volume replacement with packed red blood cells (RBCs) and crystalloids. Goals of blood and volume replacement are to maintain the hematocrit at or above 30% and the urinary output at more than 0.5 mg/kg/hour. Platelet count, fibrinogen level, and serum potassium level should be checked with every 4 to 6 units of packed RBCs administered. If DIC is suspected, the institution's massive transfusion protocol should be activated. If fetal demise has occurred and maternal status is stable, vaginal delivery should be attempted.
    - **Nonsevere abruptions:** Maternal and fetal status should be continuously monitored. This includes continuous fetal heart rate monitoring and tocometry, continuous monitoring of maternal vital signs, securing at least one (preferably two) large-bore intravenous lines, and placement of an indwelling catheter to allow for close monitoring of urinary output. Appropriate laboratory tests (see later) should be performed and the blood bank notified. Finally, all providers should be prepared for potential decompensation and the need for emergency caesarean delivery. Vaginal delivery may be attempted as long as maternal and fetal statuses remain reassuring.
    Other considerations:
    - The patient should be tested for DIC every 4 hours until delivery. Fibrin degradation products (D-dimers) are the most sensitive laboratory test, but once levels are elevated, they are not helpful in guiding therapy.
    - The ultimate therapy of DIC is delivery.

- If a cesarean delivery needs to be performed and the platelet count is lower than 50,000 or the fibrinogen level is less than 100 mg/mL, these components should be replaced individually.
- Fibrinogen may be replaced with fresh frozen plasma or cryoprecipitate, although it is present in greatest concentration in cryoprecipitate.

31. **Which laboratory studies should be ordered in cases of suspected abruption?**
Complete blood count, blood type, Rh status, and Kleihauer-Betke stain (to identify and quantify fetal and maternal hemorrhage) should be ordered, as well as coagulation studies (prothrombin and activated partial prothrombin time, fibrinogen, and D-dimers).

32. **What is Couvelaire uterus?**
Couvelaire uterus describes a finding at the time of laparotomy in which blood dissects into the myometrium and gives the uterus a mottled, bluish color. It is a significant risk factor for uterine atony.

33. **When should a pregnancy complicated by abruption be delivered?**
The method and timing of delivery depend on the gestational age of the fetus and the severity of the abruption. In cases of severe abruption, expeditious delivery is recommended at any gestational age. If the fetus is immature and the status is reassuring, mild abruptions can be managed expectantly in consultation with experts in high-risk pregnancies. Administration of corticosteroids to promote fetal lung maturation is recommended between 24 and 34 weeks of gestation because these patients are at risk of developing a sudden severe abruption. The development of coagulopathy, nonreassuring fetal status, or intrauterine growth restriction is a possible indication for delivery.

34. **What is the risk of recurrence of abruption in subsequent pregnancies?**
The risk of recurrence has been reported to be 5% to 15%. After two consecutive abruptions, the risk of a third rises to 20% to 25%. In cases of placental abruption resulting in fetal death, the recurrence rate of repeat abruption resulting in the same outcome is approximately 11%.

KEY POINTS: PLACENTAL ABRUPTION

1. Placental abruption is detachment of the placenta from its implantation site prior to delivery of the fetus.
2. Classic symptoms of placental abruption include vaginal bleeding, abdominal pain, and non-reassuring fetal status or fetal demise.
3. Bleeding from an abruption is mostly maternal.
4. The method and timing of delivery depend on the gestational age of the fetus and the severity of the abruption.

BIBLIOGRAPHY

1. Abenhaim HA, Azoulay L, Kramer MS, Leduc L. Incidence and risk factors of amniotic fluid embolisms: a population-based study on 3 million births in the United States. *Am J Obstet Gynecol.* 2008;199:49.e1–49.e8.
2. American College of Obstetricians and Gynecologists. Medically indicated late-preterm and early-term deliveries. ACOG committee opinion no. 560. *Obstet Gynecol.* 2013;121:908–910.
3. Ananth CV, Smulian JC, Demissie K, Vintzileos AM, Knuppel RA. Placental abruption among singleton and twin births in the United States: risk factor profiles. *Am J Epidemiol.* 2001;153:771–778.
4. Breathnach FM, Donnelly J, Cooley SM, et al. Subclinical hypothyroidism as a risk factor for placental abruption: evidence from a low-risk primigravid population. *Aust N Z J Obstet Gynaecol.* 2013;53:553–560.
5. Crane JM, van den Hof MC, Dodds L, Armson BA, Liston R. Neonatal outcomes with placenta previa. *Obstet Gynecol.* 1999;93:541–544.
6. Crane JM, Van den Hof MC, Dodds L, Armson BA, Liston R. Maternal complications with placenta previa. *Am J Perinatol.* 2000;17:101–105.
7. Cunningham F, Leveno KJ, Bloom SL, et al. Obstetrical hemorrhage. In: *Williams Obstetrics.* 24th ed. New York: McGraw-Hill; 2013.
8. Dashe JS. Toward consistent terminology of placental location. *Semin Perinatol.* 2013;37:375–379.
9. Faiz AS, Ananth CV. Etiology and risk factors for placenta previa: an overview and meta-analysis of observational studies. *J Matern Fetal Neonatal Med.* 2003;13:175–190.
10. Gabbe SG, Niebyl JR, Galan HL. *Obstetrics: Normal and Problem Pregnancies.* 6th ed. Philadelphia: Saunders; 2012.
11. Gemer O, Segal S. Incidence and contribution of predisposing factors to transverse lie presentation. *Int J Gynaecol Obstet.* 1994;44:219–221.
12. Mendola P, Laughon SK, Männistö TI, et al. Obstetric complications among US women with asthma. *Am J Obstet Gynecol.* 2013;208:127.e1–127.e8.

13. Olive EC, Roberts CL, Algert CS, Morris JM. Placenta praevia: maternal morbidity and place of birth. *Aust N Z J Obstet Gynaecol*. 2005;45:499–504.

14. Oyelese Y, Ananth CV. Placental abruption. *Obstet Gynecol*. 2006;108:1005.

15. Pariente G, Wiznitzer A, Sergienko R, Mazor M, Holcberg G, Sheiner E. Placental abruption: critical analysis of risk factors and perinatal outcomes. *J Matern Fetal Neonatal Med*. 2011;24:698–702.

16. Rosenberg T, Pariente G, Sergienko R, Wiznitzer A, Sheiner E. Critical analysis of risk factors and outcome of placenta previa. *Arch Gynecol Obstet*. 2011;284:47–51.

17. Salihu HM, Li Q, Rouse DJ, Alexander GR. Placenta previa: neonatal death after live births in the United States. *Am J Obstet Gynecol*. 2003;188:1305–1309.

18. Sheiner E, Shoham-Vardi I, Hallak M, Hershkowitz R, Katz M, Mazor M. Placenta previa: obstetric risk factors and pregnancy outcome. *J Matern Fetal Med*. 2001;10:414–419.

19. Tikkanen M. Placental abruption: epidemiology, risk factors and consequences. *Acta Obstet Gynecol Scand*. 2011;90:140–149.

20. Warshak CR, Eskander R, Hull AD, et al. Accuracy of ultrasonography and magnetic resonance imaging in the diagnosis of placenta accreta. *Obstet Gynecol*. 2006;108:573–581.

21. Yamada T, Yamada T, Morikawa M, Minakami H. Clinical features of abruptio placentae as a prominent cause of cerebral palsy. *Early Hum Dev*. 2012;88:861–864.

CHAPTER 67

MALPRESENTATION

Jared Roeckner, MD

1. **What is the definition of "fetal lie"?**
   Fetal lie refers to the orientation of the fetal spine in relation to the maternal spine. A fetus may be in a longitudinal lie (fetal and maternal spines are oriented in the same direction), oblique lie, or transverse lie. Normal fetal lie is longitudinal, which can be further divided into breech or cephalic depending on the presenting part.

2. **What are the possible types of cephalic presentations?**
   Most cephalic presentations are **vertex** (back of the fetal head as the presenting part). Occasionally, **face** presentations occur. A **brow** presentation is an intermediate head position between vertex and face presentation. It is rare and usually converts to another presentation.

3. **Describe the various breech presentations.**
   - Frank breech: most common breech presentation, occurring when the fetal hips are flexed and the knees extended
   - Incomplete breech: incomplete flexion of one or both knees or hips
   - Complete breech: when both the fetal knees and hips are flexed
   Figure 67-1 contains illustrations of the breech positions.

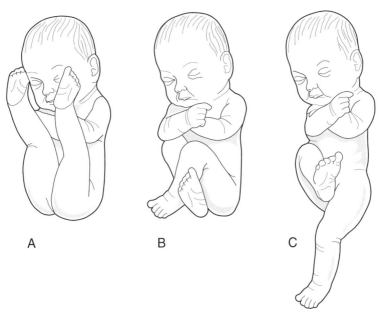

A   B   C

Figure 67-1. Breech presentations. **A,** Frank. **B,** Complete. **C,** Footling. *(From Baskett TF. Breech delivery. In: Baskett TF, ed. Munro Kerr's Operative Obstetrics. 12th ed. London: Elsevier; 2014.)*

4. **How is fetal lie determined?**
   Ultrasound examination and Leopold maneuvers are commonly used. Leopold maneuvers are often difficult to perform in obese patients.

5. **What is an unstable lie?**
This term is used to describe a situation characterized by frequent changes of either fetal lie or presentation, or both.

6. **What is the definition of fetal malpresentation?**
Fetal malpresentation describes any presentation other than vertex.

7. **How common is fetal malpresentation?**
In preterm fetuses, malpresentation occurs quite often; approximately 25% of fetuses are breech before 28 weeks of gestation. At term, the rate of malpresentation is 3% to 4%.

8. **What delivery complication is more common with abnormal axial (also known as transverse) lie?**
Compared with a longitudinal lie with vertex presentation, prolapse of the umbilical cord occurs approximately 20 times more often with an axial lie.

9. **What factors have been linked to malpresentation?**
   - Maternal: pelvic tumors, uterine malformations, high parity
   - Fetal: prematurity, multiple gestations, polyhydramnios, placenta previa or a fundal placenta, chromosomal abnormalities (e.g., trisomies), myotonic dystrophy. Among fetuses with malpresentation, fetal malformations are found more frequently.

10. **What are the options for managing a patient at term with a singleton breech pregnancy?**
Options are expectant management (wait for the fetus change of a cephalic presentation), cesarean delivery, external cephalic version (ECV), or breech vaginal delivery. Out of concern for increased neonatal morbidity and mortality from breech vaginal delivery, cesarean delivery is the standard of care. In cases of advanced labor, breech vaginal delivery may be considered. Breech delivery is also an option for delivery of a second twin in appropriately selected patients.

11. **What is external cephalic version (ECV)?**
ECV is a procedure in which one or two people manually apply pressure to the maternal abdomen to manipulate the fetus into a vertex presentation. Tocolytic agents and regional anesthesia are sometimes employed to relax the uterus and increase the patient's comfort. ECV is usually offered as an option to patients at 36 to 37 weeks of gestation; attempts at later gestational age have lower success, and earlier attempts carry a risk that the fetus will revert back to the previous position. Rarely, ECV can cause fetal distress necessitating emergency delivery.

12. **How successful are attempts at ECV?**
The rate of success varies widely (35% to 85%) and averages approximately 58%. Low success rates have been reported in nulliparous, obese women.

13. **What are the absolute and relative contraindications to ECV?**
Absolute contraindications are the same as those for vaginal delivery (e.g., placenta previa, human immunodeficiency virus [HIV] infection with high viral load). Relative contraindications are not well established and include active labor, fetal distress, multiple gestation, and amniotic fluid abnormalities (polyhydramnios or oligohydramnios). A history of previous cesarean delivery or myomectomy is not a contraindication.

14. **What are the general steps to vaginal breech delivery?**
   1. Allowing the fetus to emerge spontaneously to the level of the umbilicus
   2. Flexion of the fetal knee and delivery of the legs **(Pinard maneuver)**
   3. Gentle rotation of the fetus to make the sacrum anterior
   4. Gentle rotation of the trunk to allow the arms to be delivered by sweeping the elbows down across the fetal chest
   5. Supporting the trunk to allow for delivery of the shoulders and head
   6. Application of suprapubic pressure by an assistant to promote flexion of the fetal head while the delivering provider reaches into the vagina and gently applies pressure to the fetal maxilla to maintain fetal head flexion during maternal expulsive efforts (Mauriceau Smellie Veit maneuver)

   Aside from emergency situations involving imminent delivery, breech vaginal delivery should be attempted only by an experienced, trained provider after extensive counseling of the patient.

15. What are potential complications of vaginal breech delivery?
Fetal limb injury, head entrapment, spinal cord injury, asphyxia, and death.

16. What is meant by "compound presentation"?
Compound presentation is when a fetal extremity (e.g., hand or arm) is located beside or in front of the main presenting part. It occurs most frequently in premature infants and most often consists of a combination of vertex position and an upper extremity. Vaginal delivery may still be possible, but an experienced provider should be present. In general, compression or reduction of the compound part should not be attempted.

KEY POINTS: MALPRESENTATION

1. Malpresentation is common early in pregnancy, but at term only 3% to 4% of fetuses are nonvertex.
2. Malpresentation at term is associated with an increased risk for fetal, placental, and uterine anomalies compared with vertex presentation.
3. Cesarean delivery of a breech fetus is the standard of care out of concern for increased neonatal morbidity and mortality from breech vaginal delivery.
4. External version is a technique in which one attempts to maneuver a fetus from breech to cephalic presentation.

BIBLIOGRAPHY

1. American College of Obstetricians and Gynecologists. External cephalic version. ACOG practice bulletin no. 13. *Int J Gynaecol Obstet.* 2000;2:198–204. Reaffirmed 2014.
2. American College of Obstetricians and Gynecologists. Mode of term singleton breech delivery. ACOG committee opinion no. 265. *Int J Gynaecol Obstet.* 2002;77:65–66. Reaffirmed 2014.
3. American College of Obstetricians and Gynecologists. Mode of term singleton breech delivery. ACOG committee opinion no 340. *Obstet Gynecol.* 2006;108:235–237.
4. de Hundt M, Velzel J, de Groot CJ, Mol BW, Kok M. Mode of delivery after successful external cephalic version: a systematic review and meta-analysis. *Obstet Gynecol.* 2014;123:1327–1334.
5. Fruscalzo A, Londero AP, Salvador S, et al. New and old predictive factors for breech presentation: our experience in 14,433 singleton pregnancies and a literature review. *J Matern Fetal Neonatal Med.* 2014;27:167–172.
6. Gabbe S, Niebyl J, Simpsom J, et al., eds. *Obstetrics: Normal and Problem Pregnancies.* 6th ed. Philadelphia: Saunders; 2012.

CHAPTER 68

POSTPARTUM HEMORRHAGE

Shant Ashdjian, MD

1. **What is postpartum hemorrhage?**

   Postpartum hemorrhage is defined as an estimated blood loss greater than 500 mL after a vaginal delivery and greater than 1000 mL after a cesarean delivery. It is one of the leading causes of maternal morbidity and mortality; approximately 140,000 women worldwide die of postpartum hemorrhage each year. Early or primary postpartum hemorrhage occurs within the first 24 hours of delivery, whereas late or secondary hemorrhage can occur anywhere from 24 hours after delivery to up to 6 to 12 weeks post partum.

2. **What causes postpartum hemorrhage?**
   - Uterine atony
   - Retained placental tissue
   - Genital tract trauma
   - Coagulation defects
   - Uterine inversion

   The most common cause of postpartum hemorrhage is uterine atony (80%), which is defined as the inability of the uterus to contract fully after delivery. Several risk factors for uterine atony have been identified (Box 68-1).

Box 68-1. Risk Factors for Uterine Atony

- History of postpartum hemorrhage
- High parity
- Impaired myometrial contractility (e.g., chorioamnionitis, magnesium infusion, large leiomyomas)
- Protracted labor
- Precipitous labor
- Overdistention of the uterus (e.g., macrosomia, multiple gestation, polyhydramnios)

---

3. **What should be considered in the initial evaluation of a patient with early postpartum hemorrhage?**

   A bimanual examination should be performed to determine whether uterine atony is present. Uterine massage or bimanual uterine compression can decrease bleeding and help expel clots. A full bladder can inhibit complete contraction of the lower uterine segment, so a urinary catheter should be placed. The patient should be carefully examined for any unrecognized vaginal or cervical lacerations. It is prudent to ensure that the patient have adequate intravenous access and fluid resuscitation, and blood replacement products should be readily available.

4. **What are the different uterotonics available to treat uterine atony?**

   Uterotonics are first-line treatments for hemorrhage secondary to atony. These agents are summarized in Table 68-1.

5. **What other options are available if uterotonics fail to stop the bleeding?**

   Tamponade techniques, embolization, and surgical intervention. Tamponade techniques include uterine packing, insertion of one or more Foley catheter bulbs into the uterus and instilling each with 60 to 80 mL of saline, or placement of the Bakri balloon (inserted into the uterus and filled with 300 to 500 mL of saline). If patients are stable, arterial embolization by interventional radiology may be considered. Surgical procedures for obstetric hemorrhage are listed in Box 68-2.

6. **What if the hemorrhage is not caused by atony?**

   Heavy bleeding in a patient with a contracted, firm uterus should raise concern for retained placental fragments, unrecognized lacerations, or uterine rupture. Placenta accreta (trophoblastic invasion past

Table 68-1. Uterotonics

AGENT	ROUTE AND DOSAGE	CONTRAINDICATIONS
Oxytocin	IV (20-40 units in 500 mL normal saline) or IM (10 units)	None; avoid undiluted rapid IV infusion
Methylergonovine	IM 0.2 mg every 2-4 hours*	Hypertension
Prostaglandin $F_{2\alpha}$	IM 0.25 mg every 15-90 minutes for up to eight doses	Reactive airway disease
Misoprostol	PR 800-1000 μg as a single dose	None

IM, Intramuscular; *IV*, intravenous; *PR*, rectally.
*Can be continued every 6-8 hours orally after initial management.

Box 68-2. Surgical Options for Refractory Postpartum Hemorrhage

- Uterine curettage
- B-Lynch compression suture
- Bilateral uterine artery ligation (O'Leary sutures)
- Bilateral utero-ovarian ligament ligation
- Hypogastric artery ligation
- Hysterectomy

the Nitabuch layer) is a rare cause of postpartum hemorrhage, and unrecognized cases are classically associated with an abnormally adherent placenta that does not spontaneously separate from the uterus after delivery. Forced removal results in rapid, brisk bleeding. Management is determined by the extent of the abnormality; curettage, oversewing, wedge resection, arterial embolization, or even hysterectomy may be necessary.

7. **Can postpartum hemorrhage be concealed?**
   Yes. Genital tract hematomas can lead to large occult blood loss. If a hematoma is noted at the time of delivery, it should be closely observed for expansion. Expanding hematomas may require exploration with either ligation of the source of bleeding (if it is identifiable) or oversewing of the involved area. Refractory cases should be packed and embolized by interventional radiology. Patients' complaints of pelvic or rectal pressure after delivery should raise suspicion of a hematoma.

8. **What is uterine inversion, and how is it managed?**
   Uterine inversion occurs after delivery when the uterine fundus descends to and sometimes through the cervix. It manifests as a firm mass at or below the cervix and failure to palpate the fundus on abdominal examination. Uterine inversion can be caused by excessive traction on the umbilical cord with a fundal placenta and can be associated with hemorrhage. Correction of the inversion is achieved by exerting firm upward pressure with a sterile-gloved hand. Uterine relaxation with terbutaline, magnesium sulfate, halogenated anesthetics, or nitroglycerine may be required. If manual replacement is unsuccessful, laparotomy is required.

9. **What are the consequences of postpartum hemorrhage?**
   If severe enough, postpartum hemorrhage can cause hypovolemic shock, disseminated intravascular coagulation (DIC), and even death. Anemia and need for transfusion are not unusual. Sheehan syndrome—failure or necrosis of the anterior pituitary—may occur in rare circumstances. This syndrome manifests over time with associated symptoms of amenorrhea, inability to breastfeed, breast atrophy, loss of axillary and pubic hair, hyperthyroidism, and adrenal insufficiency.

10. **When is blood transfusion recommended?**
    Blood loss is often underestimated during delivery, and laboratory results may not accurately reflect acute blood loss. Clinical judgment should be used to determine when to transfuse, by taking into account the nature of the hemorrhage and any ongoing bleeding. One unit of packed red blood cells is expected to increase hematocrit by three percentage points and hemoglobin by 1 g/dL. If a patient is known to have coagulation defects or requires multiple units of packed red blood cells, additional products (platelets, fresh frozen plasma [FFP], or cryoprecipitate) should be given as needed.

12. What are causes of secondary postpartum hemorrhage?

Subinvolution of the placental bed, retained placental fragments, infection, and inherited coagulation defects should all be considered.

KEY POINTS: POSTPARTUM HEMORRHAGE

1. Postpartum hemorrhage is defined as an estimated blood loss greater than 500 mL after a vaginal delivery and greater than 1000 mL after a cesarean delivery, and it is a leading cause of maternal morbidity and mortality.
2. The most common cause of postpartum hemorrhage is uterine atony, which is the inability of the uterus to contract fully after delivery.
3. Uterotonics are first-line treatments for hemorrhage secondary to atony.

BIBLIOGRAPHY

1. American College of Obstetricians and Gynecologists. Postpartum hemorrhage. ACOG practice bulletin no. 76. *Obstet Gynecol.* 2006;108:1039–1047.
2. Cunningham F, Leveno KJ, Bloom SL, Hauth JC, Gilstrap LC, III, Wenstrom KD. Obstetrical hemorrhage. In: *Williams Obstetrics.* 22nd ed. New York: McGraw-Hill; 2005:809–854.
3. Oxorn H. Postpartum hemorrhage. In: Oxorn H, ed. *Human Labor and Birth.* 5th ed. Norwalk, Conn: Appleton & Lange; 1986:479–497.

CHAPTER 69

NEWBORN RESUSCITATION

Tiffany Pedigo, MD

1. **What structures are responsible for shunting blood away from the lungs in fetal circulation?**

   Oxygenated blood entering the right atrium may be immediately shunted through the foramen ovale into the left atrium. Alternatively, after passing into the pulmonary artery, it can be diverted through the ductus arteriosus into the aorta. Figure 69-1 shows details of the fetal circulation. Following birth, as the neonate breathes, the pulmonary vascular resistance decreases and pulmonary blood flow increases.

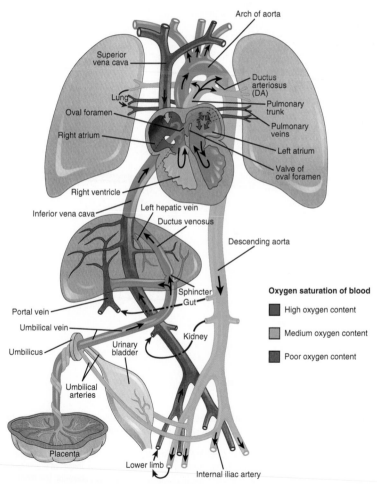

Figure 69-1. Fetal circulation. *(From Moore KL, Persaud TVN, Torchia MG. Before We Are Born. 9th ed. Philadelphia: Saunders; 2016.)*

2. **What percentage of newborns will require resuscitation at birth?**
   Ten percent of newborns will require some assistance to begin breathing at birth. One percent will require extensive resuscitation and neonatal intensive care to survive.

3. **What risk factors are associated with the need for neonatal resuscitation?**
   Box 69-1 provides a list of maternal and fetal risk factors.

Box 69-1. Risk Factors Associated With the Need for Neonatal Resuscitation

Problems Identified During Pregnancy
   Maternal diabetes
   Pregnancy-induced hypertension
   Chronic hypertension
   Chronic maternal illness (cardiovascular, thyroid, neurologic, pulmonary, or renal)
   Anemia or isoimmunization
   Previous fetal or neonatal death
   Bleeding in second or third trimester
   Maternal infection
   Polyhydramnios
   Oligohydramnios
   Postterm gestation
   Multiple gestation
   Size-dates discrepancy
   Drug therapy (e.g., lithium carbonate, magnesium, adrenergic-blocking drugs)
   Maternal substance abuse
   Congenital anomaly
   No prenatal care
   Age <16 or >35 years
   Premature rupture of membranes
   Placenta previa

Problems Identified During Delivery
   Emergency cesarean section
   Forceps- or vacuum-assisted delivery
   Breech or other abnormal presentation
   Premature labor
   Precipitous labor
   Chorioamnionitis
   Prolonged rupture of membranes (>18 hours)
   Prolapsed umbilical cord
   Prolonged labor (>24 hours)
   Fetal bradycardia
   Abnormal fetal heart rate patterns
   Use of general anesthesia
   Uterine tachysystole
   Narcotics administered to mother within 4 hours of delivery
   Meconium-stained amniotic fluid
   Placental abruption
   Prolonged second stage of labor (> 2 hours)

---

4. **What factors place preterm infants at high risk for requiring resuscitation at birth?**
   - **Surfactant deficiency**: This renders premature lungs less compliant, which in turn makes ventilation more difficult.
   - **Heat loss**: The stratum corneum (top cell layer of skin that makes keratin, which covers and insulates the skin) has fewer cell layers, resulting in increased insensible losses of water and heat. Preterm infants also have less subcutaneous fat, no brown fat, and lack shivering thermogenesis.
   - **Infection**: Compared with term infants, preterm infants are more likely to be born with an infection.
   - **Intraventricular hemorrhage**: Brain capillaries in the germinal matrix are fragile and at increased risk of bleeding during stress, hypoxia, acidosis, infection, hypotension, and hypertension.

5. **Which neonates do not require significant resuscitation?**
Those who are born at term, are breathing or crying, and have good muscle tone can receive routine care with warmth and drying. For neonates who do not meet these criteria, further resuscitative measures are required.

6. **How should newborns' body temperatures be maintained?**
The goal body temperature is between 36.5C and 37.5C after birth and through stabilization. Hypothermia is associated with late-onset sepsis, hypoglycemia, respiratory issues, and other morbidities. Preterm infants may require radiant warmers, plastic wrap, thermal mattress, warmed humidified gases, and increased room temperature in order to prevent hypothermia. Radiant warmers are typically sufficient for term infants.

7. **What are the ABCDs of resuscitation?**
In contrast to recent changes in adult guidelines, the airway remains the initial objective of resuscitation; bradycardia and other circulatory problems may resolve with appropriate oxygenation and ventilation.

Airway: Position and clear the airway with suction if needed, avoiding deep suction; stimulate by rubbing the trunk or slapping the soles of the feet.
Breathing: Establish adequate oxygenation and ventilation, whether spontaneous or assisted.
Circulation: Assess heart rate and skin color.
Drug: Epinephrine should be administered if the heart rate remains less than 60 beats per minute (bpm) after 30 seconds of positive pressure ventilation (PPV) that causes chest rise and an additional 60 seconds of chest compressions coordinated with PPV.

8. **What is primary apnea?**
When significant oxygen deprivation occurs in a newborn, a sequence of events results in abnormalities of the heart rate and respiratory pattern. As a result of this stress, the infant may have an initial period of rapid breathing associated with a decrease in the heart rate, followed by a period of *primary apnea* (no breathing or gasping). During primary apnea, stimulating the infant by drying him or her or slapping the feet will allow normal respirations to resume, and the heart rate will increase.

9. **What is secondary apnea?**
If cardiorespiratory compromise persists, the infant will have another period of irregular gasping with decreasing heart rate and blood pressure, leading to *secondary apnea*. Stimulation is insufficient to reverse secondary apnea; PPV is required.

10. **How can the infant's heart rate be assessed?**
Palpate the umbilical cord pulse, auscultate the heart, or apply a pulse oximeter or cardiac monitor. An electronic cardiac monitor is preferred for assessment of heart rate when chest compressions are being delivered.

11. **When should PPV be initiated, and at what rate should breaths be given?**
PPV, which provides both oxygenation and ventilation, should be given immediately if an infant is apneic despite stimulation. PPV is also indicated when the heart rate is less than 100 bpm. Breaths should be delivered at a rate of 40 to 60 breaths per minute, or slightly less than once per second.

12. **What fraction of inspired oxygen (FiO_2) should be used when initiating respiratory support?**
In recent years, initiating resuscitation with room air (FiO_2 21%) has been recommended for newborns greater than or equal to 35 weeks' gestation they do not gain survival benefit from resuscitation with higher levels of oxygen, and even a brief period of hyperoxia during resuscitation may lead to higher serum markers of oxidative stress. Premature infants, however, have been shown to require more FiO_2 on average to maintain appropriate oxygen saturations. For infants less than 35 weeks' gestation, resuscitation should begin with 21 to 30% oxygen.

13. **Where should oxygen saturation (SpO_2) be measured on a neonate, and what is considered normal?**
SpO_2 should be assessed on the infant's right hand. This preductal location, which is proximal to the ductus arteriosus, ensures that the measurement is not affected by shunting (e.g., congenital heart disease). The normal SpO_2 for a neonate increases gradually in the first several minutes of life (Table 69-1). If providing respiratory support during resuscitation, the FiO_2 should be adjusted to maintain values within the normal range.

Table 69-1. Normal Preductal Oxygen Saturation at Various Minutes of Life

TIME (MIN)	TARGET PREDUCTAL SPO$_2$ AFTER BIRTH
1	60%-65%
2	65%-70%
3	70%-75%
4	75%-80%
5	80%-85%
10	85%-95%

SpO$_2$, Oxygen saturation.

14. **At what point can PPV be stopped?**
    When the heart rate exceeds 100 bpm and the infant is breathing. However, if the infant demonstrates respiratory distress (e.g., grunting), oxygen should continue to be delivered by continuous positive airway pressure (CPAP). If the infant appears comfortable but SpO$_2$ is lower than the goal, supplemental oxygen may be provided by blow-by or nasal cannula.

15. **What are the indications for chest compressions?**
    After performing PPV for 30 seconds, assess for adequate ventilation (mask with good seal, equal chest rise, color change on capnography if available) if the infant continues to have a heart rate lower than 100 bpm or is still not breathing. Take corrective steps as needed; if the heart rate is lower than 60 bpm, chest compressions should be initiated using the 2-thumb technique. FiO2 should also be increased to 100% while chest compressions are being performed. They may be stopped on reassessment (after at least 60 seconds of continuous compressions) if the heart rate has risen to more than 60 bpm, and the FiO2 may be weaned.

16. **What is the ratio of chest compressions to ventilation in neonates?**
    It is 3:1 (three compressions followed by a pause for one ventilation); simultaneous chest compressions and lung inflation may impede effective ventilation. This ratio should be continued even after an advanced airway has been obtained—another key difference between adults and neonates.

17. **When is epinephrine indicated during neonatal resuscitation, and what is the dose?**
    If effective PPV (resulting in chest rise) has been given for 30 seconds followed by 60 seconds of chest compressions with PPV using 100% oxygen, and the heart rate remains below 60 bpm, epinephrine should be administered. The recommended dose is 1:10,000 concentration intravenously or intraosseously at 0.1 to 0.3 mL/kg (0.01 to 0.03 mg/kg). If given endotracheally, the dose is 0.5 to 1 mL/kg (0.05 to 0.1 mg/kg).

18. **What is the primary site of venous access for neonatal resuscitation?**
    The umbilical vein or a peripheral vein. If neither can be accessed, an intraosseous line is appropriate.

19. **When should endotracheal intubation be considered?**
    - When bag and mask ventilation is prolonged or ineffective
    - If chest compressions are needed to improve cardiovascular status
    - To administer epinephrine for persistent bradycardia
    - If the infant is known to have a congenital diaphragmatic hernia (bag and mask ventilation can distend intrathoracic intestines and should be avoided)

20. **How do you confirm that an endotracheal tube has been correctly placed in the trachea?**
    - Good and equal chest rise with each breath
    - Auscultation of equal breath sounds bilaterally
    - Mist in endotracheal tube
    - Good response to intubation (skin color and heart rate)
    - Carbon dioxide (CO_2) monitor indicates the presence of exhaled CO_2 (inaccurate in the setting of poor or absent cardiac output or a wet colorimetric device)

21. **When should hypovolemic shock be suspected?**
Hypovolemic shock should be suspected if an infant is pale or has delayed capillary refill, weak pulses, and a low heart rate that does not respond to resuscitation measures. A history of placenta previa or blood loss from the umbilical cord may be present.

22. **How should suspected hypovolemia be managed?**
Infants in hypovolemic shock need intravascular volume expansion in the form of normal saline or O-negative blood. The initial dose is 10 mL/kg.

23. **Why is albumin not used during neonatal resuscitation?**
Because of limited availability, risk of infection, and increased risk of mortality.

24. **How long should resuscitation continue if the neonate has no heart rate (asystole) despite appropriate resuscitative measures?**
The Neonatal Resuscitation Program (NRP) recommends terminating resuscitation after 10 minutes of asystole; at this point it is unlikely to obtain return of spontaneous circulation (ROSC), and outcomes if ROSC is obtained are very poor.

25. **Do circumstances exist in which noninitiation or discontinuation of resuscitation is appropriate?**
Yes. Examples include extreme prematurity (<23 weeks), very low birth weight (≤400 g), and certain known underlying conditions (e.g., anencephaly, trisomy 13 or 18). After confirmation and counseling the family, it may be appropriate to withhold resuscitation. If antenatal information is incomplete or unreliable, a trial of resuscitation with ongoing evaluation and discussion with both the family and health care team can be done. Support may be discontinued later, after further assessment and counseling.

26. **What is the Apgar score?**
An anesthesiologist named Virginia Apgar developed the Apgar scoring system to quantify a newborn's response to the extrauterine environment and resuscitation (Table 69-2). Scores are assigned at 1 and 5 minutes after birth; if the 5-minute score is lower than 7, additional scores should be given every 5 minutes for up to 20 minutes. This system can be remembered by the mnemonic APGAR: **A**ppearance, **P**ulse, **G**rimace, **A**ctivity, and **R**espirations.

Table 69-2. Apgar Scoring System (Mnemonic APGAR)

SIGN	0 POINTS	1 POINT	2 POINTS
Appearance	Blue or pale	Acrocyanosis*	Pink
Pulse	Absent	<100 bpm	≥100 bpm
Grimace	No response	Grimaces	Cough, sneeze, cry
Activity	Limp	Some flexion	Active motion
Respirations	Absent	Slow, irregular	Good, crying

*Acrocyanosis: blue extremities, pink core.

27. **Should the Apgar score be used to determine whether resuscitation is needed?**
No. It is not acceptable to use the Apgar score to determine the appropriateness of resuscitative actions, nor should intervention for a depressed infant be delayed until the 1-minute assessment. Biochemical disturbances such as acidemia and hypoxia are already significant by the time the score is affected.

28. **What is a normal Apgar score?**
A 5-minute Apgar score of 7 to 10 is considered normal. Although low 1-minute Apgar scores do not correlate with future outcomes, scores of 3 or less at 10, 15, and 20 minutes are associated with an increased risk of poor neurologic outcome.

29. What resuscitative measures should be taken in cases of meconium-stained amniotic fluid?
Intrapartum bulb suctioning has not been shown to prevent or alter the course of meconium aspiration syndrome and is no longer routinely performed. Additionally, while the 2010 Neonatal Resuscitation Program guidelines recommended that infants with poor respiratory effort, decreased muscle tone, or a heart rate lower than 100 bpm be intubated for tracheal suction, this has not significantly decreased the risk of meconium aspiration syndrome. The 2015 NRP guidelines recommend following the same pathway as previously described, including stimulation and PPV if needed.

30. What effect can magnesium sulfate have on the neonate in the delivery room?
Ineffective respirations and apnea.

31. Should naloxone be given to infants whose mothers received opioids either immediately before delivery or on a long-term basis during pregnancy?
Although it should not be given routinely, naloxone may be considered if the neonate has persistent severe respiratory depression after PPV has restored normal heart rate and color. It may precipitate neonate withdrawal in infants born to mothers who use opioids on a long-term basis.

32. What effect can β-mimetics used for tocolysis have on the neonate?
These drugs may cause maternal hyperglycemia and compensatory hyperinsulinemia, which can then result in neonatal hypoglycemia. Studies have also shown lower Apgar scores and increased need for ventilation.

33. In what situations should umbilical cord blood acid-base analysis be obtained?
Consider checking arterial and venous umbilical cord blood gases in cases of known severe intrauterine growth restriction (IUGR), multifetal gestation, intrapartum fever, maternal thyroid disease, breech delivery, and preterm birth. Umbilical cord blood gases may also be obtained when meconium staining, an abnormal fetal heart rate pattern, or a low 5-minute Apgar score complicates a delivery.

34. What are mean values for umbilical arterial blood gases?
- pH: 7.28
- Partial pressure of CO_2 (Pco_2): 50.2 mm Hg
- Bicarbonate (HCO_3) :22.4 mEq/L
- Base deficit: 2.5 mEq/L

Measuring oxygenation does not have significant clinical implications.

35. What umbilical arterial blood gas values have been associated with significant morbidity and mortality?
- **pH lower than 7.0** is associated with neonatal mortality, hypoxic ischemic encephalopathy, intraventricular hemorrhage, and cerebral palsy.
- **Base deficit greater than 12 to 16 mEq/L** is associated with hypoxic ischemic encephalopathy, respiratory complications, hemodynamic instability, and abnormal renal function.

36. What is asphyxia?
Asphyxia can be defined as significant and progressive hypoxemia, hypercapnia, and metabolic acidemia that can affect the function of vital organs and lead to permanent brain damage and death. Birth asphyxia is responsible for approximately 1 million neonatal deaths each year worldwide.

37. When may therapeutic hypothermia be beneficial to a neonate?
For term infants with hypoxic ischemic encephalopathy secondary to acute perinatal asphyxia, several studies have shown neuroprotective effects from therapeutic hypothermia that manifest as decreases in death or disability. Criteria for hypothermia or "cooling" include a pH of 7.0 or less or base deficit of 16 or greater, a 10-minute Apgar score of 5 or less, assisted ventilation for at least 10 minutes, or the presence of encephalopathy. Cooling should be initiated within the first 6 hours of life, with a goal core temperatures of 32.5° C to 34° C. Infants awaiting transfer to a facility where this can be done may be passively cooled by turning off the warmer, unwrapping the infant from any blankets, and uncovering the head. Ice should not be applied.

KEY POINTS: NEWBORN RESUSCITATION

1. Neonatal resuscitation is summarized by ABCD (airway, breathing, circulation, drug).
2. Primary apnea should be remedied with stimulation and supplemental oxygen; secondary apnea requires PPV.
3. For newborns greater than or equal to 35 weeks' gestation, start resuscitation with room air (FiO2 21%). For preterm infants born prior to 35 weeks' gestation, start with FiO2 21% to 30%. Adjust as needed to maintain normal saturation for the infant's age in minutes.
4. If the heart rate is lower than 60 bpm despite effective PPV, the infant needs chest compressions with a compression-to-ventilation ratio of 3:1.
5. Epinephrine is utilized when the infant's heart rate remains below 60 bpm despite both effective PPV and chest compressions.
6. Apgar scores are used to survey neonatal condition, but they are not used to determine need for resuscitation.
7. Neonates with meconium should not be routinely bulb suctioned intrapartum or intubated and tracheally suctioned following delivery. Although prior NRP guidelines advocated for routine intubation and suctioning of non-vigorous neonates with meconium, the 2015 guidelines no longer recommend this practice.

BIBLIOGRAPHY

1. American College of Obstetricians and Gynecologists. Fetus and newborn: The Apgar score. ACOG committee opinion no. 333. *Obstet Gynecol.* 2006;107:1209–1212.
2. American College of Obstetricians and Gynecologists. Management of delivery of a newborn with meconium-stained amniotic fluid. ACOG committee opinion no. 379. *Obstet Gynecol.* 2007;1103:739.
3. Armstrong L, Stenson BJ. Use of umbilical cord blood gas analysis in the assessment of the newborn. *Arch Dis Child Fetal Neonatal Ed.* 2007;92:F430–F434.
4. Gao Y, Raj JU. Regulation of the pulmonary circulation in the fetus and newborn. *Physiol Rev.* 2010;90:1291–1335.
5. Kattwinkel J, ed. *Textbook of Neonatal Resuscitation.* 6th ed. Elk Grove Village, Ill: American Academy of Pediatrics and American Heart Association; 2011.
6. Low JA, Lindsay BG, Derrick EJ. Threshold of metabolic acidosis associated with newborn complications. *Am J Obstet Gynecol.* 1997;177:1391–1394.
7. Mackeen AD, Seibel-Seamon J, Muhammad J, Baxter JK, Berghella V. Tocolytics for preterm premature rupture of membranes. *Cochrane Database Syst Rev.* 2014;2. CD007062.
8. Moe-Byrne T, Brown JV, McGuire W. Naloxone for opiate-exposed newborn infants. *Cochrane Database Syst Rev.* 2013;2. CD003483.
9. Rabi Y. Oxygen and resuscitation of the preterm infant. *Neoreviews.* 2010;11:130–138.
10. Shankaran S, Laptook AR, Pappas A, et al. Effect of depth and duration of cooling on deaths in the NICU among neonates with hypoxic ischemic encephalopathy. *JAMA.* 2014;312:2629–2639.
11. Wyckoff MH, Aziz K, Escobedo MB, Kapadia VS, Kattwinkel J, Perlman JM, Simon WM, Weiner GM, Zaichkin JG, Part 13: Neonatal Resuscitation: 2015 American Heart Association Guidelines Update for Cardiopulmonary Resuscitation and Emergency Cardiovascular Care. *Circulation.* 2015;132:S543–S560.

CHAPTER 70

POSTPARTUM CARE

Stephanie G. Valderramos, MD, PhD

1. **What is the puerperium?**

   The puerperium is the period of time immediately after delivery of the placenta until 6 to 12 weeks post partum. During this time, the physiologic and psychological changes of pregnancy return to the prepregnancy state. The puerperium has also been called "the fourth trimester."

2. **How long does it take for the uterus to involute completely?**

   Within 2 weeks of delivery the uterus should be approximately at the level of the pelvis. By 6 weeks post partum, it should be normal size.

3. **What is lochia?**

   Lochia is the term used for postpartum uterine discharge. Initially, it is known as lochia rubra and is a flow of blood lasting several hours, which decreases to a red-brown discharge by the third or fourth postpartum day. This is followed by lochia serosa, which lasts a median of 22 days (but can last up to 6 weeks). It is characterized as mucopurulent and may have a mild odor. Lochia serosa is followed by lochia alba, which is a yellow-white discharge. Breastfeeding and the use of oral contraceptives do not affect the duration or character of lochia.

4. **When is postpartum bleeding abnormal?**

   It is normal for lochia to ebb and flow during the postpartum period. Frequently, an episode of heavy vaginal bleeding occurs between days 7 and 10 when the placental eschar sloughs. However, an increase in postpartum bleeding that is heavy and persistent (saturating more than one pad per hour for more than 2 hours) requires evaluation for possible retained placental tissue.

5. **How is abnormal postpartum bleeding evaluated and treated?**

   Ultrasound examination is the most useful test in the evaluation of abnormal postpartum bleeding. It can distinguish between blood clots and retained placental tissue and aids in determining which patients will benefit from uterine evacuation and curettage. Patients with minimal uterine contents usually respond to methylergonovine or misoprostol therapy.

6. **What are the most common postpartum issues?**

   Perineal pain, difficulty breastfeeding, urinary incontinence, flatal or fecal incontinence, and urinary infections are all common postpartum issues that usually resolve by 6 to 8 weeks postpartum.

7. **Should any activities be restricted during the postpartum period?**

   Patients may resume normal physical activity (including walking, using stairs) at any time after delivery. No absolute restrictions on exercise exist, and instructions should be patient specific. After a cesarean delivery, it is recommended to avoid heavy lifting (>10 to 15 pounds) for 4 to 6 weeks. Sexual activity may be resumed after the perineum has healed and bleeding has diminished. Postpartum dyspareunia is common, even after cesarean deliveries, and may be related to decreased levels of estrogen.

8. **How long are patients amenorrheic after delivery?**

   Women who breastfeed are amenorrheic for longer periods than women who do not. The mean time before ovulation in nonlactating women is 70 to 75 days, and menstruation usually resumes by postpartum week 12 in 70%. In women who are breastfeeding, the length of anovulation is directly related to the frequency of breastfeeding, the length of each feeding, and the amount of supplementation that is given. The risk of ovulation within the first 6 months is 1% to 5%.

9. **How soon can patients conceive after delivery?**

   In women who are exclusively breastfeeding, ovulation can occur as early as 3 months post partum (12 weeks). In women who are not breastfeeding, ovulation can occur as early as 25 days after delivery.

10. **Why does postpartum ovulation suppression occur?**
Ovulation suppression is related to elevated prolactin and decreased estrogen levels. In lactating women, increased prolactin can last up to 6 weeks post partum, whereas estrogen levels remain low. In nonlactating women, prolactin normalizes by postpartum week 3 and estrogen rises, reaching normal levels 2 to 3 weeks after delivery.

11. **What type of care is required for perineal lacerations?**
Spontaneous lacerations of the perineum or vagina are common during childbirth, and episiotomies are sometimes performed. Routine cleansing is usually all that is necessary for uncomplicated lacerations that do not extend beyond the transverse perineal muscle, do not have hematomas or infection, and have been adequately repaired. Pain can usually be managed with ibuprofen. In patients with third- or fourth-degree lacerations or episiotomy extensions, stronger pain medication is often necessary. These women benefit from sitz baths as well as ice packs to reduce swelling, and they should use stool softeners to promote a normal bowel regimen. Any patient experiencing an inordinate amount of pain should have a physical examination to rule out hematoma or infection.

12. **What is the definition of a postpartum fever?**
A temperature of 100.4° F (38° C) or higher on two separate occasions, more than 24 hours after delivery.

13. **What is the differential diagnosis of postpartum fevers?**
- Endometritis
- Urinary tract infection
- Wound infection
- Pulmonary infection
- Thrombophlebitis
- Mastitis

14. **What is the most likely cause of infection in a patient with postpartum fevers?**
Endometritis. Symptoms include fever, chills, lower abdominal pain, and malodorous vaginal discharge. Patients have uterine tenderness on palpation, and the vaginal discharge is mucopurulent. Treatment is usually with a combination of clindamycin and gentamicin to provide coverage for most aerobic and anaerobic organisms. These organisms include group A *Streptococcus, Bacteroides,* enterococci, *Escherichia coli, Klebsiella,* and *Proteus.* Blood cultures rarely influence clinical management, but they should be obtained in cases of sepsis or poor response to treatment. Once symptoms have subsided and the patient has been afebrile for 24 to 48 hours, intravenous antibiotic therapy can be discontinued. It is not necessary to continue oral antibiotics.

15. **What is septic pelvic thrombophlebitis?**
Septic pelvic thrombophlebitis is a diagnosis of exclusion made when a patient who is receiving antibiotics for endometritis has spiking temperatures and all other potential sources have been excluded. Treatment consists of adding therapeutic doses of heparin to the patient's medications. Although magnetic resonance imaging (MRI) may show obstructed pelvic veins, it is usually not necessary. Defervescence usually occurs within 72 hours of starting heparin, and most patients do not need anticoagulation on discharge.

16. **What are the maternal health benefits of breastfeeding?**
Breastfeeding mothers experience decreased postpartum bleeding and more rapid uterine involution, earlier return to prepregnancy weight, and decreased risk of breast and ovarian cancers.

17. **Do breastfeeding women need additional nutrition?**
A woman who is breastfeeding needs approximately 500 extra calories per day. With the exception of zinc and calcium, almost all other nutrients necessary for breastfeeding can be obtained through a balanced diet.

18. **What is mastitis?**
Mastitis is a localized infection of the breast that occurs in approximately 1% to 2% of breastfeeding women. It can develop at any time, but it is most common between postpartum weeks 1 and 5. Symptoms include a sore, erythematous area on one breast, which may become indurated. The patient may also experience fevers, chills, and malaise; 3% to 4% of cases of mastitis progress to abscess formation.

19. **How is mastitis treated?**
    The most common cause of mastitis is *Staphylococcus aureus*. Other common causes include *Haemophilus influenzae, Klebsiella pneumoniae, E. coli, Enterococcus faecalis,* and *Enterobacter cloacae*. First-line treatment is dicloxacillin. If methicillin-resistant Staphylococcus aureus is a concern, clindamycin or Bactrim can be used. Women who are allergic to penicillin should be given erythromycin. Encourage patients to stay well hydrated and use acetaminophen for discomfort and fever. Abscesses may require drainage and inpatient treatment with intravenous antibiotics.

20. **Is mastitis a contraindication to breastfeeding?**
    No. It is important to empty the affected breast, and patients should be encouraged to continue breastfeeding or use a pump.

21. **Do any contraindications to breastfeeding exist?**
    Yes. Although most women can breastfeed safely, exceptions include any who:
    - Are infected with human immunodeficiency virus (HIV; in the United States)
    - Have active, highly communicable infections such as untreated tuberculosis, varicella, or herpes simplex with breast lesions
    - Are taking antineoplastic, thyrotoxic, and immunosuppressive agents
    - Use street drugs or abuse alcohol
    - Have an infant with galactosemia
    - Are undergoing treatment for breast cancer

22. **How can patients suppress lactation if they do not plan on breastfeeding?**
    Breast support, ice packs, and analgesic medications are helpful to relieve breast engorgement. Expression of milk or nipple stimulation should be avoided. Breast engorgement and pain usually subside within a week.

23. **What medications are contraindicated while breastfeeding?**
    For a full list, refer to the American Academy of Pediatrics Guidelines for Drugs and Breastfeeding. Some important examples are bromocriptine, cyclophosphamide, cyclosporine, doxorubicin, ergotamine, lithium, methotrexate, phencyclidine, and radioactive iodine. "Lactmed (available at: http://toxnet.nlm.nih.gov/cgi-bin/sis/htmlgen?LACTMED) is a valuable resource for up-to-date information on the safety of medications in lactation.

24. **Can breastfeeding women use birth control?**
    Yes. Although breastfeeding postpones the time to first ovulation, it should not be relied on for contraception. The U.S. Centers for Disease Control and Prevention (CDC) recommends that estrogen-containing contraceptives be avoided in women who are breastfeeding until at least 6 weeks post partum because of an increased risk of venous thromboembolism. (For nonlactating patients, these drugs are contraindicated for at least 3 weeks if no other risk factors are present.) Progestin-only methods can be started immediately post partum. For more information on contraception, see Chapter 14. Data on the effect of hormonal contraceptives on lactation and milk production are controversial.

25. **What is an ideal interpregnancy interval?**
    The interpregnancy interval is defined as the time from delivery to conception of the next pregnancy. Although the World Health Organization (WHO) recommends an interpregnancy interval of at least 24 months after a live birth to decrease the incidence of perinatal complications such as preterm delivery and low birth weight in the subsequent pregnancy, more recent data suggest that an interval of at least 18 months is sufficient.

26. **What is postpartum thyroiditis?**
    Postpartum thyroid dysfunction is an autoimmune disorder characterized by destructive, lymphocytic thyroiditis. Often underdiagnosed, it can be found in as many as 5% to 10% of postpartum women. Symptoms usually begin 1 to 4 months post partum and include features of hypothyroidism, hyperthyroidism, or both. Sometimes a goiter may be noted on examination. The diagnosis is confirmed with thyroid function tests. The most common outcome is spontaneous resolution, although 10% to 30% of patients will develop permanent hypothyroidism.

27. **How common is postpartum depression?**
    The incidence of true postpartum depression is 10% to 15%; signs and symptoms are no different from those in the rest of the population. Women with an earlier history of depression or a related

mood disorder are more prone to postpartum depression, and it has a 50% to 100% recurrence rate in subsequent pregnancies.

Approximately 70% of women experience a period of mood symptoms (also known as "baby blues") that begin during the first week after delivery and spontaneously resolve by postpartum day 10. These mood symptoms include tearfulness, anxiety, irritation, and restlessness. No treatment is necessary, but emotional support and rest are beneficial.

28. What is the treatment for postpartum depression?

Depression is a serious illness, and medical treatment should be strongly considered. Serotonin reuptake inhibitors such as fluoxetine, paroxetine, and sertraline have been found to be effective and have few side effects. If symptoms do not response to monotherapy, consultation with a psychiatrist is advised.

KEY POINTS: POSTPARTUM CARE

1. The physiologic changes of pregnancy return to the prepregnancy state during the first 6 to 12 weeks after delivery.
2. The most common cause of postpartum fever is endometritis.
3. Breastfeeding is associated with decreased postpartum bleeding, more rapid uterine involution, and earlier return to prepregnancy weight. It has very few contraindications.
4. Women who are breastfeeding may experience prolonged ovulation suppression and amenorrhea, although this should not be relied on as a form of contraception.
5. Estrogen-containing contraceptives should not be initiated until 6 weeks post partum because of an increased risk of venous thromboembolism. Progestin-only contraceptives can be initiated at any time.
6. Postpartum depression is a serious illness that affects 10% to 15% of women and has an extremely high recurrence rate.

BIBLIOGRAPHY

1. American Academy of Pediatrics and the American College of Obstetricians and Gynecologists. *Guidelines for Perinatal Care.* 7th ed. United States: American Academy of Pediatrics and the American College of Obstetricians and Gynecologists; 2012.
2. American College of Obstetricians and Gynecologists. Optimizing support for breastfeeding as part of obstetric practice. ACOG committee opinion no. 658. *Obstet Gynecol.* 2016;127:e86–92.
3. American College of Obstetricians and Gynecologists. Thyroid disease in pregnancy. ACOG practice bulletin no. 148. *Obstet Gynecol.* 2015;125:996–1055.
4. Centers for Disease Control and Prevention.. Update to CDC's US medical eligibility criteria for contraceptive use 2010: revised recommendations for the use of contraceptive methods during the postpartum period. *MMWR Morb Mortal Wkly Rep.* 2011;60:878–883.
5. Katz VL. Postpartum care. In: Gabbe SG, Niebyl JR, Simpson JL, et al., eds. *Obstetrics: Normal and Problem Pregnancies.* 6th ed. Philadelphia: Saunders; 2012:517–532.
6. Shachar BZ, Lyell DJ. Interpregnancy interval and obstetrical complications. *Obstet Gynecol. Surv.* 2012;67:584–596.

INDEX

Page numbers followed by "*b*", "*t*", and "*f*" refer to boxes, tables, and figures respectively.